UNDERSTANDING LANGUAGE DISORDERS

THE IMPACT ON LEARNING

Vivienne L. Ratner, Ph.D. • Laura R. Harris, M.S., CCC-SLP

Thinking Publications
Eau Claire, Wisconsin

© 1994 **Thinking Publications®**   *A Division of McKinley Companies, Inc.*

03   02   01   00   99   98   97   10   9   8   7   6   5   4

Ratner, Vivienne L.

  Understanding language disorders : the impact on learning / Vivienne L. Ratner, Laura R. Harris.

     p.   cm.

  Includes bibliographical references (p.) and index.

  ISBN 0-930599-90-X

  1. Learning disabled children—Language. 2. Language disorders in children—Treatment. 3. Learning disabled children—Education. 4. Language acquisition. I. Harris, Laura R., II. Title.

LC4704.5.R38 1994

371.91'4—dc20   93-23636

Printed in the United States of America

Table 4.1   Age (Years-Months) at Which Children Master Speech Sounds in Five Studies from *Introduction to Communication Disorders* by M. Hegde, 1991, Austin, TX: Pro-Ed. ©1991 by Pro-Ed. Reprinted by permission.

Table 9.1   Final DSM-IV Draft Criteria for Attention Deficit Hyperactivity Disorder from *DSM-IV Draft Criteria (3/1/93)* by the American Psychiatric Association, 1993, Washington, DC: APA. ©1993 by the American Psychiatric Association. Reprinted by permission.

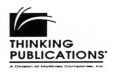

THINKING PUBLICATIONS®
A Division of McKinley Companies, Inc.

424 Galloway Street
Eau Claire, WI 54703
(715) 832-2488
FAX (715) 832-9082

DEDICATION

To my husband,
Irving M. Ratner, M.D.,
physician, teacher, and
human being of the
highest caliber.

Vivienne Ratner

To my husband and
dearest friend,
Lawrence S. Harris,
for his love and
encouragement.

Laura Harris

TABLE OF CONTENTS

TABLES

PREFACE

Understanding Language Disorders: The Impact on Learning is written for adults who enjoy observing children as they develop and begin to express thoughts about the world in which they live. We reach out especially to classroom teachers and other educators who are perplexed and frustrated when individual children are not learning as expected. We want to help educators understand the vital role language plays in the child's academic, social, and emotional development.

This textbook also addresses the needs of teachers and all professionals who are concerned with children who, for known and unknown reasons, do not acquire language at the stages that their peers acquire language. Included in this group of youngsters are those with language disorders and/or sensory, cognitive, and minimal cortical impairments that impede and curtail normal language development and learning.

In the past 25 years, the use of new electronic devices has exposed many secrets of brain functioning hitherto only suspected. Research techniques involved in the testing of children have been refined. Knowledge about language development has been enriched by extensive, valuable research. The intervention techniques currently used to remediate language disorders are built upon the knowledge gleaned from the theories of professionals from many fields of expertise.

We have presented a number of different viewpoints. Children exhibiting language difficulties do not present a consistent and clear picture of a specific disorder. How convenient it would be if that were the case. There are many different approaches to the same disorder, each one affecting the selection of intervention techniques to be used with individual children.

We realize that communication skills and disorders involve complex systems that affect a child's ability to learn, to interact, and to behave. These systems generally are grouped into four categories:

1. articulation and its disorders, which concern control and motor ability for sound production;

2. fluency and its disorders, which include stuttering, stammering, and the phrasing and rhythm with which speech is expressed;

3. voice and its disorders, which concern vocal abuse, hoarseness, loudness, pitch, and the general quality of speech;

4. language and its disorders, which involve the understanding and expression of appropriate ideas in context.

Of these components, it is language which most directly affects a child's ability to learn. This textbook concentrates on the acquisition of language, the factors which impede language acquisition, the impact of language on learning and academic achievement, and those pervasive disorders (e.g., cognitive disabilities, autism, etc.) in which language is one major factor among more global deficits.

ACKNOWLEDGMENTS

Many people have been sources of inspiration and support in the development of the ideas presented in this book. However, it was our students at the Graduate School of Special Education at the College of New Rochelle who planted the idea to write this textbook. Our students, who were pursuing graduate degrees in special education, wanted to learn about the impact of language on learning. Year after year they encouraged us to write a textbook which would elucidate the particular language and learning issues that affected them professionally. We thank these students for their interest, prodding, and intellectual contributions.

Writing a textbook entails extensive research and endless revisions. The rewriting process was aided significantly by our patient editors, Linda Schreiber and Nancy McKinley. They deserve our special thanks for their extraordinary concern and care as they supervised the writing process and facilitated the transformation of ideas into text. We also appreciate the expert comments, criticisms, and contributions by our colleagues, Susan Anderson, Dagney Bergstrom, Linda Carpenter, Barbara DeLoretto, Thea Eichler, Katheryn Hathaway, Loretta Holland, Julie Johnson, Adele Lafferty, Michelle Langus, Vicki Lord Larson, Roni Liebowitz, Elaine Masket, Joyce Olson, Jeanine Optman, Andy Papineau, Maria Polignano, Lou Rosetti, Judith Schaffer, Karen Schlesinger, Nancy Smith, and Marie Stadler. We are most grateful to Kim Gallagher, the Interlibrary Loan librarian at the University of Hartford, who obtained many volumes and articles during the research process. Special thanks is also given to Linda Seigle for her typing and retyping of endless drafts.

The hundreds of children with varying language abilities with whom we have worked over the years have taught and inspired us immeasurably. We recognize the efforts that they, their parents, and others have exerted to help them to become the special individuals that they are.

Needless to say, this work would not have been possible without the encouragement of our families and friends, who showed patience and understanding during the many months that were devoted to writing this book. We love them and are grateful to them.

ABOUT THE AUTHORS

Vivienne L. Ratner, Ph.D. holds certification in the fields of education of deaf and hearing impaired individuals, special education, with a specialization in learning disabilities, and speech-language-hearing. Her doctorate is from New York University, Departments of Communication Disorders and Deafness Education and Rehabilitation. She has had many years of experience teaching in the classroom, therapy room, and resource room with individuals who are deaf, hearing impaired, learning disabled, language disordered, or multihandicapped. She has done considerable research on learning disabilities, and has published a test to identify visual perceptual learning disabilities, with versions for hearing impaired and hearing children. She is Adjunct Associate Professor at the Graduate School, Department of Special Education, College of New Rochelle, NY. In her private practice, she acts as consultant to school districts, advocate for children with special needs, learning disabilities specialist for both hearing and hearing impaired children and adults, aural rehabilitation counselor for individuals with hearing impairment, and vocational rehabilitation counselor for adults who are deaf.

Laura R. Harris, M.S., CCC-SLP graduated from Brandeis University and received her masters degree in speech and hearing rehabilitation from Adelphi University. She is a speech-language pathologist and an advocate for children with special needs and disabilities. She developed and worked in a model program for early elementary school children with severe communication disorders and was later chief diagnostician for a speech center. She spent several years helping youngsters with all forms of disabilities by advising families and professionals working with these children when they sought appropriate programs and services. As an Adjunct Assistant Professor in the Department of Graduate Special Education at the College of New Rochelle, she has taught experienced teachers and graduate students who are training to be special education teachers about language disorders in children. Her interests center on the impact of language on social and academic growth in children and on the way each child learns most effectively.

INTRODUCTION

Language is the primary tool for both incidental and academic learning. Whether the reader is a regular classroom teacher, a special education teacher, a speech-language pathologist, a special therapist, a child psychologist, an educational evaluator, a school administrator, a psychosocial worker, a nurse, a pediatrician, a student, or a parent, this textbook introduces those language issues which impact on every aspect of educational, social, and emotional development. Children who have language deficiencies as toddlers are at high risk for learning disabilities as they mature. Their linguistic deficits may later be manifested as serious reading difficulties, inability to express their thoughts in oral and written form, inability to understand nonverbal communication, and inability to understand and express emotions.

At present, there is a trend toward even greater inclusion of children with language disorders into regular school settings. Educational professionals who develop learning environments require adequate training. Professionals and parents need to understand language development and language disorders to enrich their social and educational interactions with children. Sharing knowledge among the disciplines facilitates the implementation of appropriate educational settings.

Chapters 1 and 2 discuss the terminology and historical framework for language disorders. Chapters 3 and 4 explore normal language acquisition and its effect on educational and social development. The importance of early and intensive experiences and interactions with others is emphasized.

The United States is composed of people with diverse cultures and languages. Chapter 5 examines the issue of language differences versus language disabilities. Chapter 6 considers the current progress and limitations regarding the assessment of children's language and communication.

Chapters 7 through 14 explain some of the ways in which underlying linguistic, conceptual, and cognitive deficits can affect the ability of children to learn. Each chapter emphasizes the impact of language on the student's educational success. Since eligibility for program placement and state and federal funding continue to be etiology-based, Chapters 7 through 14 are arranged in this way.

In Chapter 9, three disorders have been separated from the learning disabilities described in the previous chapter: dyslexia, attention deficit hyperactivity disorder (ADHD), and nonverbal information processing disorder. Although many students with language disabilities exhibit attentional deficits, social problems, and/or severe reading disabilities, they do not necessarily each have dyslexia, ADHD, or the debilitating social imperception observed in children with a nonverbal information processing disorder.

Each child is unique and possesses special abilities and weaknesses. Therefore, intervention "techniques" have not been listed that would be appropriate for all children exhibiting the behaviors of a specific disorder. Individuals who are familiar with children who have language deficits find that some are intellectually superior, some are sociable, some understand, and some can verbalize, while others are extremely limited. Chapter 15 introduces intervention principles rather than specific tasks. More recent legislation is summarized that has generated discussion as well as different approaches to educational intervention.

This is an exciting era with rapid growth of knowledge regarding language development and its impact on learning. Recent approaches to education for children with language disabilities have provided improved learning opportunities. The most recent theories have been included in this text. The authors also have contributed original theories based upon many years of collective experience in the fields of speech-language pathology, learning disabilities, sensory impairments, and special education. These theories are presented so that the readers may draw their own conclusions.

1 THE LANGUAGE OF LANGUAGE

Every professional specialty has its own vocabulary, that is, technical terms used to describe or discuss specific conditions that are relevant to those who work in the field. Frequently, an ordinary English term is "stretched" to encompass a broader meaning more clearly applicable to a particular situation or condition. These terms are appropriate and acceptable as long as they are used in a manner agreed upon by the professional community. Unfortunately, interpretation is often very subjective on the part of the reader or listener, and confusion results unless the specific terms are clearly defined by the individuals who are using them. Journals and textbooks on language disorders contain different interpretations of terms commonly used to discuss the conditions of concern. The purpose of this chapter is to define the more important "general" terms so that there will be no confusion regarding the authors' intended meaning in this text.

LANGUAGE—WHAT IS IT?

Language is a consistent, rule-regulated, coded system with which one can convey and exchange thoughts, ideas, and feelings regarding people, situations, and events in the world. The code of each language has been agreed upon by the speakers of the language. The fact that language is a consistent and rule-regulated code enables children to acquire the sounds that form words and words that form sentences that are understood by others in their language community. If everyone haphazardly strung together sounds and phrases, the result would be incomprehensible and would have meaning only for the speaker.

3

Children with normal hearing usually acquire language by listening to the language users in their immediate environment. They imitate and experiment initially with sounds, then words and phrases, and finally with grammatically structured sentences repeated for a variety of purposes and in a variety of contexts. The thoughts and ideas expressed by language are also influenced by the environment and culture in which the child lives. Chapter 5 describes cultural influence in detail.

When the ability to hear is diminished, sign language is an alternative, rich, consistent, rule-regulated, and coded means of expressing thoughts, ideas, and feelings. The code can be visual and still be considered a language, even though no one is "talking." Manual language is acquired naturally through the visual sense by children who imitate sign language users in their immediate environment. The culture of the deaf community has a strong influence on the ideas and thoughts manually expressed by the deaf child. Sign language and hearing impairment will be discussed in detail in Chapter 12.

Expressive Language

Expressive language is the symbolic system used to convey one's thoughts, attitudes, emotions, and needs. Expressive language can be conveyed by speaking, signing, writing, and also by body positioning, gesture, tone of voice, facial expression, and forms of art.

Receptive Language

Receptive language is oral speech that is perceived and processed; signed expressions that are seen and comprehended; and printed language that is read with understanding. It also refers to the analysis and interpretation of the message expressed by dance, painting, sculpture, and music.

WHY DO WE NEED LANGUAGE?

Humans are social beings. When deprived of human contact and opportunities to share feelings, they become emotionally and physically ill. Humans need to communicate and receive feedback about how their messages are being understood and about how much they are loved, wanted, needed, and appreciated. They need to share their ideas and their impressions about events in their environment. These reactions and emotions are conveyed by language. Body language, facial expressions, and tones of voice also provide effective nonlinguistic cues for conveying emotions.

Humans also need a means of expressing an opinion, asking for something, protesting, pointing out something of interest to another, influencing someone, and describing experiences and ideas. Without language to plan, create, and organize thoughts and experiences, humans would be disorganized and without motivation, having no control over their lives (Johnson and Myklebust, 1967; Lerner, 1985).

SPEECH

Speech is an oral means of expressing language. It involves the motoric functions that control the tongue, larynx, diaphragm, and other specific organs to create words and sounds. However, language does not have to be expressed by spoken words. Thoughts and emotions can be expressed by means of manual signs, art, dance, or written expression.

COMMUNICATION

Communication is the purpose and the function of language. By means of communication, humans can exchange information, control or influence others, and express their attitudes and feelings to others. Communication can be very effective without language.

Newborn infants can communicate and animals can communicate. However, language cannot be considered without communication. Language must be communicated to others.

DOESN'T SPEAK YET: SO WHAT?

Understanding what constitutes age-appropriate language is important for teachers. The ability to acquire language is innate in humans (Bower, 1982; Meltzoff, 1985a). Nevertheless, human infants are active, hard-working language learners during the first 24 months of life. The fact that within such a short period of time, infants acquire most of the elements of the language of their society is rather awe-inspiring.

Children who do not acquire language as expected are considered to be **language delayed**. Children who fail to produce 50 words and two-word combinations by 24 to 34 months may be considered delayed in expressive language development and are "at high risk for language disorders" (Capute, Palmer, Shapiro, Wachtel, Schmidt, and Ross, 1986; Catts, 1991; Coplan, Gleason, Ryan, Burke, and Williams, 1982; Paul, 1991; Rescorla, 1989; Resnick, Allen, and Rapin, 1984).

Long-range studies indicate that a large percentage of preschoolers with language delays do not outgrow their difficulties (Aram, Ekelman, and Nation, 1984; Aram and Nation, 1980; King, Jones, and Lasky, 1982; Miller, 1981a; Paul, 1991; Wallach and Liebergott, 1984). Even if those difficulties appear to be resolved by school age, their language deficiencies have been found to reveal themselves later on in the form of disabilities in reading, writing, and narrative expression. Moreover, there is evidence from these studies that, despite intervention, their language problems persist throughout their school years and even through adulthood.

Classroom teachers and other specialists working with children cannot evaluate normal language acquisition unless they understand what it is that children should be acquiring. They cannot implement remedial strategies, no matter which technique or educational approach is used, unless they can break the linguistic task into basic components or elements in their own minds. These components of language are discussed in the next section and then followed by a discussion of nonverbal communication, inner language, and written language.

COMPONENTS OF LANGUAGE

Specific components of language are defined and discussed in this section. Components included are phonology, morphology, syntax, semantics, and pragmatics.

Phonology

Phonology is the study and description of the sounds of language. Each spoken language has specific rules that regulate the order of sounds in the words and the pronunciation of these sounds. **Phonemes** are the smallest units of sound that, when combined, form the words in a language. When in written form, phonemes are represented by phonetic symbols within slash marks. A phoneme has no meaning by itself, but when combined in a specific order, phonemes create words and contribute to meaning in a sentence. They contribute to meaning by recombining in a variety of ways to form different words in a sentence, e.g., /m/, /k/, /b/, /f/, /æ/, /t/, /s/ form words such as *m-a-t, c-a-t, b-a-t, f-a-t, t-a-b, s-a-t,* depending upon their arrangement. *The cat sat on a mat* has a different meaning from *The cat sat on a hat.* By combining the phonemes differently in similarly constructed sentences, the meaning can be changed entirely and different inferences deduced.

Phonological rules are the rules of the English language that govern sounds and their arrangements in words. These rules regulate the order of the consonants and vowels within words. A word can begin with the consonants *spr, str,* and *scr* (e.g., *spr*ing, *str*ing, *scru*mptious), but not with the consonants *psr* or *ngs*. In addition, words in the English language cannot consist of only consonants; they must contain a vowel. These are examples of phonological rules.

Morphology

Morphology is the study of word formation and its effect on meaning. **Morphemes** are the smallest "meaningful" units in words. English words are composed of one or more morphemes. For example, the word *dress* is one morpheme; it has a meaning and it cannot be broken down any further. The prefix *un*, as in *undress*, is also one morpheme because it has meaning indicating reversal. The word *undress* consists of two morphemes. Thus, words consist of morphemes combined in a variety of ways to express specific meanings.

Morphological rules are the rules for forming words with morphemes. Each morpheme in a word has a specific meaning. By interchanging the morphological elements of words, the speaker can form an infinite variety of meanings. For example, by adding morphemes to the ends of words, we can express plurality, present tense, past tense, and ongoing action (e.g., shoe*s*, walk*s*, walk*ed*, go*ing*). By adding morphemes to the beginnings of words, we can express negation and temporal information (e.g., *un*natural, *non*verbal, *re*organize, *pre*arrange). When *s* is removed from the end of a verb, such as *walk*, the speaker is indicating that more than one person or animal is doing the walking (e.g., The man *walks*, The cat *walks*, He *walks*, It *walks*, but *They walk*).

These examples of morphological rules apply only to speakers of Standard English. There are several dialects that are considered legitimate languages because they are consistent, coded systems, and they are rule-regulated. These include Black English, a dialect used by some African-Americans in the United States. The morphologic and syntactic rules of Black English require different endings for verbs than those used in Standard English (e.g., She *walk*, The boy *walk,* I *walks,* You *walks,* He *walking* home, She *be walking* home after dinner for years) (*be* is used in the habitual sense). Like most languages and dialects of language, Black English is flexible, with many variations depending upon the context, the social environment, and the people engaging in the communication (Owens, 1992).

Syntax

Syntax is the part of grammar which regulates the arrangement of words to form meaningful sentences. The sentences of language are also regulated by **syntactical rules**. A speaker cannot link words in a sentence in a haphazard order or the sentence will have no meaning and, more important, recalling the definition of language, no "consistent" meaning. Various types of words have specific functions in a sentence. For example, only pronouns and words or phrases acting as nouns can be subjects or objects. Only verbs can convey action and they must relate to the nouns and pronouns that are the subjects and objects of the sentence (i.e., they cannot be singular and in the present tense when the subject is plural and the action occurred in the past). Only adverbs can describe the how, when, or where of the verb (e.g., *quickly, then, now, here*).

The arrangement of the parts of speech in a sentence is also determined by the syntactical rules of the language. In English, the adjective usually precedes the noun (e.g., *black* cat, *funny* story). The subject usually precedes the verb (e.g., *He* works). The adverb usually follows the verb (e.g., He ran *quickly*). The object of the sentence usually follows the verb (e.g., The boy hit the *ball*). The arrangement of the subject, verb, and object is the means of determining the meaning of the sentence (e.g., *The ball hit the boy* as opposed to *The boy hit the ball*). The syntactical rules of other languages may place their verbs, nouns, adjectives, and adverbs in other arrangements within the sentence.

Semantics

The **semantic** component of language is concerned with word meanings and relationships between words. Semantics also relates to multiple word meanings, figurative language, and underlying meanings of words in specific contexts. The meanings of words are arbitrary decisions by the members of a language community. Meanings of words change over time. New words and idioms are added to a language constantly and enrich its quality.

Many words have similar meanings, and speakers select one that applies best to a specific context. Initially, children overgeneralize new words in a variety of contexts, some of which are inappropriate. Later in their development, children's decisions about word meanings become more specific and well-defined. The child is then able to retrieve from the vocabulary stored in memory the precise word or phrase that is most appropriate in a particular context. Very important in this process are children's opportunities for direct experiences with their world and the acquisition of knowledge related to these experiences. Vocabularies are related to experiential knowledge. The more experiences that children have, the more refined their vocabulary, the broader their points of view, and the deeper their insights. This kind of intellectual growth leads to greater semantic understanding.

The understanding of multiple-meaning words is a semantic skill which requires children to be flexible and to accept the fact that one word can have different meanings depending on context and situation (e.g., the *running* brook, *run* out of money, The boy *runs* faster than his father, There is a *run* in the woman's nylon stocking, His nose is *running*). In addition, multiple-meaning words require that the speaker has a knowledge of the rules of phonology, morphology, and syntax (Pease, Gleason, and Pan, 1989; Wiig and Semel, 1984).

Idioms and metaphors require semantic understanding. If they are taken literally, they are meaningless. Many **idioms** contain multiple-meaning words, such as *time flies, tickled pink, hold your tongue,* and *raining cats and dogs.* These phrases must be interpreted figuratively, not literally. **Metaphors** compare the actual subject with an image of something very different, yet similar to the subject in some aspect (e.g., *hard as nails, black as night,* and *fit as a fiddle*). Metaphors require that the child develop **imagery**, or the ability to retrieve from the mind's eye the contours, configurations, movements, colors, qualities, particular smells and sounds, and also feelings and emotions associated with specific objects, situations, and events. To interpret a metaphor, children must compare the image retrieved from their mind's eye with the image described in the phrase and then find the similarities.

Most of the words we use belong to **semantic categories**, such as persons, objects, actions, attributes, and feelings. *Butterflies* can belong to categories including insects, things having many colors, living creatures, creatures that fly, etc. *Bananas* can belong to fruit, things to eat, and yellow objects. *Synonyms* are words that have a similar meaning. For example, synonyms for the word *wait* are *pause, tarry, stay, dally, procrastinate, hesitate, stall,* and *mark time. Antonyms* are words that are often referred to as opposites. Examples of antonyms are *near/far, tall/short, hot/cold, love/hate.*

The meanings of children's words, thoughts, and perceptions gradually increase in complexity. Their ability to express their thoughts and to comprehend both the obvious and abstract meanings of verbal or written expressions used by others is based upon their semantic understanding.

Pragmatics

The ability to use language for a purpose while interacting with other human beings is generally referred to as **pragmatic ability**. Children start to learn the role of communicator from the first day of life. This early development process will be described in detail in Chapter 3. The child who can successfully use pragmatic skills will not only develop socially and emotionally, but also academically. On the other hand, pragmatic disability is one aspect of every language disorder in this text. Therefore, it is important to examine this essential component of language development carefully and in-depth.

Pragmatic abilities are not being used unless at least one speaker and one listener are interacting. A "need" or "motivation" to interact with another individual is present. The speaker might want to request something, or attempt to influence or change the listener's opinion. There also would be motivation to communicate if the individual needed to ask questions to gain information or to focus the listener's attention on an object or ongoing activity that is relevant and important. The rules underlying pragmatic activities are established by the society in which an individual lives. Individuals find that socially acceptable behavior can be quite different when they travel to other countries with different cultures.

To be successful as a communicator, one must be able to take the role of either the speaker or the listener. Both roles are complex and require continuous effort and attention.

Topic

Oral communication requires a speaker, a listener, and a message. The message has to be expressed in a language that is understood by both listener and speaker. The subject matter of the message being discussed is referred to as the *topic* of discussion. The topic is a reference point agreed upon by both speaker and listener that has to be carefully monitored during the communication. If there are signs of confusion or strong disagreement regarding the topic, both speaker and listener have the responsibility to repair the damage and prevent communication breakdown. In addition, topics change rapidly during communication by mutual consent, and pragmatic ability includes the understanding of when and how the topic has been switched or altered.

The Role of the Speaker

The rules of pragmatics require that the speaker understand what is appropriate language and behavior with regard to the status, age, and relationship of the listener and also with regard to the context and the setting of the conversation. Children learn very early that they cannot speak to their grandmother or to their teacher in the same way they can speak to their brother, sister, or peer on the playground. Children also learn early that they cannot behave in the same manner when in church as they do when fooling around at home.

A speaker must continuously monitor the facial expressions of the listener for signs of confusion. The speaker must make rapid inferences about the listener's linguistic abilities and store of knowledge regarding the topic. The speaker must also rephrase the statement quickly if necessary so that the listener can understand the message.

The process of getting a listener to respond to a request for something or to do something that the speaker wants to have done is a complex communicative skill. The speaker must express clearly what action he or she wants the listener to take. The person who is making the request must take into account the listener's needs and the listener's motivation to comply with the request (Becker, 1982, 1990; Bruner, Roy, and Ratner, 1982; McTear and Conti-Ramsden, 1992).

The Role of the Listener

A listener must sustain attention to the speaker, while keeping track of the current topic being discussed because topics often change rapidly during a conversation. If the message is not clearly stated and causes confusion, the listener must express to the speaker the need to have the message rephrased. The listener must be attuned to pauses between the speaker's utterances and differentiate between a pause required for taking a breath and a pause indicating that it is time for the speaker to take a turn as a listener; the listener must then take the role as the speaker.

Turn-taking is an essential component of conversation. To monitor the discussion so that the time to exchange roles will not be missed, the listener has to have knowledge of syntactic structure and nonverbal cues involving tone of voice, inflection, and pitch; the pitch is usually lowered at the end of a sentence. Some children have good pragmatic turn-taking abilities, but have difficulties with the linguistic and nonverbal requirements involved in the exchange of roles (Craig and Evans, 1989). Investigations of early interaction between infants and caregivers indicates that most children are able to engage in activities involving turn-taking before they have acquired any verbal language at all (Kysela, Holdgrafer, McCarthy, and Stewart, 1990).

To be successful socially, a person must understand how to enter a communication already in progress between two or more individuals. Learning the appropriate manner in which to enter a room where activities between individuals are ongoing and to join a group activity are also important. These are pragmatic skills.

To be an effective communicator, an individual must also observe the communication partner's body language and facial expressions and interpret the expressed feelings and emotions, e.g., sadness, fear, anxiety, fatigue, excitement, confusion, pleasure. At the same time, the listener must perceive by the person's tone of voice, loudness of voice, and inflection, the emotions underlying the words that are being expressed. These nonverbal communication behaviors are discussed in the next section.

NONVERBAL COMMUNICATION

Often, listeners require more information than can be gleaned from the spoken message alone. This additional information is important to help them understand the meaning of the speaker's message. They will need to use vocal (not verbal) cues, body (including gestural) language, and contextual clues, as well.

Paralinguistics

Additional valuable clues to the meaning of an oral message and the emotions contained in the message are conveyed by the speaker's tone of voice, rate of speech, volume, emphasis, and pitch. These deliberate vocal modifications carry information essential to the understanding of an oral communication and are generally referred to as **paralinguistics**.

Kinesics

Kinesics refers to nonverbal behaviors which by themselves carry important message value. Most often these behaviors (e.g., the manner of walking or standing, the ways the shoulders and head are held, and the tension of the body actually visible to the observer) convey emotions or feelings. Kinesics includes gesturing and eye gaze. Examples are nodding or shaking of the head to indicate yes or no, lifting the eyes toward the sky indicating exasperation, shaking an index finger from side to side when wanting to indicate an emphatic no, stamping a foot to express frustration, and turning away to indicate that no further conversation is desired. Gestures are often culturally bound in that they are understood by the language users of particular societies. The movements and expressions of the face and eyes convey emotions, such as anger, happiness or pleasure, fear, confusion, annoyance, and even hatred. These emotions, conveyed through facial expressions, are described as **affect**. Affective expressions carry valuable information and are essential components of a successful communication between human beings.

Proxemics

The purposeful use of space conveys very clear messages without the necessity of a single word or sign. Such communications are referred to as **proxemics**. The distance we maintain when standing or sitting next to another person expresses clear intention and love, attraction, dislike, or abhorrence. The extent of "private space" maintained by an individual is influenced by culture and a particular society's mores.

INNER LANGUAGE

Inner language is the language used for thinking, planning, problem solving, and self-monitoring. It is a means by which a person can transcend the restrictions of time. **Inner language** requires the ability to represent things, people, and events in one's mind when they are not actually present. Individuals can then think about events that have taken place in the past and anticipate events that will take place in the future. When verbal symbols can represent actual objects, people, and events, then thoughts and ideas can be used to plan, organize, create, develop, and alter reality. We can think about future events based upon our experiences of the past.

WRITTEN LANGUAGE

In this section, aspects of written language are discussed with regard to the essential role of linguistic abilities. The three aspects considered are decoding, reading comprehension, and written expression.

Decoding

Decoding is the process of extracting sufficient information from a printed word to recognize that it is, indeed, a distinct, meaningful word. The first step in the process of decoding an unknown word is recognizing each of the printed symbols that represent spoken speech sounds within a word. A reader must understand the sound/symbol relationship. To do this, a reader must have an understanding of phonological rules and discriminate the various sounds of the language. The second step in the process of decoding is blending the sounds together until the word and its meaning are recognized. The understanding of morphological rules is also essential because sometimes it is necessary to divide large words into smaller, pronounceable parts, or syllables. Then the word components must be blended together. Vocabulary is important also because if the word is altogether unknown to the reader, then it cannot be recognized once the sounds are blended together. The printed word is mapped onto the child's existing language. This analysis of and reflection on sounds, symbols, and their relation to words and their meanings are essential parts of decoding (Tunmer and Cole, 1991). Decoding is different from reading comprehension. Decoding is the synthesizing of all the elements of an individual word until the word is recognized.

Reading Comprehension

Reading comprehension is the process by which a reader understands the meaning of an entire passage, paragraph, or portion of text and can draw appropriate conclusions and inferences from the text itself. There is a significant relationship between listening skills and reading comprehension skills (Carlisle, 1991; Danks and End, 1987; Sinatra, 1990). Both skills are components of receptive language (i.e., the gleaning of meaning from a spoken, signed, or written message). The reader and the listener must have knowledge of syntactic rules, semantic understanding, and also an age-appropriate vocabulary.

Reading comprehension also interacts with readers' cultural backgrounds, interests, experiences, and attitudes (Anderson, Hiebert, Scott, and Wilkinson, 1985). In addition, when reading stories the child has to think about the setting, anticipate what may happen, consider the motives of the characters, and consider why an event occurred or a character reacted in a particular way (Paris, 1991). These very necessary analytical skills are referred to as **metacognitive abilities**.

Children must also perceive emotions in characters as they interact in a fictional story. Children's ability to comprehend the effect of the events on the characters in a story is often a reflection of the child's awareness of relationships in the world and a reflection of the child's own ability to interact socially with adults and peers (Kronick, 1981; McTear and Conti-Ramsden, 1992).

Written Expression

The process of **encoding** is the translation of thought into a coded system so that it can be expressed, either by an oral or signed form of language or by a written form of language. Encoding skills include speaking, signing, and expressive writing. Writing skills are closely related to children's narrative or storytelling abilities. All of the language abilities that are necessary for expressing thoughts and impressions orally or manually are required for expressing these thoughts in written form. Writers must consider the audience and the purpose of the narrative. They must plan, organize, and monitor the content, using syntactic, semantic, and pragmatic knowledge.

Cultural influences, basic attitudes, and world knowledge also play important roles in the process of writing. In addition, phonological abilities and morphological abilities are essential to spell the words that have to be written. Vocabulary not only has to be available for use, but has to be carefully selected so that the meaning of the content is clear to the reader. The writer is now the speaker in a communication with the reader, and the reader of the written text has to be considered. All possible problems that might cause confusion for the reader have to be anticipated and eliminated from the written content. Expressive language is more difficult for an author than for a speaker in a face-to-face interaction. There is no opportunity for the author to perceive facial expressions of the reader indicating confusion, and no opportunity for the reader to ask questions for clarification. Metacognitive skills described earlier, play an important role when writing.

SUMMARY

Language is a complex process. It is the essential component in the social, emotional, and academic development of a child. Learning will be curtailed and encumbered by a language deficit. Reading, writing, and communicating require language knowledge. Teachers should understand how language develops normally. The following chapters will describe the "ingredients" of a rich linguistic environment in which a youngster can grow and thrive.

SUGGESTED READINGS

Bower, T. (1982). *Development in Infancy* (2nd ed.). San Francisco, CA: W.H. Freeman.

McTear, M., and Conti-Ramsden, G. (1992). *Pragmatic Disability in Children*. San Diego, CA: Singular Publishing Group.

McCormick, L., and Schiefelbusch, R. (Eds.). (1990). *Early Language Intervention: An Introduction* (2nd ed.). New York: Charles E. Merrill.

2 THE HISTORICAL CONTEXT OF LANGUAGE INTERVENTION

An examination of the many facets of language clarifies the critical relationship between language and a child's social, emotional, academic, and cultural development. Awareness and acceptance of this interdependence have emerged only in the last few decades, although interest in child language development has existed for hundreds, if not thousands, of years. Chapter 2 explores this interdependence and the more recent advances in understanding language development.

SCHOOL INTERVENTION

During the early part of the 20th century, children's language was evaluated primarily by observational studies of their grammar and parts of speech. Researchers judged a child's language development by the number of nouns, verbs, adjectives, and other parts of speech that were included in an utterance. "Count studies" would tally the grammatical errors a child made to determine language proficiency (Smith, 1933).

In the 1930s, the members of the American Speech-Language-Hearing Association (ASHA), the professional organization for speech-language pathologists and audiologists, which was organized in 1925 as the American Academy of Speech Correction, began to look at brain function and physiology to determine speech production. Practitioners in the field created a new institution known as the speech clinic. It tended to be university-

or hospital-based and resembled a medical clinic in that a professional made a diagnosis based on the patient's symptoms. Therapeutic interventions were designed to remediate the problems. Patients were seen, one at a time, in a therapy room at the clinic. Parents sat in the waiting room and were not involved in the therapeutic regimen. The intervention strategies initiated in these clinical settings often did not transfer easily to the client's natural everyday environment (Miller, 1989).

This "medical" model of intervention was utilized in school settings as well (Bennett, 1971; Myklebust, 1971). The speech correctionist became a "therapist" or "clinician." He or she sought physical or organic origins for a child's difficulties. After assessing a child, an **etiology**, or cause, for the disability was determined. A diagnostic label was attached to the child's difficulty such as aphasia, anomia, agnosia, or dyslalia. Ideally, in school, the child had an appointment with the speech therapist once or twice a week for individual therapy. This "pull out" model removed the child from the classroom environment for intervention.

By the 1940s and 1950s, speech therapists were an integral part of support staff in many urban schools. The caseloads consisted primarily of children with speech or "articulation" problems, who had difficulty producing speech sounds such as the *r* sound or the *s* sound. Therapy was provided, as well, to children who stuttered or who had other dysfluency. Youngsters who couldn't form clear sentences, or whose narratives seemed confusing, or who couldn't follow directions, or who struggled at reading and writing, were rarely referred to the speech therapist for a language evaluation. Yet, child language proficiency was recognized as being related to cerebral palsy, mental retardation, hearing impairment, or other disorders. Children who had received head trauma with resulting memory and/or language loss were also treated by speech therapists. Language problems were viewed primarily as difficulty with vocabulary, limited ability to produce adequate sentence length, or problems creating a particular type of sentence like a question form.

THE LANGUAGE REVOLUTION

The publication of two books in 1957 sparked debate in the area of child language acquisition. B.F. Skinner's book, *Verbal Behavior*, viewed language as one of many learned behaviors that could be controlled and modified. Noam Chomsky's book, *Syntactic Structures*, published simultaneously, regarded language acquisition as a universal process common to almost all people.

Language as a Learned Behavior

Skinner's work is rooted in psychology and the notion that a stimulus can create a response. A child cries and someone reacts to the cry. Thus, the child learns that crying behavior produces a bottle. In a similar way, Skinner expressed language learning as the adult response to random vocalizations. Those utterances that are positively reinforced by another person will be produced often by the youngster. The parent also models sounds and words. As the child imitates and approximates these models, the adult responds positively.

Language imitation and reinforcement were embraced by school speech therapists as a way to develop language. Children were given practice drills for a targeted sound, word, or sentence. Reinforcement in the form of check marks, happy-face drawings, candy, or prizes was provided for positive change. By tallying correct responses, specific goals could be met. This structured intervention interfaced well with the "medical" model already established in education settings. The system was "scientific" in that tracking correct responses could measure the child's progress.

Skinner's theory viewed the child as a blank slate whose language development could be molded by proper stimuli. Because language acquisition depended upon adult models and reinforcement, the child was seen as a passive language learner. Early language behavior was shaped by the child's environment.

Language Learning as a Process

Chomsky's 1957 theory was derived from biology and **psycholinguistics,** the study of language structure and meaning in relation to human development. He stated that infants have an innate capacity to acquire and apply the rules of language. Although languages differ substantially, the apparatus to develop the underlying principles of language was a biological component in each person's brain.

Chomsky's theory viewed children as active and creative language learners. He argued that the early word groupings, or grammars, of toddlers are not simply imitations of adult models (Chomsky, 1959). Young children create utterances that they have never heard before by selecting and rearranging words that others have spoken. They also blend sounds and words in their own unique way, such as *bye-bye car* or *all gone bus.* These utterances are not random. They follow rules that are universal to all languages.

In an effort to explain linguistic processing, Chomsky developed hypotheses primarily for language form, or structure. He called these structures *transformational grammar.* Language meaning, or semantics, was limited to the sense or nonsense the words created. For example, he explained how parts of speech such as nouns, verbs, and objects of the verb assume specific positions in sentences. *The boy kissed the baby* is a possible utterance. Yet *The flower kissed the baby* is not possible, although the grammatical parts of speech are aligned identically in both examples. The child discovers how universal linguistic rules are used in the language of the environment or the culture.

Chomsky's theory caused researchers to look at language development in new ways. Language is acquired not simply by imitation and reinforcement. Children experiment with and explore linguistic rules. As they accumulate experiences in using language, they refine the rules. Processing information and experiences in apparently complex ways provides the child with the ability to generate an infinite variety of utterances, most of which have never been heard before.

Semantics and Language Learning

The Skinner-Chomsky debate intensified research into child language development and disability. Emphasis on the form or syntax of language spread to include semantics. The research of Bloom (1970) acknowledged the nonverbal events as well as actual words that occur between conversational partners. She understood that underlying meanings of words, as well as word placement in an utterance, affects the effectiveness of communication. For example, a child may state the words *Mommy sock* several times. In one instance, the child may find mother's stocking. In another situation, the child could be commenting as the mother is putting a sock onto the child's foot. The meanings of words children use are affected by the context. Looking at syntax alone could not express the various intended meanings a particular utterance could convey.

Contemporary Views of Language

Today, some schools acknowledge that Skinner's behavior theory and the use of behavior modification does not always encourage communication skills. Behavior modification can respond to a child's good behaviors in a positive way. Conversely, bad behaviors are not rewarded and may even be countered with negative responses. For example, youngsters who continually shout inappropriately to express themselves might be ignored or given negative consequences, such as being placed in the hall or a "time-out" room. More recently, educators have regarded shouting as attempts by some children to communicate. If these children had the ability to utilize more socially acceptable communication modes, they would. Therefore, facilitating development of appropriate communication skills is viewed as preferable to ignoring or isolating children. Youngsters are taught to talk through problems.

This problem-solving strategy is a conscious and systematic verbalization of steps to solve the problem. Language becomes a tool to change behavior.

COGNITION AND LANGUAGE

The word *cognition* became well known in North America in the early 1960s as Skinner's behavioral psychology began to give way to new information processing theory. Definitions of cognition ranged from simple explanations such as "awareness" or "intelligence" to broader views encompassing all higher mental processes. **Cognition** is the act of knowing. It can be described as those mental faculties which allow the individual to absorb knowledge. Those faculties include skills in attending, discriminating, sequencing, remembering, classifying, integrating, analyzing, and retrieving information. These skills are needed by the individual to think, reason, problem solve, create, and use language. Cognitive skills can be used for linguistic knowledge and nonlinguistic knowledge (Maxwell and Wallach, 1984; Muma, 1983).

One of the earliest researchers in the field of cognition was James Mark Baldwin in the 1890s. His theory of intellectual development was based on observations of infants and young children. He found that attention was the underlying mechanism in obtaining information. The information is organized and attached to prior knowledge. Children's ability to manipulate information and adjust their understanding of the world so that knowledge is applied to new situations depends on the maturation of the brain. Therefore, children pass through developmental cognitive stages (Case, 1985).

Cognitive Hypothesis

Jean Piaget, the Swiss psychologist, used Baldwin's theory of intellectual development as the basis for his work which began in the 1920s. As Piaget analyzed the way children manipulate knowledge, he became interested in the relationship between language and cognition. He believed that language is a part of general symbolic abilities and that cognition precedes and accounts for language acquisition. That is, children acquire the ability to represent in their mind experiences and things from their environment. First the child encounters the experience of rolling a ball under a chair. The event of the rolling ball is stored in the mind. Language learned at a later time expresses the knowledge that the ball can roll. The utterances produced by a child reflect that youngster's understanding of an object or event as well as the way the concept or experience has been processed by the brain. This view was later characterized as the strong cognitive hypothesis (Bruner, 1975; Nelson, 1974a; Rice, 1983).

Cognitive Hypothesis in Question

Rice (1983) discusses the issue of how cognition relates to language. She cites Piaget's notion of **mental representation** or the ability of children to picture or recreate in their minds experiences or objects that are no longer present. Young children also become adept at the use of symbols so they can use gestures and objects to stand for real elements in their environment. For example, a spoon placed at the child's ear might represent a telephone. Children are ready to utilize symbol systems such as language or drawing at this stage.

Yet the cognitive hypothesis, which states that language acquisition is "dependent" on general cognitive knowledge, has been questioned. Analysis of studies undertaken in the 1970s and 1980s suggests that children's acquisition of language is not always dependent on cognitive development. General mental representation mechanisms can be functioning adequately in the presence of a language disorder. The same cognitive systems are used whether the child uses language or other symbol systems such as music, mathematics, or gestures (Gardner, 1983). Furthermore, factors such as the age of the child, the linguistic abilities in question, and the type of cognitive skill involved may have greater impact on the relationship between cognition and language development (Rice, 1983).

Many state departments of education continue to view language and cognition as two distinct entities with cognitive skills being a prerequisite to language skills. This translates to providing language services only to those youngsters whose language level is significantly below their cognitive functioning.

IQ tests usually are the assessment instruments for determining a child's cognitive level. Yet traditional intelligence tests tend to explore a child's potential school success rather than how the mind manipulates information. In addition, a child's world knowledge varies according to each culture and the child's experience. Youngsters living in certain social and educational environments are inclined to achieve higher scores on IQ tests if their knowledge corresponds to the specific words or group of facts about the world that appear in the test (Gardner, 1983).

Therefore, schools today should recognize that cognitive development is not necessarily the prime prerequisite to language development. Dale and Cole (1991) have reviewed the research in the last decade and suggest that some children may develop language skills that exceed their general cognitive ability as measured on intelligence tests. Additional factors viewed as positive influences on language development include social interaction and varied worldly experiences. Schools must account for the complexities of language as well as normal variation in child development when determining appropriate educational services. They should recognize that cognition is not necessarily the major prerequisite for language development. This challenges the current practice in approximately 31 states of deciding eligibility for language intervention based on language skill lagging behind cognitive skill (Casby, 1992).

PRAGMATICS AND INTERVENTION

By the early 1970s, communicative intentions of children were recognized as critical to language. That is, a child might know how to pronounce words and might know the meanings of words. But some children don't know under what circumstances to use the language they know. The focus of language study centered on children's pragmatics (i.e., the use of language in specific contexts or situations). The components of language (phonology, morphology, syntax, and semantics) were expanded to include pragmatics. Effective communication, speaker/listener relationships, perspectives of the listener, and elements of conversational etiquette were researched (Bates, 1976; Dore, 1975; Halliday, 1975; Miller, 1978).

The pragmatic framework to understand language affected the educational setting. For younger children, the interactions between the parent and the child, even before the child could utter understandable words, were seen as the origins of communication skills. The parent or caregiver might respond to a baby's gesture or random sound by talking or giving the baby attention. The baby gestures and coos again. This interchange is the forerunner of true conversation. Educators began to recognize that parent participation in child language acquisition was crucial (Lieven, 1984; McDade and Varnedoe, 1987). The therapist might work with the child several hours a week, but an informed parent could provide language stimulation several hours a day. Numerous articles were written outlining intervention programs promoting parent participation in the education of children with delays. The medical model of "therapist" providing "treatment" evolved into an educational model of language facilitation in natural settings. The "speech therapist" became known as a speech-language clinician, specialist, or pathologist.

By the late 1970s and early 1980s, with the impact of the Education for All Handicapped Children Act (PL 94-142), collaboration between speech-language clinicians, teachers, and parents emerged. By mandate, educational plans for children with disabilities had to be compiled by a team which included a parent, one or more specialists, and/or a teacher. Accountability and required reports informed team members of the child's goals and progress.

In 1986, a report to the Office of Special Education of the U.S. Department of Education (Will, 1986) proposed a movement to place special education students back into the regular classroom and avoid traditional "pull out" therapy. This report initiated efforts to establish the Regular Education Initiative (REI). More recent progress toward including youngsters with special needs and disabilities in regular activities and settings is an outgrowth of the initiative.

COLLABORATIVE/CONSULTATIVE SERVICE

The federally mandated initiatives cited in the last section, coupled with the impact of pragmatics and cognitive research in language intervention, merged to create a cooperative model of language service. By the late 1980s and early 1990s, some school systems were adopting a collaborative/consultative service delivery model to augment the "pull out" clinical model that isolated children and prevented the application of intervention strategies in real or natural environments like the classroom (Ferguson, 1991; Moore-Brown, 1991). In this model, intervention staff examine the various contexts, attitudes, and policies encountered by a particular student to see how these can promote better learning. Thus, the students' environments become as critical as the students themselves in discovering solutions to learning problems.

Such an orientation suggests at least five classroom-based types of collaborative/consultative models for the language specialist. These include actually teaching a self-contained language class; teaching with the regular classroom teacher or special education teacher; providing one-to-one, classroom-based intervention with a specific student; consulting with the classroom teacher or special service provider; and offering staff, curriculum, or program development to the school district (Miller, 1989). The intent of the collaborative model is to enhance the communication skills and academic experiences of students by fostering sharing and consultation of all individuals involved with the child exhibiting problems (Ferguson, 1991).

THE DESCRIPTIVE APPROACH

As schools began to redefine the medical or clinical framework for providing intervention to children with disabilities and to incorporate the collaborative approach, classrooms that had been created for specific disorders were also reexamined. Special education services usually had been developed to accommodate children with defined etiologies such as autism, mental retardation, hearing impairment, or cerebral palsy. Those youngsters with language and learning problems without a confirmed organic etiology were difficult to place. Sometimes the language deficit was too complicated to define using the terminology mandated by the regulating agencies such as the state education departments. Frequently, children could not be placed in preexisting programs because they exhibited several etiologies. For example, a child might have been diagnosed with emotional disability and mental retardation. The descriptive approach in explaining language disorders rectified some of these barriers to appropriate service. Instead of placing a label on a child, a particular youngster's capabilities and deficits were described (Bloom and Lahey, 1978). Children with similar educational needs and learning styles could be grouped together regardless of any confirmed etiology. A child whose language abilities were the result of mental retardation might be in the same class as a child whose etiology was neurological dysfunction.

To comply with PL 101-476 (i.e., IDEA), state education departments continue to require disability labels before a child can be placed in special services and programs. This federal mandate has limited the acceptance of the descriptive model. Yet the descriptive approach has instructional relevance. It allows the speech-language specialist and other school professionals to focus on specific strengths and weaknesses. Greater flexibility in program options can be promoted, since the student no longer must fit a specific preestablished program. However, when adopting a descriptive approach, the child must be provided with relevant linguistic and educational environments to function effectively.

As child language has been better understood during the last decade, viewing it as an isolated skill has been recognized as inadequate. Language competence affects school success, both academically and socially (Wallach and Miller, 1988). It impacts on the acquisition of literacy. It affects the child's experiences out of school as well. Therefore, to fully understand a child's language competence, language processing in a variety of contexts in the youngster's life must be examined. The whole child becomes critical to the evaluation/intervention process. Classroom-based programs for children with language difficulties (sometimes referred to as *inclusion* or *immersion*) have promoted integration of academic, social, and language proficiency.

THE "METAS" AND INTERVENTION

Various studies of the language skills of school-aged children have explained the importance of language proficiency for academic success (Simon, 1991; Wallach and Butler, 1984; Wallach and Miller, 1988). Children in the early stages of language acquisition are most concerned with the ability to communicate their message to a listener. If particular words are not known, the child tries to substitute other words, or use gestures, or point, or modulate the tone of voice. The child's focus of attention is on what is being said and understood.

"Meta" Skills Defined

Between the age of four to eight years, children begin to deliberately reflect on language, how it is structured, and how to say specific words in various ways to denote different meanings. When a youngster thinks about the language and words being uttered and then manipulates and controls what is being said, the behavior is known as **metalinguistic awareness** (Tunmer and Cole, 1991).

During the late 1970s, a proliferation of language research examined the development of language awareness in children (i.e., metalinguistics) (Cazden, 1974; Leonard and Reid, 1979; Slobin, 1978a; van Kleeck, 1984a). Studies described how children begin to think about and discuss language. They might recite words that rhyme or figure out the number of syllables in words. The youngster who has not developed some metalinguistic skill will have difficulty with reading. That is, when a child has no understanding that the string of sounds flowing from a person's mouth forms words, and that these words can be written down with specific squiggles called *letters*, this child is not ready to decode letters for reading.

Children's understanding of how to talk to people in various situations has been labeled **metapragmatics**. The child who reflects on how to remember a long list of names, or how to pay attention more effectively in class, or how to solve math problems correctly and with consistency, is employing metacognitive skill.

"Meta" Impact on Education

"Meta" (referring to a change or transformation of language or thinking) research has impacted educational practices for children with language disability. By making a child aware of language forms, meaning, and use, and by helping the child verbalize about specific linguistic situations, the educator can determine language breakdown and facilitate better language learning. Students become more facile at using language in various contexts, understanding the linguistic code, acquiring literacy, and developing social skills (van Kleeck, 1984a).

Metalinguistic skill requires basic linguistic skill. Cognitive growth is a prerequisite for more advanced metalinguistic skill. However, there is considerable variability in the development of children. Thus, in order for children to consider how to convey a message effectively, they must attain competencies both in manipulating language and in cognitive reasoning ability. Because all of these factors affect a child's ability to succeed in academic and social environments, it is important to evaluate each child's language and cognitive development to determine the optimum period to engage in various academic activities.

AUGMENTATIVE SYSTEMS

With the plethora of language research in recent years came recognition that children with more serious disability could have inner language and no means to express their knowledge and feelings. In addition, speech-language pathologists began to explore ways to develop language using nontraditional modalities. For example, some youngsters with motoric impairment do not have the physical ability to form words to communicate. Others seem to demonstrate some understanding of their world but do not speak. Alternate forms of communication have been expanded and new systems have been developed. Their purpose is to stimulate language understanding and expression in children. Alternate forms of communication other than speech are known as **augmentative systems**.

Sign Language

One such augmentative system is *sign language.* Sign language is considered augmentative when it is used with children who have normal hearing. Some educators are encouraged particularly by very young hearing children with other disabilities who use sign language because it seems to stimulate speech (Reich, 1978). Sign language as an educational tool has been used in the United States since the early nineteenth century when it was introduced by Thomas Hopkins Gallaudet. Yet its use has proliferated in the last two decades with hearing children who have autism, mental retardation, and other disabilities. Although a number of these youngsters have developed a means for expressive language by using signs, they have considerable difficulty in maintaining educational and language development. Most school systems only have staff who use sign language in the programs for children with hearing impairments, and the hearing child who uses signs has few communication partners.

Communication Board

A second type of augmentative system is the *communication board*. It comes in many forms and has been widely accepted because it does not limit the user to communication only with individuals who are familiar with sign language. It does, however, become cumbersome because it must be available to the child at all times if it is the sole means of communication. Communication boards can contain letters, words, pictures, photographs, symbols, or whatever is suitable for a particular youngster. An example of a communication board system is *Blissymbolics*, an international picture language (McNaughton, 1975). In this system, symbols represent words. For example, a small circle is the symbol for mouth. A heart designates feeling. A heart accompanied by another symbol such as an arrow pointing down indicates sadness.

The items on communication boards are placed in rows on the board and children express themselves by pointing to the appropriate symbol. As the language level of the child matures, the number of symbols on the communication board increases. Even 500 symbols on a board can limit a more proficient language user from expressing ideas fully. Also, a board that contains hundreds of symbols becomes quite large and unwieldy.

Computer Technology

Computer technology has generated a number of hand-held and desktop augmentative devices. Some instruments print words, others create graphics, and some utilize prerecorded or synthesized speech. For the nonverbal youngster, this technology has expanded communication opportunities considerably. The user can either type a message or scan on a computer screen with a pointer until the desired symbol appears. In integrated school sites, the computer can be disruptive to regular education programs and generate problems in the transportation and storage of the machine. Many students are not able to utilize the computer without ongoing training and supervision. Furthermore, appropriate software for children with more severe disabilities is limited (Schery and O'Connor, 1992). Yet computer technology does provide better opportunities for the child with severe disabilities to communicate and participate in the classroom community.

Individual Needs Considered

In the last decade in school environments, augmentative systems have been used simultaneously or individually. Each child must be thoroughly assessed to determine the most appropriate selection of systems at any given time or age. Consideration of the child's language environment at home as well as at school is crucial. Alternate forms of communication should reflect the child's needs, routines, and interests so that they enable the youngster to participate more in mainstream or regular education and community activities. Innovative school systems have equipped students who cannot speak effectively with their own personal computers and voice synthesizers. This technology has also provided more focused, individualized instruction to the specific student. Whatever augmentative system or systems are chosen for a child, meaningful use of language must be encouraged. In addition, the speech-language pathologist should continue to educate those youngsters utilizing alternate forms of communication for speech production.

SUMMARY

The advances in understanding language development and disability in the last few decades are reflected in the educational setting. Speech therapy as a medical model, which emphasized specific, quantitative causes and treatment, has evolved into an educational model of language facilitation carried out in real situations. Removal of children with language problems from their classrooms for infrequent therapy with language goals possibly unrelated to the school curriculum or home environment is being replaced by more collaborative and consultative intervention. More children with severe disabilities are integrated into regular educational environments. Youngsters with significant language disorders not associated with other disabilities are recognized as being at risk for reading, academic, social, and emotional difficulties. Youngsters with the inability to verbalize orally can be introduced to alternate forms of communication such as sign language, communication boards, and computers to enable greater integration into the mainstream school setting.

Today, the field of communication disorders looks beyond "speech" as the basis of communication. Language encompasses the way the child views the world, integrates and understands knowledge and ideas, interacts and communicates with other people, refines concepts based on expanded experience, comprehends directions and stories, and expresses thoughts and narratives. The professional who facilitates these skills has evolved from therapist to speech-language pathologist, specialist, or clinician. Instructional practices concentrate on teaching language in natural contexts and during real language interactions. This places the educational focus on both the individual child and the instructional environment. All significant communication partners, including family members, teachers, and classmates, form a cooperative framework around the child with language impairment.

SUGGESTED READINGS

Miller, L. (1989). Classroom-Based Language Intervention. *Language, Speech, and Hearing Services in Schools, 20*(2), 153–169.

Rice, M., and Kemper, S. (1984). *Child Language and Cognition.* Baltimore, MD: University Park Press.

Simon, C. (Ed.). (1991). *Communication Skills and Classroom Success: Assessment and Therapy Methodologies for Language and Learning Disabled Students.* Eau Claire, WI: Thinking Publications.

3 EARLY LANGUAGE DEVELOPMENT

To plan an education program or to analyze the problems children appear to be having academically and socially, the teacher and other educational specialists need to identify linguistic factors that ordinarily contribute to the development of language. By learning about these factors, educators can then consider which of the factors are lacking or deficient.

Chapter 3 examines the following factors in the context of language development from birth to approximately age two:

1. the innate abilities that influence normal language acquisition;

2. the relationship between symbolic thought and language;

3. important milestones that are considered by a number of researchers to be precursors of pragmatic and expressive language;

4. environments that contribute to the quality, quantity, and variety of child language; and

5. the role of caregivers in facilitating language growth.

INNATE COMMUNICATION ABILITIES

The newborn infant with all biological, chemical, and neurological systems intact is predisposed, or born with the abilities necessary for language acquisition. The newborn is ready, motivated, and equipped to communicate with other human beings (Meltzoff, 1985a). The remarkable innate abilities of newborn infants to communicate require nurturance and stimulation to continue to develop normally.

Reflexive Behaviors

The human infant is born with specific reflexes such as sucking, grasping, and crying. A **reflex** is a response behavior that is unlearned and automatic. By means of these reflexes, neonates (i.e., newborns) are able to communicate their needs and learn about their environment.

Crying is the means of communication through which the infant's needs and wants are expressed. The various cries in the infant's repertoire can be easily differentiated by the caregiver (i.e., hunger, pain, discomfort, and request for attention) (Lester and Zeskind, 1982; Zeskind and Lester, 1981). Paralinguistic information can be perceived in the infant's cry (e.g., intonational patterns, inflection, stress, and intensity). These paralinguistic components of language also convey emotions such as happiness, anger, or fear.

Visual Recognition

Visual recognition of mother appears to occur within hours after birth (Barrera and Maurer, 1981; Masi and Scott, 1983). Ability to discriminate facial expressions, such as happy, sad, and surprised, has been reported in healthy prematurely-born infants (Field, Woodson, Cohen, Greenberg, Garcia, and Collins, 1983). These findings indicate that the ability to perceive differences in the expressions on human faces is innate; in other words, the infant is born with this ability.

Auditory Perception

A surprising degree of auditory perceptual ability is present at birth (Aslin, Pisoni, and Jusczyk, 1983). Infants are able to localize and orient to (i.e., turn to) sources of sound from a very young age (Clifton, Morrongiello, Kulig, and Dowd, 1981; Field, Muir, Pilon, Sinclair, and Dodwell, 1980; Mehler, 1985). One-hour-old infants will orient to the sound of a gentle human voice (Alegria and Noirot, 1978; Gibson and Spelke, 1983; Sherrod, 1981).

The emotion transmitted by the human voice has been shown to be clearly perceived by infants (Murray and Trevarthen, 1987; Trevarthen, 1983a, 1983b).

Face-to-Face Interaction

The infant appears to be fascinated by the human face from the first days of life (Izard, Huebner, Risser, McGuiness, and Dougherty, 1980). Infants make eye contact with caregivers in the first hours of life (Bower, 1982). Early responses by mother or caregiver are encouraged by the infant's gaze and intense attention to the adult's face (Fernald, 1984). When the adult responds to the cry of discomfort by cuddling or holding the infant closely, a definite social interaction takes place between infant and caregiver. Infants learn many of the rules of communication used in their environment by the face-to-face interaction and the exploration of the caregivers' affect during these interactions (Lester, 1984; Lester and Zeskind, 1982; Maskarinec, Cairns, Butterfield, and Weamer, 1981; Tronick, Als, and Brazelton, 1980; Zeskind, 1980; Zeskind and Lester, 1981). By the third week of life, the infant begins to smile in response to the human voice and the human face, a smile that involves the whole face, including the eyes (Bower, 1982).

To be a good communicator, an individual must take the role of speaker or listener. During conversational exchanges, the listener must be attuned to pauses between the speaker's utterances, indicating that it is time for the listener to take a turn as a speaker. In addition, to be an effective conversational participant, an individual must observe the communication partner's body posture, facial expressions, tone of voice, loudness of voice, and inflection to interpret the feelings and emotions underlying verbal expression. In the case of an individual who communicates with a manual language, emphasis of movement and facial expression indicate the underlying emotion. Do children between the ages of birth and nine months have these abilities, even though they have not uttered or signed their first true word? Research indicates they do (Bates, O'Connell, and Shore, 1987; Bruner, 1981; Dore, 1983, 1986; Feagans, Garvey, and Golinkoff, 1984; Fernald, 1984; Field and Fox, 1985; Golinkoff, 1983; Golinkoff and Gordon, 1988; Greenfield, 1980; Harding, 1983; Miller and Byrne, 1984; Wetherby, Cain, Yonclas, and Walker, 1988).

Relationship of Attachment

In this newborn period, there is a beginning of reciprocal, turn-taking in the communication between the infant and the adult. All the abilities described earlier serve to establish a relationship of attachment to a particular caregiver immediately after birth. The interaction and close relationship that develops quickly between a newborn infant and an adult are "precursors" of pragmatic development. A **precursor** in this context is a condition, ability, or behavior that ensures by its presence that the child will more likely progress through subsequent developmental stages, although it is not an actual requirement for such future development. Precursors facilitate the child's progress.

Communicative Intentions

Immediately after birth, infants begin to express their needs by crying. At that point, their crying is reflexive. Within the first three months of life, they begin to cry intentionally. There are distinct differences between the cries denoting hunger, pain, discomfort, anger, and the request for attention. Early social interactions involving face-to-face experiences lead to the infant's awareness of the effect that his or her behavior can have on others (Bruner, 1981; Dore, 1986).

Long before children use a distinct language to communicate their intentions or desires, they engage in topics of conversation through the use of gesture, crying, and eye gaze. At one month, attention-getting is the limit of infants' communicative abilities (Foster, 1985). They can initiate a topic with the adult by expressing their discomfort or hunger and thus draw attention to themselves. Most caregivers have no difficulty determining that the infant is making a clear statement.

True Intentions

By three months of age, infants can interact in a more complex fashion by cooing, gurgling, squealing, and smiling. The topic of conversation is infant-oriented (i.e., the child may initiate the interaction by burping or sneezing). The adult treats these behaviors as true communications and may respond to the burp by saying, *My what a big burp! I'm so glad you enjoyed your bottle,* with a great deal of inflection. The gentle, musical response soothes the infant who may be alarmed by the noise of the burp. It was mentioned previously that newborn infants will orient to the sound of a gentle voice. The awareness that someone is speaking or communicating by sign language alerts the child to the fact that an interaction is beginning, information that is so important when acquiring pragmatic skills.

Social Referencing

During the second three months of life, face-to-face play between mother and infant becomes increasingly meaningful. The infant can then tolerate more sustained eye contact (Malatesta, 1982; Malatesta and Haviland, 1982). It is also during this period that distinct turn-taking behaviors take place. The infant learns to appreciate the relationship between mother's feelings and emotions and her facial expressions and behaviors. These emotions often mirror those of the infant. When a baby is happy, contented, and smiling, the caregiver smiles in response. If babies are unhappy, irritable, or ill, their expressions of distress are mirrored on the adults' faces. Infants have been shown to recognize the relationship between the way they feel and the expressions on the caregivers' faces (Malatesta and Izard, 1984; Meltzoff and Moore, 1985). Both the face and the voice convey social signals that also express emotion (Locke, 1993).

The infant will continue to seek mother's face for information during times of uncertainty (Campos and Stenberg, 1980). This process is referred to as *social referencing*. Particularly when the context and the environment are unfamiliar, young children will try to "read" their mothers' affect for clues as to whether the situation warrants their becoming frightened (Cicchetti and Pogge-Hesse, 1980).

Parentese (Previously Referred to as Motherese)

The adult's speech to a young infant is unique, automatic, highly specialized, and significantly affects the child's language acquisition. The particular type of communication used by an adult who is speaking to a young child is referred to as **motherese** or currently **parentese**. Deaf mothers also use motherese when communicating with their infants in sign language (Erting, Prezioso, and Hynes, 1990; Papousek and Papousek, 1987; Rea, Bonvillian, and Richards, 1988). The same characteristics of parentese apply to spoken language and to manual language.

Infants usually initiate the interactions between caregivers and themselves. The infant may look at an object and possibly reach out and attempt to grasp it. The adult labels the object, explains what it is, and comments on its qualities. During this interaction, adult and infant make eye contact, and the adult, using parentese, is heard to exaggerate the rhythm and inflection of speech or sign. The speech is much slower and simpler than that used when communicating with an older child. Articulation is more precise. There is a great deal of repetition of phrases and labels used by the adult. There is also a great deal of smiling observed on the part of the adult.

When playing with adults, infants use vocalization and recognizable, deliberate gestures, such as pointing, reaching, and giving. The child is using language, albeit nonverbal language, for a distinct purpose with a distinct goal in mind. During these interactions, the adult will frequently pause and attempt to elicit a response from the infant, such as a smile, a gaze, or a vocal sound. Very young infants learn to listen for this pause, indicating a realization that it is their turn to respond.

The communicative use of nonverbal language in this early period enables the child to influence and actually regulate the behaviors and social interactions with important adults in the environment (Adamson and Bakeman, 1985; Foster, 1985; Prizant and Wetherby, 1990; Stern, 1985).

By nine months of age, children are seen to shift eye contact from adult to object deliberately and persistently until their vocal and gestural communications result in the desired response from the adult (Bates, 1979; Sachs, 1989; Scoville, 1983).

THE TRANSITION TO SYMBOLIC THOUGHT AND LANGUAGE

Piaget has made a tremendous impact on modern educational, psychological, and developmental theories of how children acquire symbolic language and develop intellectually. Piaget conducted extensive testing on children and adolescents and drew specific conclusions through observations of children's behaviors under testing conditions.

Concept Development

According to Piaget (1950, 1952), a child's intellectual development proceeds in distinct stages as children interact with their environment. His theory emphasizes that children learn about people, objects, and events in their environment by means of active interaction with the environment. At first, this interaction consists of reflexive responses to external stimuli, such as crying, sucking, and grasping. Quite rapidly, the child's behaviors become less reflexive and more deliberate.

Sometimes children succeed in accomplishing unexpected or accidental results which provide important sources of information. These actions then are repeated deliberately to obtain results similar to the one accidentally discovered. When children physically manipulate, explore, and transform objects in the environment, they acquire knowledge about them, their functions, their qualities, and the ways they can be manipulated to obtain a goal. As infants learn to coordinate visual, auditory, and tactile sensations with motor activity, they have more success in their attempts to manipulate the objects in their environment. They squeeze the objects, stroke them, bang them, push them, and put them in their mouths. Tactile awareness in the mouth is highly sensitive. The tip of the tongue particularly is an extremely sensitive instrument for exploring the surface texture and consistency of an object, as well as its taste, if it has a taste (Bower, 1982).

The hardness, acoustic qualities, specific size, shape, and color of an object are perceived by the baby. If the object is bright, colorful, shiny, and makes a noise, it attracts greater attention. The child stores the image of the object, with all its characteristics, in memory. The next time a similar object is encountered, the child recognizes its qualities. With each new experience in different contexts, the child modifies and adds to the knowledge of that particular object and stores the new information in memory. Thus, a concept is developed. A **concept** is a perceived category of related information regarding specific objects and events. Concepts enable the young child to organize the continuous stream of information received through the senses. When concepts are stored in memory in an organized fashion, they can later be retrieved and possibly modified as more related information is acquired through personal experience.

Precursors of Symbolic Thought

During the process of developing language with which to communicate effectively, infants progress through sequences of accomplishments, both biological and intellectual. The progress of this development is facilitated by a number of precursors.

Perceptual Integrity

The five senses should be functioning adequately for children to detect or become aware of the qualities of the objects in their world. However, it is not enough that the eyes, ears, nose, taste buds, skin, and muscles of the body can detect the visual, auditory, olfactory, gustatory, and tactile stimuli. These stimuli must be carried by an intact neurological system to the cortex of the brain where they will acquire meaning and be stored in memory in an organized fashion. In addition, internal sensory systems (e.g., kinesthetic perception, proprioceptive perception, and vestibular perception) must also be functioning. The importance of a well-functioning, well-coordinated perceptual system cannot be under-estimated when analyzing the components of an environment from which a child will glean knowledge about objects, people, and events. These components must be recognized, interpreted, and stored in an organized fashion for the child to derive meaning from an otherwise disorganized array of stimuli.

Eye-Hand Coordination

Grasping is initially a reflex. Bower (1982) describes reaching and grasping as behaviors of tremendous importance to human experience and learning. The unborn fetus is already reaching and grasping in the womb at 14–16 weeks of gestation (Bower, 1982). Initially, infants reflexively grasp objects that touch their hands. Very soon, they become aware of near and far objects and reach for them. Within several weeks, finer coordination of motor movements and the ability to perceive depth in space enable the infant to reach out and deliberately grasp a specific object. Bower, Broughton, and Moore (1970a, 1970b) conducted studies indicating that newborn infants deliberately reach for objects and intend to grasp them because they mold their fingers appropriately while they direct their arms toward various objects. The tactile information received from grasping an object contributes understanding about its shape, texture, form, and position in space. The response by an adult to the gesture of reaching constitutes positive reinforcement for the communicative intention on the part of the infant. A social interaction has taken place.

Before children can express their thoughts with speech or by another form of symbolic language, such as a manual code, they must retain a mental image of objects and people when they are no longer in view and of events after they have occurred. Only then can the stored images of objects, people, and events become symbols that are expressed as words, signs, or pictures. The following four precursors described are indices of the child's retention of mental images. Use of first words coincides with development of symbolic images.

Object Permanence

Object permanence refers to the ability to understand that things and places continue to exist when they can no longer be seen. Sometimes a toy rolls out of sight. A young infant less than one year of age will probably not go after it; in fact, once the toy is out of sight, it apparently no longer exists. However, by the end of the first year, children usually begin to look for the toy after it has disappeared from view, indicating that its image has been stored in memory and they can "see" it in their mind's eye. By about 18 months of age, however, children look intently for the toy, even in locations where the toy might be. If they find it, they recognize it as the toy that was missing and can match the found object to the image in their mind's eye. That is what makes 18 month olds different from younger children (Meltzoff and Gopnik, 1989).

Object Constancy

Object constancy is the ability to perceive objects accurately even though they become distorted as they move in space or if the child moves while viewing them. The child tries to make the world consistent and predictable. As indicated previously, very young infants can identify and discriminate forms, sizes, and contours, both dynamic and static. Objects become familiar to children through their active experiences with them (i.e., banging, stroking, squeezing, grasping, mouthing). When an image of an object is stored in memory in such a fashion that the child can recognize it even though it is distorted or partially occluded by another object, there is clear indication that the child has acquired object constancy. The image in his mind's eye can represent the real object in its entirety.

Deferred Imitation

Deferred imitation is the ability to store images of people's actions and speech sounds in memory and to imitate them in the child's own unique manner after a considerable time interval. The ability to store images of actions and speech sounds for retrieval and later use is thought to facilitate representational or symbolic thought.

Before children can duplicate actions or speech of others after a time interval, they must be able to duplicate these actions immediately after seeing the model. Meltzoff and Moore (1977, 1983a, 1983b) found newborn infants imitate the actions of adults when they make funny faces and stick out their tongues. Their findings have been replicated in at least seven independent studies (Abravanel and Sigafoos, 1984; Field, Woodson, Greenberg, and Cohen, 1982; Fontaine, 1984; Heimann and Schaller, 1985; Jacobson, 1979; Kaitz, Meschulach-Sarfaty, Auerbach, and Eidelman, 1988; Vinter, 1986). To imitate these actions, the infant must focus on, attend to, accurately perceive, and then immediately reproduce all the specific features of an adult's behavior.

Meltzoff's research (1985b) revealed that infants as young as nine months of age reproduced sequential actions of an adult after a 24-hour delay. In subsequent studies by Meltzoff (1988a, 1988b),

14-month-old infants remembered and imitated multiple complex actions they had seen only once after a one-week interval (e.g., manipulation of particular toys).

Means-Ends Behavior

At about 12–18 months of age, children begin to actively explore their environment. They experiment through trial and error in an attempt to solve problems they encounter, such as when they cannot reach something, cannot find something, and cannot move or change something. They are observed to use objects as tools to rake in toys that have rolled beyond their reach. At this stage, children have been described as "little scientists designing spontaneous experiments" (Bernstein, 1989).

When abilities such as object permanence, object constancy, and deferred imitation are in place, the children can be observed "thinking about" possible actions rather than physically acting by trial and error. They can actually "anticipate" the results of their actions with objects because they have stored their experiences and perceptions regarding these objects in their memories. They can retrieve these images and manipulate the objects in their mind's eye. This behavior is referred to as **means-ends behavior**, which reflects the children's ability to think about and anticipate results of their actions on objects.

Pretend Play

Much of the child's language develops within the context of play with an adult or with other children. Play is an ideal vehicle for language acquisition (Sachs, 1984a, 1984b). Play is also a vehicle for concept development and social development (Garvey, 1990).

Precursors of Symbolic Play

Garvey (1990) emphasizes that object play requires certain abilities, such as visually directed grasping and adequate eye-hand coordination so that the child can pick up, hold, and turn objects. Object play depends upon the achievement of object permanency, the understanding that an object continues to exist even though it is not within view. It also requires the knowledge that one can perform different actions with an object. In addition, the child must be able to imitate an action someone else has performed several minutes, hours, or even days before (i.e., deferred imitation). These are important precursors of later symbolic play (Garvey, 1990; McCune-Nicolich and Carroll, 1981).

Early Play

According to McCune-Nicolich and Carroll (1981), children proceed through five stages before reaching the stage of symbolic play and its accompanying symbolic language. Children must first learn the functions of objects as a basis for later pretending. When they can take an object in hand and perform an action with it, such as combing hair or drinking from a cup, they are ready to proceed to the next stage of development.

Gestural Naming

The next two stages progress as the child is seen to mime an action, such as drinking from an empty cup or eating from an empty spoon, with a gleeful expression showing that this is a make-believe game. These actions are referred to as **gestural naming** and often predict the emergence of single words (Bates, Bretherton, and Snyder, 1988). Gradually, by the beginning of the second year, the child performs pretend actions on dolls, stuffed animals, and people, and accompanies these actions by the use of single words.

Fourth Stage Play

The fourth stage of pretend play usually appears during the second year (Nicolich, 1977). At this time, the child can perform different pretend activities with the same object, e.g., feed the doll, scold it for some imaginary misbehavior, and then put it into a toy stroller for a pretend outing.

Symbolic Play

The final stage of development is symbolic play, which becomes evident late in the second year. Children can now substitute one object for another. They can also use one object or toy as an agent to act on another object, e.g., a doll serving tea to a toy elephant, or Mommy's pendant being used as a stethoscope on the doll's chest. According to Nicolich (1977), after children have been pretending in this way for several months, they can be observed to search for missing objects needed to complete a pretend activity. This accomplishment usually occurs at about 18–26 months of age. Eventually, the child will symbolize or represent the object with a word or label while role playing or telling a narrative.

Interaction During Play

Play provides an ideal situation in which adults can teach children to comprehend and to express vocabulary (Masur and Gleason, 1980). During the activity of pretend play, the adult gradually increases expectations regarding the quality of the child's vocal commentary. At first, when playing with an infant, a smile alone is a response that motivates the adult and is all that is expected. Gradually, more is required of the child. The adult pauses in the activity expecting some comment. When the child is a young infant, babbling, squealing, or gurgling is acceptable. As the child grows older, adults positively respond to more complex forms of vocal participation during play activities, and indirectly help to improve the child's verbal skills (Sachs, 1984a). Solitary play or play without child/adult interaction excludes very important components essential for learning and language development. (See a detailed discussion of adult linguistic input later in this chapter, pages 67–68.)

LANGUAGE COMPREHENSION

Perception of Speech by Infants

The comprehension or understanding of the components of language begins while the infant is still a developing fetus. Babies are predisposed to process voice information (Locke, 1993). For example, they are born with the ability to perceive sound differences (Burnham, Earnshaw, and Quinn, 1987; Sachs, 1989; Werker and Tees, 1984). Infants are able to identify their mother's voice before birth while still in the womb (Benzaquen, Gagnon, Hunse, and Foreman, 1990; Spence and De Casper, 1982). They will actively respond to this voice while in the womb. De Casper and Fifer (1980) found that at one or two days of age, infants will suck to produce their mother's voice and can recognize their own mother's voice as distinct from the voices of other women.

The neonate can recognize mother's face and discriminate that face from other faces soon after birth. By the end of the second day after birth, most neonates recognize the face and voice of their mother. To understand language, a child must first focus on the parts of the human physiology that are involved in speaking and communicating (e.g., the whole face, the eyes, the moving mouth accompanied by vocalization). It has been pointed out previously that newborns only hours old can focus on the face and imitate movements by researchers, such as sticking out the tongue and puckering the lips. These behaviors indicate that newborns can focus and sustain attention to the parts of the face having to do with speech. "Infants who see the maternal face 'talk' are likely to notice aspects of her speech" (Locke, 1993, p. 82). Also, when an adult signs to a neonate, an integral part of the meaning of the message is read in the facial expression and movement of the eyes (Meier and Newport, 1990).

Bloom (1974) described two types of comprehension: children's knowledge of language and their knowledge of the world.

Children have at least three sources of information available: the events they witness, the speech they hear, and the gestural and manual language they see. A one-year-old has a fairly sophisticated understanding of events. The child has stored memories of events that are likely to happen and recur. The people identified with these events are also stored in memory. Children under a year of age begin to reveal by their behavior some indication that they understand the relationships between events, people, and words or phrases that are repeatedly used in a familiar context. For example, mother's taking out the carriage is associated with going outside. In addition, she will usually make a comment such as, *Let's get your jacket. It's time to go out now.* Sitting in the high chair in the kitchen is associated with eating and an adult's statement, *Let's see what will we have for lunch today. How about some spaghetti?*

In the second year, children should understand the meaning of words apart from a specific context. By two years of age, children usually reveal understanding of the additional information conveyed by the tone of voice (e.g., an emphatic "NO!" by mother when the infant is attempting to grasp a $200 vase).

Comprehension involves the need to attend to more information than speech alone. Natural interactive situations provide important nonverbal clues to aid the child in understanding what is being said and what is happening (e.g., emphasis, inflection of the voice, facial expression, body language, ongoing activity, and physical objects in the immediate environment that are the focus of attention). These communicative situations contribute to comprehension. Failure to use the various communicative cues is a real cause for concern (James, 1989). Children who fail to show the comprehension skills described above by 16 to 18 months are possible candidates for intervention (Bricker and Schiefelbusch, 1990).

LANGUAGE PRODUCTION

At birth, the infant's anatomy does not permit speech. During the time it requires the child to develop the anatomical structures necessary for speech, about three months, the child is busy learning. Although language production does not start immediately after birth as language comprehension does, the infant is born with effective means of communication.

Physiological Basis for Speech

Newborn infants are born with the reflexive ability to cry. Crying is their primary mode of communication. Newborns do not have the anatomical structures in place to produce all speech sounds voluntarily. Their anatomy is similar to a nonhuman primate (Lester, 1984). The newborn's tongue, epiglottis, larynx, rib cage, and lungs cannot produce the sounds necessary for speech or vocalizations other than crying. At about three months of age, the anatomical structures change their form and position in the infant's body. Only then are infants ready to produce the sounds that are similar to the sounds in the language used by their linguistic communities.

Precursors of Language Production

Crying

Crying is important for survival as well as for drawing attention to the need for feeding, changing, and social play. Adults must understand infants' specific types of cries and respond to them. Equally important, the interactions between infant and caregiver that are conducted during these activities will help to establish a relationship of attachment (Goldberg, 1982).

Awareness of Visible Articulators by Infants

Kuhl and Meltzoff (1982, 1988), Meltzoff and Kuhl (1989), and Studdert-Kennedy (1986) noted that the facial expressions newborn infants can imitate are related to the movements used in speech production (e.g., mouth opening, tongue movements). Their research revealed that five-month-old infants could imitate the shape of the lips that corresponded to a particular vowel sound. The infants could match the wide open mouth with the short *a* sound production, and the slightly opened mouth, similar to a faint smile, with the short *i* sound production. Further research by Kuhl and Meltzoff (1982, 1988) and Papousek and Papousek (1981) revealed that infants six months of age can imitate some aspects of adult speech productions, such as inflection and melody in the voice and some individual phonemes. Kuczaj (1987) suggested that the ability to reproduce specific oral configurations that resemble the visible articulations of the speaking adult when the model is no longer present and after a considerable period of time (i.e., deferred imitation) is a precursor of language acquisition.

Babbling

Normal infants begin to babble around the age of five months (Bower, 1982). Initially, the child appears to engage in **babbling**, or sound play, just for sheer enjoyment. The child does not seem to be "talking" to anyone, and there does not appear to be any relationship between the baby's vocalizing and a particular object or event (Menn, 1989). When vocalizing for attention, the child is often observed to vary the pitch, volume, and rate of babbling.

Jargon

Gradually, the characteristics of sound play begin to change and appear to become more meaningful. This different type of babbling is referred to as **jargon** or **conversational babbling**. These vocalizations sound as though the child is actually having a conversation, and they are accompanied by eye contact, gesture, facial expression, stress, and rise and fall of pitch. However, the words are unintelligible. Conversational babble clearly conveys the child's communicative intent (e.g., requests for help, attention, food, or toys) (Menn, 1989). The infant assumes the adult understands and often becomes annoyed if the jargon is not correctly interpreted. The adult has to look at the infant's direction of gaze or pointed finger to interpret the intended meaning. Also, body language and facial expression may indicate discomfort, fatigue, hunger, or illness. The adult cannot rely on the jargon itself for meaning.

Phonological similarities between babbled utterances and the first recognizable words have been demonstrated (Stoel-Gammon and Cooper, 1984; Vihman and Greenlee, 1987; Vihman, Macken, Miller, Simmons, and Miller, 1985). Furthermore, during the period of transition to intelligible speech, infants from different countries and language communities tend to include in their babbling the sounds of the language used by their caregivers or heard most frequently in their immediate environments (Blake and deBoysson-Bardies, 1992; deBoysson-Bardies, Halle, Sagart, and Durand, 1989). Research by Vihman, Macken, Miller, Simmons, and Miller (1985) has revealed that the baby's choice of early words contains the sounds that the child preferred when babbling. Early speech develops gradually out of babbling and coexists with it for several months (Blake and deBoysson-Bardies, 1992; Levitt and Aydelott-Utman, 1992; Menn, 1989; Owens, 1992).

First Words

Children usually acquire their first set of 10 words by 15 months (McCormick, 1990; Reich, 1986). Research indicates that the child's first words are not poorly constructed replicas of an adult's verbal language (Harris, Barrett, Jones, and Brooks, 1988). First words are usually names for specific objects or persons, but the child does not use the names simply to label or identify things. Initially, children talk about what they are doing or what they want to do using these single words (Carrow-Woolfolk and Lynch, 1982; Lahey, 1988; McCormick, 1990; Nelson, 1973). Most important, these first words reflect the child's understanding of the concepts they acquired through previous experience.

Relationship to Symbolic Thought

Research by Gopnik and Meltzoff (1987a, 1987b) has shown that around the time when children reveal that they have mastered object permanence, or the notion that objects that disappear from view continue to exist in some unseen location, they begin to express understanding of this phenomenon with words such as *gone*.

Bates, Bretherton, and Snyder (1988) observed that children who used means-ends cognitive behaviors and improvised tools to obtain objects that were out of reach also began to use objects, vocal means, and gestures to gain adult attention (e.g., giving or pointing) with a view to using an adult to obtain an object. First words are often names for the objects they want the adult to help them obtain.

The earliest words acquired are usually labels for the salient things in the child's world (de Villiers and de Villiers, 1978). Predominant among these early words are labels for objects that children can manipulate or act upon (Ross, Nelson, Wetstone, and Tanouye, 1986). Also, important persons like Mommy, Daddy, Grandma, and Grandpa, and the family pet are represented in early lexicons.

Categorical Organization

Early labels also express the child's categorical knowledge. Research studies indicate that preverbal children have the ability to categorize specific objects in their world (Freeman, Lloyd, and Sinha, 1980; Ross, 1980; Sugarman, 1981, 1983). Long before young children can use words or specific signs, they indicate by their actions with objects that they have categorized them according to function (e.g., cuddle a teddy bear, roll a ball, push a toy truck) (Pease, Gleason, and Pan, 1989; Reznick and Kagan, 1983).

When children begin to use single words to name objects, they are actually labeling the objects that they have classified as belonging to categories. The child has selected common attributes or features of objects, and on the basis of these common attributes has grouped them under a single label. For example, the word *bird*, will be used to refer to a categorical class of objects that includes all creatures that have two legs, two wings, a beak, and feathers. Some children classify objects in terms of the actions associated with them (e.g., all things that roll, all things that bounce, all things that move by themselves) (Nelson, 1974a, 1974b). Clark (1983) suggested that some children categorize objects on the basis of shared defining features (e.g., roundness, hardness, four legs, furriness, ability to move). Thus, when a child labels his pet as *cat*, he is incorporating all the qualities of this object (e.g., fur, whiskers, four legs, a tail, and the ability to purr and meow) into a *cat* category.

Overextensions

Bowerman (1977) suggested that when children extract not just one but many properties or attributes of an object and apply the label to other objects that share any one of these attributes, they are **overextending.** For example, the child will say *cat* when looking at a cat, cow, or elephant. Sometimes, the child will extend the label *cat* even further to include butterflies, beetles, and spiders, and it is not always clear which attributes the child is generalizing. Nancy, age 14 months, called a plane a *bird*; only the feathers were missing from the necessary components. Also, young children can often be heard calling all men *Daddy*. Clark (1973, 1975) suggested that children may use the words in their vocabularies that most closely fit the object they want to discuss, even though they know the word is not quite right; however, it is the only one they have at their disposal. Children may also employ this strategy to learn the correct labels for objects, since overextensions of a word frequently elicit a correction from the parent (de Villiers and de Villiers, 1978).

Underextensions

Early labels are not always overextensions. Sometimes, the child has an inadequate understanding of the range of meaning of a word, an

underextension. Tommy, 15 months of age, referred to his pet terrier, Max, as *dog*. However, he did not call his neighbor's collie *dog* or his grandmother's spaniel *dog* or any other animal *dog*. That was a term only used for Max. Tommy was 20 months of age before he pointed to an abstract illustration of a dog in a storybook his mother was reading to him and said *dog*. Very soon after, he began to use the label for his neighbor's collie and his grandmother's spaniel. Through repeated experiences with a variety of animals, Tommy finally categorized and conceptualized the word *dog*.

When a child uses the word *dog* only for a particular dog or in response to one particular picture in a book, the word is considered *context bound*. If the child uses the word *dog* to label different canine animals in a variety of contexts, the same word is classified as *context flexible* (Bates, Bretherton, and Snyder, 1988). "Children with a high proportion of context-flexible object names in their vocabulary have probably passed an important milestone in language acquisition: They have obtained some insight into the idea that things have names" (Bates, Bretherton, and Snyder, 1988, p. 46).

All Encompassing One-Word Utterances

One-word utterances also express whole thoughts. During the stage of development when youngsters have only a limited number of words in their lexicons, they use a single word to express whole thoughts and whole events. For example, when a child says *up*, it could mean *Pick me up, Look up, Mommy get up, Daddy get up, Put me in my high chair,* or *I want my truck on the top shelf.* During these interactions, the caregiver has to rely on the child's gestures and focus of attention to interpret the meaning of one-word/one-thought utterances (Bretherton, McNew, Snyder, and Bates, 1983).

Successive Single-Word Utterances

Successive single-word utterances are different from later two-word utterances. At about 16 months, the child uses multi-word utterances that are really successive single-word utterances. The child uses two, sometimes three words together, but they are separate one-word utterances and do not necessarily refer to a single event. Careful listening will reveal a distinct pause and a drop in pitch between the words.

Two-Word Utterances: Syntactic Development

By 15 months of age, the average expressive vocabulary size is 10 words (Reich, 1986). At the point at which the child's expressive vocabulary reaches about 50 words, generally at about 18 months, there is usually a spurt of vocabulary growth (Reich, 1986).

In the latter half of the second year, children reach another milestone. They begin to combine words to form the first "sentences" (Tager-Flusberg, 1989). Two year olds who are developing language according to expectations are using at least equal numbers of one- and two-word utterances (Bloom, 1973; Miller, 1981b). Children who fail to produce 50 words and two-word combinations at 24 months can be considered delayed in expressive language development (Capute, Palmer, Shapiro, Wachtel, Schmidt, and Ross, 1986; Coplan, Gleason, Ryan, Burke, and Williams, 1982; Rescorla, 1989, 1991; Resnick, Allen, and Rapin, 1984).

The first two-word utterances are combined in a specific rule-oriented fashion, not in a haphazard fashion. How do children acquire syntactic knowledge? How do they learn about the use of nouns, verbs, and adjectives? On what basis do they combine their first two-word utterances?

Studies of children from different areas in the world who use two-word utterances reveal that they all talk about similar things. They talk about objects, where they are, what they do, who owns them, and who is doing things to them. Their sentences are composed primarily of nouns, verbs, and adjectives. Certain topics, such as possession (e.g., *Daddy shoe, baby bed*), location (e.g., *there Tommy*), disappearance (e.g., *bye-bye doggie, all gone*), and recurrence (e.g., *more milk*) are prevalent in the child's sentences (Pease, Gleason, and Pan, 1989; Tager-Flusberg, 1989). An important feature of children's two-word utterances is their consistent word order, an indication that the child understands the basic rules of syntax. The order of the words in these early two-word utterances usually does not resemble adult language and they are not imitations. They are unique and universal combinations (e.g., *more juice, allgone car*). As children grow older, their sentences become more complex as they add morphological endings, such as plurals and tense markers (Tager-Flusberg, 1989). Table 3.1 summarizes normal language development birth through 24 months.

Table 3.1

Normal Language Development in Toddlers

Age	Behavior
Birth–3 mos.	Communicates through crying and gaze, uses some vowel sounds.
3–6 months	Uses vocal play, such as cooing, gurgling, squealing.
5 months	Begins to babble.
12 months	Exhibits communicative intentions using gestures and unconventional vocalizations (jargon) to express requests and protests and to call attention to themselves before their first word is said (12 months) (Chapman, 1981).
15 months	Uses an average expressive vocabulary of 10 words; receptive vocabulary size exceeds the number of words produced. First word understood is not necessarily the same as the first produced. (Reich, 1986).
12–18 months	Acquires first words a word or two at a time. When expressive vocabulary reaches 50 words (18 months), there is a spurt of vocabulary growth.
20 months	Uses a spoken vocabulary of over 150 words on average (Dale, Bates, Reznick, and Morisset, 1989).
24 months	Vocabulary may increase to over 200 words (Reich, 1986).
	Combines words into simple two-word sentences, e.g., *allgone milk, my cookie* (Brown, 1973).
	Produces 70 percent of consonants correctly (Stoel-Gammon, 1991) and a variety of syllable types (Stoel-Gammon, 1987).
	Speech is at least moderately intelligible to those in their immediate environment.

Continued

Table 3.1—*Continued*

24 months	Produces frequent intentional communicative acts and has begun to put together multi-word utterances. Ninety percent have a vocabulary of 50 or more words (Coplan, 1987).
	Uses at least equal numbers of one- and two-word utterances (Miller, 1981a).

Factors Contributing to the Quality of Language Production

When adults make appropriate responses to the child's overextensions, underextensions, and one-word utterances, they are contributing to vocabulary growth (McCormick, 1990). Correct interpretations by the caregiver offer positive feedback to the child and motivate further attempts at communication.

The ability to communicate verbally is learned in the context of interaction between children and their caregivers (Nelson, 1985; Ninio, 1983, 1992). A child's utterances cannot be interpreted apart from the context in which they are expressed.

The context includes the physical environment, the objects and people in that environment, the events occurring in that environment; the culture that has contributed to and controls the child's attitudes, behaviors, and language usage; the structure of the child's family; the child's personality and learning style; and the preferences and personal communicative style of the adults who interact with the child.

Physical Environment

The physical environment influences the topics being discussed. The objects, people, and on-going activities discussed in the kitchen of a suburban home are different from those in the bedroom of a city apartment, at the beach, on a farm, in a jungle community, or in a war-torn area in a makeshift shelter. The first words used by children to communicate in these very different environments will not be the same (Nelson, 1985).

Various activities in different contexts provide unique opportunities for specific language acquisition (e.g., playing with toys, reading, eating, dressing, playing with siblings and peers, and listening to nursery rhymes) (Nelson, 1981a, 1981b). Book reading appears to be more conducive to acquiring labels for objects than playing with blocks or trucks (Ninio, 1980; Ninio and Bruner, 1978).

Cultural Environment

The cultural contexts also determine to a great degree the objects, people, and activities that are important and appropriate for the child to discuss (Nelson, 1985). The type of behavior, language usage, and childcare practices that are considered appropriate by different cultural groups in the United States and throughout the world will determine the words young children select and the manner in which they are expressed.

An important cultural influence that is changing rapidly in many societies of the world are the attitudes regarding males and females. DeFrancisco (1992) points out clearly that through language, children are taught the attitudes, behavior, and social status considered by their society as being appropriate for a man and for a woman. The type of play activities conducted with little girls is quite different from those selected for little boys, and the language associated with these activities and particular toys or objects vary greatly (Rakow, 1986). In a study of parent-child interaction, O'Brien and Nagle (1987) found that more lengthy discussions were conducted when interacting with dolls than when playing with trucks. Little girls are expected to have more so-called "proper speech" (Quina, Wingard, and Bates, 1987) and more polite speech (Spender, 1980) than little boys. The one-word utterances of little girls that are reinforced by female caregivers are different than those reinforced for little boys; this tendency is even more pronounced in the communications of male caregivers.

Social Environment

In addition, the structure of the child's family, or social context, influences early word acquisition (Nelson, 1985). The family structure includes the presence or absence of father or mother, the number of siblings, the position of the child in the order of siblings' births, the gender of the child, the gender and age of siblings, parental education, and socioeconomic status of the family. In the varying contexts within the particular family structure, children learn the different ways of interacting and talking with parents, siblings, grandparents, and other adults; pragmatic rules are learned in this social context (Garcia, 1992; Saville-Troike, 1982, 1989).

Differences Among Children

Individual preferences and personalities of children also influence the selection of words to include in their early vocabularies. In a classic study of early vocabulary development, Katherine Nelson (1973) found that there are important differences in children's learning style. Referential children (i.e., those who have a higher proportion of nouns in their total vocabularies) enjoy playing with objects. The first words they use, for the most part, are names of the objects in their world and words that describe their specific locations. Expressive children enjoy social activities and interactions with people. Their early words include a high proportion of personal pronouns, proper names, greetings, and expressions of feeling.

Children who are referential in their expressive speech have been observed to be more advanced in overall vocabulary development, with referential children acquiring a total of 50 words weeks or months earlier than children with more heterogeneous vocabularies (Nelson, 1973; Snyder, Bates, and Bretherton, 1981). Moreover, research by Bates, Bretherton, and Snyder (1988) showed that "the more precocious referential children were also more likely to use their words for common objects in a context-flexible way" (p. 46).

The Language a Child Hears

Studies of conversations between expressive and referential children and their mothers indicated that these interactions reflected the mothers' own preferences and language styles. Olsen-Fulero's research findings (1982) indicated that at least some aspects of maternal communicative style appear to influence children's acquisition of early lexicons. **Referential language** is associated with maternal utterances that refer to and describe objects and that request and reinforce names for things. Mothers of referential children seem to use more descriptive words and fewer directives (Della Corte, Benedict, and Klein, 1983; Tomasello and Todd, 1983). The topics of mutual interest, interaction, and conversation involve objects in the immediate environment (Bates, Bretherton, and Snyder, 1988; Goldfield, 1985, 1987). **Expressive language** in this context is associated with maternal utterances that refer to persons rather than objects and that direct or regulate the child's behavior. The early vocabulary of children is strongly influenced by the topics and purposes of caregivers' communications (Goldfield, 1987; Goldfield and Snow, 1989).

The words adults use when they label objects for children are also reflected in children's vocabularies (Pease, Gleason, and Pan, 1989). Dunn, Bretherton, and Munn (1987) noted in their studies that when talking with their young children, mothers routinely labeled a number of the child's feelings and emotional states (e.g., bored, happy, tired). By the age of two years, the children used many of these labels to express their own feelings (Bretherton, Fritz, Zahn-Waxler, and Ridgeway, 1986).

Maternal input also reflects the culture of the child's family. American mothers will often reinforce the child's naming of objects and events because they consider this style of interaction as instructive. A Kaluli mother from Papua, New Guinea, does not value the child's naming of objects, and naming activities are discouraged (Schieffelin, 1986). Kaluli children are instructed to imitate modeled utterances; this is acceptable social behavior and the culturally appropriate means of learning language in these societies (Goldfield and Snow, 1989; Schieffelin, 1986).

ADULTS AS LANGUAGE FACILITATORS

The role of the caregivers is not to give specific language instruction, but rather to facilitate communication. Adults facilitate child language acquisition using several types of language extension techniques.

Modeling and Expansion

Modeling is a form of parentese. Adults who use parentese are not aware that they are teaching language to the child. During a natural conversation while sharing materials and interests, they make language and speech modifications to correct and expand the child's utterances. The adult may begin by asking a question regarding an object of mutual interest. When the child responds with a gesture and any verbal comment, even if it is not intelligible, the adult will supply a label for the object. Gradually, the adult requires more clearly formed labels from the child and will prod the youngster for more acceptable responses. The child's verbalizations are not immediate imitations of the adult's label or comment (Owens, 1992). The child's statement is a very personal, unique, individualized rendition of the word the adult uses. As part of a natural dialogue, the adult is shaping the child's speech. For example, a conversation may progress as follows:

Child: *That blue car.*

Adult: *Yes, that is a pretty blue car. A lady is driving the car. Do you see she is wearing a pretty blue dress?*

Child: *Blue dress.*

Adult: *Yes, it is a pretty blue dress and a pretty blue car.*

The above dialogue is an example of an adult modeling and also a type of **expansion** technique; the adult repeats the words used by the child and elaborates the child's utterance to make it longer and more grammatically correct. It has been observed that children tend to imitate the expansions of the adult, and the imitations are more likely to approximate syntactically correct phrases than the original utterances (Hirsh-Pasek, Treiman, and Schneiderman, 1984; Owens, 1992).

Prompting

Prompting is also used by adults when conversing with young language-learning toddlers. This technique usually requires a response from the child. For example, the adult may attempt to hide a stuffed toy and say, *Where is the teddy bear?* The adult's facial expression and gestures will indicate a game or teasing.

Prompting also serves as an attention-getter. Often the prompt is a question such as, *What is that?* when the doorbell rings. *Is that the doorbell? Is someone coming to visit? Let's go and see.* Unanswered or incorrectly answered questions are usually expanded and rephrased by the adult (Owens, 1992). When asking questions, the adult pauses and waits for an answer. Children learn to listen for these pauses and how to shift from speaker to listener roles. When the child responds to a question, the adult either confirms and reinforces the child's utterance or requests more information or clarification from the child.

Adults do not consciously teach the child language using these techniques. They evolve in the course of conversation and interaction while sharing some activity. It has been observed that toddlers who interact with adults who use a conversational style with less obvious instructing and who encourage child participation in the interaction, learn language more quickly (Wells, 1985).

SUMMARY

Newborn human infants enter the world with a vast array of abilities that enable them to learn the cultural and linguistic rules they will have to know to communicate their intentions and needs to others in their language community. By the middle of the first year, long before they can express their first one-word utterances, they have actively explored their environment and have acquired a considerable world knowledge. They can initiate complex communications with other human beings, and they have acquired social skills that are considered appropriate by their cultural communities. Very young infants have been shown to be active learners regarding their environment, the events in their lives, and the important people in their world.

Children learn to comprehend the messages addressed to them and to others in their environment if these messages are associated with events, objects, or activities that are familiar in their daily lives. In language development, the earliest uses of language are tied to a physical context. When children begin to produce their own utterances, their choices of words for their lexicons depend upon the social and linguistic restrictions imposed by their cultural communities. Over time, the child begins to reveal increasing independence from the immediate context involving specific things, environments, and people.

By the age of two years, children should produce frequent intentionally communicative acts; have an expressive vocabulary of at least 50 words, and a substantially larger receptive vocabulary; have begun to put together two-word utterances; and be generally intelligible to those who know them well. Twenty-four months of age appears to be the point at which delays in these areas can be identified.

SUGGESTED READINGS

Owens, R. (1992). *Language Development: An Introduction* (3rd ed.). New York: Charles E. Merrill.

Schwartz, S., and Heller-Miller, J. (1988). *The Language of Toys.* Rockville, MD: Woodbine House.

Nelson, K. (1985). *Making Sense: The Acquisition of Shared Meaning.* New York: Academic Press.

Locke, J. (1993). *The Child's Path to Spoken Language.* Cambridge, MA: Harvard University Press.

4 THE IMPACT OF LANGUAGE ON LEARNING

By the age of two, most children have acquired symbolic thought. A child's mind can picture or represent an object, relation, or concept that has been encountered even when it is no longer present. Language as we know it, which is also a symbol or representation of reality, can now develop in more complex ways. The child elaborates the structure, the meanings, and the use of language.

Two-year-old children are most interested in communicating needs, wants, and information. However, by the time children are six years old, they become consciously aware of the sound, symbol, and social aspects of language. They appreciate language for its own sake. Children become conversationalists and understand some of the language rules for social interaction. Language development continues throughout adulthood. Individuals continue to learn more word meanings, to converse in more appropriate ways, to speak and write more effectively, and to select more suitable words when expressing themselves.

This chapter has four goals:

1. to explore the relationship between language development and cognition;

2. to examine language development as its structure, word meaning, and usage become more complex;

3. to explore the impact of language and communication ability on the experiences of preschoolers, the educational and social development of children and adolescents, and the special significance of language and its social ramifications during the teen years;

4. to contrast the language expectations of the home with school language requirements by clearly exploring the impact of language on academic growth.

COGNITION AND LANGUAGE

As stated in Chapter 2, a relationship between language development and cognition exists (Rice, 1983). However, the effect of one on the other as the child matures has engendered considerable discussion. Cognition involves those mental skills which organize knowledge that is attained when a child encounters experiences relating to people, objects, and events. Intellectual functions, which include reasoning, analyzing, and problem solving, develop as children attend, discriminate, remember, sequence, classify, integrate, and associate acquired knowledge. The knowledge helps youngsters to make sense of their world and to use the information effectively to manipulate their environment and to solve problems.

Language becomes more closely linked to cognition as the child matures. At first the young infant knows a little about the world but has no language. As children age, linguistic knowledge begins to overlap with general world knowledge (Rice and Kemper, 1984). Language becomes a cognitive tool. It is a means to express the child's thoughts. Children talk about what they know. Language becomes increasingly important because it draws attention to events and categorizations that the child might not otherwise notice, which expand the knowledge repertoire (de Villiers and de Villiers, 1978).

It is through cognition that concepts are formed. Concepts are the aggregate of a person's experience. If a child has seen five different chairs, a composite of the characteristics of those chairs forms the mental representation or concept. At some later date, the child may see other chairs of different styles such as a rocking chair or a stool. The concept may have to be refined. Through cognitive processes, the child perceives, organizes, integrates, and analyzes the new information regarding chairs. The amalgam of the child's various experiences with chairs forms the internal concept of *chairness*. Language helps to define concepts. If the youngster has begun to form the concept of *chair* and calls a sofa a chair, the child is told, "No, this has three seats and is called a sofa." Thus, language helps children to refine their notion of objects and events in the world.

Cognitive Theory

Some theorists (Piaget, 1955; Slobin, 1978b; Westby, 1980) regard language development as being dependent on cognitive maturity. If a child has not attained certain cognitive milestones, more complex aspects of language cannot develop. Other theorists (Christie, 1989; Vygotsky, 1962) challenge this theory and state that certain mental skills as well as social skills are dependent on mastery of linguistic patterns. Rice and Kemper (1984) discuss the various theories including the notions that both language and cognition are interactive or that the relationship between both systems depends on the age and linguistic ability of the child and which aspect of cognition is involved at any given time.

Researchers agree that cognition and language both impact on meaningful and significant learning when children are encouraged to enter into genuine inquiry, develop skills of questioning and speculation, and control and extract meaning from their experiences. This implies a very intimate relationship between the actual language that a child understands and uses and the nature of knowledge that can be processed. New experiences constantly reshape the child's view of the world and language provides organizational options for the knowledge obtained in these experiences by categorizing, associating, and integrating them with prior experience. Language provides the capacity to structure the world of experience and knowledge (Shafer, Staab, and Smith, 1983).

By studying the way information is processed, stored, and retrieved, cognitive psychologists discuss several approaches. One is the "top-down" (cognitive) model where the individual looks at the larger picture first and then examines the details that make up the general framework. Other individuals begin with the details to arrive at the big picture. This "bottom-up" (data driven) model involves arriving at a general conclusion after analyzing individual details (Wallach and Miller, 1988).

Cognition and Education

Reading instruction can be viewed in this information processing framework. The **whole language approach** emphasizes reading purposeful and meaningful language texts like signs, directions, stories, and lists. Learning about and analyzing the parts of words occurs after the language as a whole functional unit is understood. This is a top-down reading model. In contrast, some **phonetic approaches** to reading introduce sounds and letters first. These language parts are combined to make words, sentences, and then stories. Skill development for reading is a bottom-up model. Information processing is the larger context for language processing, since words and their meanings are also processed, stored, and retrieved.

Butler (1984) discusses levels of processing and states that deeper and more complex levels of knowledge require greater analysis by the child. Duchan (1983) views the processing of language associated with knowledge as being multidimensional. That is, she challenges the notion that language processing is like an elevator that stops at floor one for certain types of information and floor two for others. Rather, processing occurs on several levels simultaneously. The listener takes the incoming language and connects it in many ways with higher order knowledge to create meaning and make sense.

The more the child knows about people, objects, events, and social categories, the more accurately new information can be associated with prior concepts. Meanings can be redefined more precisely. Conversely, the more language children acquire, the more their thoughts are shaped by the finite vocabulary and grammar of the language. The vocabulary and grammar of any native language will influence the thought of its speakers. Language and cognition can be viewed as being linked in specific areas. Each can influence the other at various connecting points. Factors affecting the relationship between cognitive development and language acquisition include the cognitive and linguistic competencies involved, the child's mental development, and the nature of the task (Rice and Kemper, 1984).

THE DEVELOPMENT OF THE STRUCTURE OF LANGUAGE

As children progress through the preschool years, tremendous language growth occurs. When two-word combinations emerge, language evolves into a rule-governed grammar which begins to approximate adult language by kindergarten and continues to develop more complexity throughout life. This language development reflects a child's cognitive and interactional skills.

Young language learners are like scientists. They try out a word or words they have come to understand to convey a message. If the combination of chosen words produces the intended result, it confirms their notion of the words. Children begin to learn that individual words can represent many meanings. A simple word like *cup* can be used for a little plastic container with a handle, a fancy porcelain container with a handle, or a styrofoam container with no handle. Meanings are expanded and refined. The multiple meanings of words are gradually learned as well, particularly between the ages of seven and eleven when children develop significant increases in the comprehension of logical, spatial, temporal, and other relationships (Owens, 1988). *Block* can initially be a toy and later refer to the place in which your house is located. At another juncture, the child understands that the word can pertain to the action taken by football players.

Developing Syntactic Rules

Rules for grammar also develop and change to reflect the child's advanced understanding of the language code and how it is used in conversation. Slobin (1978b) examined the structural aspects of language that influence children as they engage in strategies to learn language. He examined 40 different language groups and concluded that there are universal language-processing schemes used by children in their attempt to express themselves. These schemes, he argued, stem from the child's general cognitive development. Early on, children have ideas about language and as they listen to utterances they try to discover meaning. Their strategies for language learning include operating principles such as paying attention to the ends of words. This means that markers signifying plurals *(s)*, or past tense *(ed)*, are learned before prefixes (e.g., *dis, un*). Another strategy presented is the way children avoid exceptions in language. This means that if plurals tend to be formed by a final *s*, then *man* becomes *mans* and *foot* becomes *foots*. Slobin's theories developed seven operating principles that explain how a child scans language input to discover meaning and rules for language expression.

Developing Morphological Rules

Brown (1973) studied the sequence of child acquisition of language form by examining morphological and syntactic development. He stated that children do not understand all the rules of language form at once. Rather, they pass through language stages that seem to correspond to a child's typical sentence length during that period. **Mean length of utterance** (**MLU**) is used to determine a child's language stage. MLU is computed by counting the number of morphemes or meaningful units in each utterance and dividing the grand total by the number of utterances the child generated during a given period. For example, if a youngster says *Boys run fast,* there are 4 morphemes. The *s* in the word *boys* designates plurality creating more than one meaning unit in that word. Young children vary the length of their utterances so that an

MLU of 3.0 does not exclude the possibility of producing longer and shorter utterances.

Developing Grammatical Morphemes

Brown outlined five linguistic stages of children between the ages of 12 to 48 months. By examining Stage II, the notion that children gradually use and understand morphological rules is seen. Brown (1973) states that children reach this stage at approximately 27–30 months of age and have developed an MLU of between 2.0 and 2.5 words. He identified 14 morphemes that emerge at various times during these five stages. For example, regular plurals (e.g., *cats, balls*) appear before the regular past tense (e.g., *walked, played*). Contractible auxiliary verbs (e.g., *Mommy is/Mommy's, you are/you're*) develop even later.

Brown (1973) considered the reasons that language forms emerge at different ages. He tested the notion that the morphemes heard most frequently would appear earliest. The frequency hypothesis compared parental use of words before they were produced by the child. Articles (e.g., *a, the*) were most frequently used by parents although they were among the latest forms acquired by children. No relationship was found between the forms heard most and earlier acquisition by the child. Brown also considered linguistic complexity and a child's order of acquisition of language. He demonstrated that both semantic complexity and syntactic complexity predict a child's sequence of language development with the most complex linguistic forms emerging last.

Developing the Question Form

The way in which children develop the interrogative or question form is another example of consistency among youngsters in the acquisition of linguistic rules. Questions can be divided into at least three groups: those that begin with a wh-question word (e.g., *who, what, when, where, why*), those that require a yes/no answer, and tag questions which are composed of a statement with a short question such as ...*can't I?* at the end. The earliest examples of children's questions consist of saying a word or group of words and raising the pitch of their voice as the utterance ends. *Mommy is sleeping?* could be a statement or a question depending on the intonation when the words are spoken. The next stage is characterized by a statement with a wh-question word preceding it as in, *Where Mommy is sleeping?* Later the child begins to invert the subject and auxiliary verb to generate a question. Generally, the youngster will produce questions of this type omitting the wh-question word first. For example, the question *Is Mommy sleeping?* will appear before *Where is Mommy sleeping?* (Lindfors, 1987; Tager-Flusberg, 1985). Klee's research (1985) has produced some contradictory results regarding the way in which children invert auxiliary verbs and subjects in the question form. However, he discusses various studies where the data were collected using different methodology as an explanation of conflicting findings.

The general order in which children use wh-question words corresponds to their cognitive maturity. *Who, what,* and *where* tend to appear before *when* and *why* (i.e., by approximately two years versus three years).

Who, what, and *where* question words often relate to a youngster's immediate environment and responses can be short and uncomplicated. The word *when* requires understanding of temporal, or time, concepts which begin to develop later. Time concepts are based on the child's understanding of the future and the past, which is abstract and removed from the immediate context.

Comprehension of the words *why* and *how* requires more developed semantic relationships. When a child is presented with a *why* or *how* question, it necessitates the formulation of more than a one-word response. Although very young children often use the word *why* as a general question form that functions semantically as a *what* question, its meaningful use occurs when the child attains more mature linguistic and cognitive abilities (i.e., cause-effect relationship). Owens (1988) discusses *why* questions that require cause-effect understanding (e.g., *Why did you hit your brother?*). The child must explain the events that preceded the action to answer the question. The ability to reverse the order of sequential events requires a level of thinking that is difficult for most children younger than seven and even for some children who are nine or ten. Thus, understanding of semantic complexity such as causal or temporal relationships, knowledge of syntactic changes, and commensurate cognitive development all interface to affect the child's ability to understand and formulate questions (Bernstein, 1989; Owens, 1988).

Developing Phonological Rules

Children's phonological development progresses in stages just as morphological and syntactic aspects of language. Spoken words or speech sounds should approximate adult models for the communication attempts of a child to be understood. Therefore, a child's ability to discriminate between the different sounds of a language and then to produce those sounds accurately affects language use.

Certain speech sounds are related because they are produced by positioning the tongue and lips in a similar manner. Other speech sounds are grouped together because of similar flow of breath or air through the nose or mouth. Some sounds are **voiced** because they require the larynx to vibrate (e.g., *v, z*) and others are **unvoiced** (e.g., *f, s*). Thus, sounds are classified by the way in which they are produced. The position of the lips, teeth, tongue, roof of the mouth, and throat to one another for a particular sound is referred to as the **place of articulation**.

There are sounds formed in some languages that are not used in English. Conversely, sounds used in the English language do not appear in all other languages. English sounds can only be arranged to make words in specific ways. For example, an English word cannot begin with *ng* but might end with that sound sequence as in *running* and *talking*. Children acquire accurate production of speech sounds progressively because some of them require more mature musculature; others are rarely heard and used; and still others are difficult to pronounce when they occur alongside of other sounds (e.g., *street*). Some children have difficulty with the position of articulation and others have difficulty with voicing (use of the vibrating larynx). In general, if youngsters are having difficulty with a sound, they use some features of a sound correctly and then work toward standard production. Children who totally omit many sounds from their utterances have the greatest hurdles toward attaining adult speech.

Children utilize varying strategies when learning how to produce sounds in words. As they begin to combine a greater variety of sounds, they might substitute one sound for another in certain instances (e.g., *cwow* for crow) or omit the sound elsewhere (e.g., *fist* for first). Usually, the child is reducing the complexity of the consonant structure in the word. This may occur as the omission of a final consonant (e.g., *ba* for ball) or reduplication of a syllable (e.g., *bah bah* for bottle). However, if a word is produced in an oversimplified fashion, the message may not be understood by the listener (Edwards and Shriberg, 1983).

Speech sounds develop over time. Those that occur in the initial position in words are acquired first. In general, vowels appear before consonants. Research has suggested that for 75% of children, consonant sounds are acquired over a span of three to four years (Hodson and Paden, 1983; Owens, 1988). According to Owens (1988), certain sounds like those in the /s/ family may not be produced correctly in all positions in words until age seven for even normally developing youngsters. The earliest sounds to be used are /m/, /n/, and /p/. Yet children naturally strive to produce speech sounds correctly because of their need to have more complex ideas understood by greater numbers of people. Table 4.1 outlines five studies which present the mastery of speech sounds by children.

Table 4.1

Age (Years-Months) at Which Children Master Speech Sounds in Five Studies

Speech Sounds (Phonemes)	Wellman et al. (1931)	Poole (1934)	Templin (1957)	Sander (1972)	Prather et al. (1975)
m	3	3-6	3	before 2	2
n	3	4-6	3	before 2	2
h	3	3-6	3	before 2	2
p	4	3-6	3	before 2	2
f	3	5-6	3	3	2-4
w	3	3-6	3	before 2	2-8
b	3	3-6	4	before 2	2-8
		4-6	3	2	2
j	4	4-6	3-6	3	2-4
k	4	4-6	4	2	2-4
g	4	4-6	4	2	2-4
l	4	6-6	6	2	2-4
d	5	4-6	4	2	2-4
t	5	4-6	6	2	2-8
s	5	7-6	4-6	3	3
r	5	7-6	4	3	3-4
	5		4-6	4	3-8
v	5	6-6	6	4	4
z	5	7-6	7	4	4

Adapted from *Introduction to Communication Disorders* (p. 107) by M. Hegde, 1991, Austin, TX: Pro-Ed. © 1991 by Pro-Ed. Reprinted by permission.

THE DEVELOPMENT OF MEANING IN LANGUAGE

Young children develop language meaning or semantic knowledge primarily from communicative interactions with others and from involvement in everyday experiences and play. These activities help to deepen the understanding of the words they produce and to introduce multiple word meanings. They also provide a platform to test their hypothesis about what language means. For example, children begin to generate conversational **narratives** or stories, concerning their real experiences. Between the ages of four and six, narratives evolve from a listing of events, often out of sequence, and which don't always relate to one another, to well-formed stories that orient to a listener and outline a logical sequence of events (Dickinson and McCabe, 1991).

As youngsters engage in more experiences, their conceptual under-standing of words increases. For example, foods may be categorized into groups such as vegetables and meats. A trip to a supermarket might expose a child to varieties of lettuce not seen at home, or new packaging. A trip to a farm might introduce a child to carrots with long green tops or foods actually growing. At home, the child begins to differentiate those foods eaten hot or cold, foods eaten at various times during the day, foods that require chewing, and a myriad of tastes in food. All of these experiences provide the child with greater differentiation among food classes. Associations among specific foods are developed. This information is stored and used as a basis for greater language variety and complexity during conversation. Experience also provides the child with multiple meanings of words and more precise application of specific words.

Developing Language During Play

It is through play that children express themselves. Play allows others to observe the ways in which children see their world (McCune-Nicolich and Carroll, 1981). It allows children to use toys and objects as they wish. There is total freedom from all but personally imposed rules which can be changed at will. Fantasy and discovery are encouraged. Self-expression can be verbal, gestural, or dramatic. For example, a child can use a pot in the kitchen to pretend to make a meal. In midstream, the child can then take the lid to the pot and transform it into a steering wheel and pretend to be driving a car. These activities provide an observer with an opportunity to view the child's understanding of the activities which are based on prior experiences that have been internalized by the youngster.

Play develops cognitive, motor, social, and emotional abilities. It allows the child to express stored thoughts and ideas, promotes physical dexterity as the child interacts with objects and toys, provides practice opportunities to engage in communicative exchanges such as, *Come, baby, let's go to bed,* and provides a venue to express feelings such as anger and fear.

Games differ considerably from play and don't become part of a child's activity plan until after play is established. Whereas during play, each child establishes his or her rules such as pretending lids are steering wheels during a particular play session, games have specific rules that are mutually agreed upon by two or more people engaged in the game. Furthermore, games usually are designed to be competitive with winners and losers, which can create considerable stress for children (Sachs, 1984a).

Symbolic play is one mechanism for assessing a child's symbolic thought and language. The way in which a child mentally represents reality is expressed in both pretend play and language (Ogura, 1991). Westby (1980) researched stages of child play and their relationship to cognitive and linguistic development. She charted these stages to determine which semantic concepts, language structures, or communication functions should be given priority when interacting with specific youngsters. She stressed that language training can only assist children in expressing what they already understand. By age three, most children are able to create sequential events in symbolic play. That is, events are not isolated. The child might pretend to mix a cake, bake it, serve it, and wash the dishes. Linguistically, children begin to use both past and future tense verbs to express these sequential stories, but the props tend to remain realistic. At age three years, the child's awareness of perceptual attributes of objects permits substitution of materials for real objects during play. At this stage, the child begins to think about language, comment on it, and modify it to suit the character being represented during play. That means having the baby say, *goo goo,* or speaking in a firm, loud voice when impersonating a scolding mother (McCune-Nicolich and Carroll, 1981). By age five, children have moved to full cooperative play with one another. Play sequences can be planned in advance between two or more children. Imaginative scenes are created and language reflects the temporal concepts now internalized such as *when, first,* and *next.*

Pellegrini and Galda (1990) elaborate the notion that the language of children's social make-believe play and the language of literacy are similar because they serve similar functions. That is, in both contexts children redefine and transform reality, integrate and organize themes, and convey meaning. They accomplish these goals in the absence of shared knowledge and meaning with the immediate context. Children using language in inappropriate ways during play or who find it difficult to interact with others or who cannot create a sequence of related events suggest characteristics of language difficulty (Blank, Rose, and Berlin, 1978).

Temporal Knowledge Development

Conceptual understanding can reflect cognitive development. Consequently, comprehension of concepts is expanded gradually. **Temporal concepts** (those related to time) depend on a child's ability to symbolize the future and past. They also relate to the child's conceptual knowledge of temporal terms. For example, a young child is told to *wait a minute.* Within seconds, the child's demands recur. The adult becomes annoyed because the child isn't complying with the directive. Yet the child may have only a vague concept of *minute*. Terms such as *in a while, later, soon,* or *not yet* must be experienced many times in concrete situations to be internalized. Discussing the time it takes for the bread to brown in the toaster or the light to turn green at the crossroad are concrete examples which clarify temporal terms for young children.

The temporal uses of *before* and *after* begin to emerge between the ages of three and five (Pease and Gleason, 1985). These concepts are particularly difficult linguistically as well as conceptually. Structurally, the words *before* and *after* can introduce a clause or a prepositional phrase. Children use these terms initially as prepositions (e.g., She ate *before* me). Later, they produce them in clauses (e.g., *After you eat your dinner,* do your homework). Use of *before* and *after* in clauses can be confusing because the initial clause may not indicate the first event. When examining the utterance "Put your books away after you complete your math assignment," it is evident that the first task is the math assignment and yet in the linguistic format that instruction is subsequent to putting books away. Owens (1988) observes that even six year olds have difficulty interpreting these clauses. An actual order of events is best understood when it is presented in order linguistically (e.g., *After you wash your hands, brush your teeth*).

Children usually are well into the primary grades before days, months, and years are understood. Ben, in kindergarten, talked about "a long time ago when George Washington and the dinosaurs were alive." Distant past and future merge and blur. Youngsters often benefit from concrete time lines that pinpoint specific events or periods.

Understanding temporal concepts and relationships is essential in the academic setting. The ability to plan ahead and set realistic time goals depends on temporal knowledge. Specific school subjects also rely on an understanding of time. Reading comprehension depends on the ability to manipulate past, present, and future verbs and the durational distinctions expressed by progressive and present tense (e.g., *He is walking; He was walking; He will be walking*). Cause-effect relationships are also related to time. In social studies, one event can impact on a subsequent event. Students also will compare, classify, categorize, and predict outcomes in science as conditions change over time. Although temporal relationships should be stabilized by age 13 or 14, some adolescents only know how many days there are in a month, or a year, or how many years there are in a decade, or a century. Others can project theories regarding man's place in the universe and formulate the future role of mankind (Britton, 1972).

Later Semantic Development

Individuals expand their depth of understanding of words, concepts, and ideas throughout their lives. When youngsters are in elementary school, literate forms of language as well as experience contribute to semantic development. Miller (1990a) describes **literacy** as more than the ability to read and write. It involves being able to think, manipulate knowledge, and understand how language is used so that the person can organize knowledge, evaluate events and issues, and know how to effectively communicate with other people. The literate medium can be the printed form or oral language. Literacy is related to the acquisition of an abstract knowledge of meaning. Class discussions, teachers' lectures, and the printed word all separate language from concrete, here-and-now contexts.

During the elementary school-age period, children begin to shift their cognitive processing from a nonlinguistic visual-perceptual mode to linguistic categorization (Owens, 1988). Decreasing reliance on visual input for memory and recall allows the child to process greater amounts of linguistic information. An outgrowth of this new organization of semantics is the use of figurative language. **Figurative language** moves beyond using words in their concrete or literal sense to expressing an imaginative or creative sense of the word. Idioms, metaphors, similes, and proverbs are examples of figurative language. Meanings are understood and inferred from the context. For example, when a person says, *I will throw a party,* the listener must move beyond the traditional definition of *throw.* People cannot take an event such as a party, place it in their hand, and toss it. The context of the communication determines the creative use of the word *throw.* Nippold (1985, 1988) suggests that the mastery of figurative language goes beyond the school years and adolescence and continues through life as individuals encounter or create new linguistic expressions through written or spoken contexts.

Extensive reading and writing contribute to the child's ability to manipulate language in more abstract and imaginative ways. Greater semantic knowledge results in more accurate communications. Nelson (1988) states that children develop greater literacy skills as they proceed through adolescence by relying more on conceptual and linguistic processes than on perception. Conceptual and linguistic processes become the primary tools for efficient acquisition of knowledge.

PRAGMATIC DEVELOPMENT

During preschool years, children become increasingly aware of what their listeners need to know during conversational exchanges. Yet children at this age find spontaneous utterances easier to produce than verbal utterances in response to a conversational partner. Thus, self-selected statements are not as difficult for the preschooler as speech that is influenced by and dependent upon the comments of the conversational partner (Owens, 1988). Most conversation during this period centers on everyday activities that occur in the immediate setting. More conversational exchanges between the child and other adults transpire than between the child and peers (Kaye and Charney, 1981). If the preschooler is not successful in transmitting a message, repeating the utterance is the typical means of clarification.

At about age four, **indirect request forms** begin to emerge. The child can request something in a more subtle way. The goal of the utterance doesn't match the literal meaning. Instead of saying, *I want cookies,* the child can now state *M-m-m. Those cookies sure look good!* These more advanced linguistic forms also reflect politeness to the conversational partner (de Villiers and de Villiers, 1978). Also at this age, the child begins to learn to speak differently to different people. Depending on whether the conversational partner is a stranger or a younger sibling, the child alters vocabulary, loudness, tone, and length of sentence. Speaking style changes.

Between the ages of four and five, awareness of humor emerges. Children understand that words can cause people to laugh. Usually, they don't understand the subtleties and double meanings of words that make them amusing. Therefore, children will tell preriddles that are in the correct structural format but which do not have the linguistic humor (Wolf and Dickinson, 1985). Ben, at age five, said *I have a joke. Why did the rooster cross the street? Get it? Because he wanted to catch a little ball.* This utterance was followed by gales of laughter. He enjoyed the social value of the verbal interchange but could not generate the semantic nuances in words that a true joke requires.

During the elementary school years, children continue to develop the ability to use language appropriately in a variety of situations. They are able to adjust conversational styles and content when speaking to adults and other youngsters. Stephens (1988) indicates that most research on the pragmatic development of the school-age child tends to assess oral language in the classroom. The section of this chapter on home versus school language discusses classroom discourse and narrative ability in greater detail.

Teen Language and Social Development

Once youngsters reach adolescence, they interact more frequently with strangers and peers. The content of each communication is now competing with the manner in which it is spoken. Language is used to establish and maintain relationships with others (Larson and McKinley, 1987). Verbal jousting becomes a popular way to win approval from the observers of a conversational exchange. Teenagers who can't think of suitable responses to a verbal gibe will mentally review the conversation later only to realize all the clever remarks they could have generated. Wolf and Dickinson (1985) discuss the adolescent practice of trading insults within a framework of rules set up by the group. The participants might bring up obscene topics, often in front of the peers, who act as evaluators of the conversational exchange. Audience reaction determines approval and can enhance an adolescent's stature within the group. The most skillful speakers receive the greatest admiration.

The teen language used in social situations is not always appropriate for the school environment. The vocabulary might be different as well as the manner of speaking. Furthermore, versions of teen language change over time. For example, words that express favorable acknowledgment might change from *awesome* to *cool* to *bad* to *yes*. Students need to be aware of the vernacular of the moment to identify with their peer group. Those youngsters who don't conform to the language code are often ostracized. Youngsters who move from one locality to another sometimes use a different version of adolescent language. Their utterances reveal an identity which contrasts with the crowd.

Gender also affects the way in which some children speak. Craig and Evans (1991) found that boys as young as 8 years were more assertive conversationally than girls. In reviewing recent research, they found that as children approach adulthood, males interrupt females significantly more, produce more direct requests, and generate more factual information. Conversely, females use more question forms, especially tag questions, and produce more emotional and interpersonal items. Because self-identity is so critical during the adolescent years, conformity to gender-specific peer group norms regarding language and behavior is typical. Young men often produce language reflecting confidence and strength whereas young women are denied interactional control. Thus, men appear more argumentative, make more interruptions, and exert greater topic control (Cooper and Anderson-Inman, 1988). Discussions among same gender peers are reported to be more restricted for close male friends than for close female friends. Intimate problems were topics in more female conversations than in their male counterparts. Cooper and Anderson-Inman (1988) also note that the primary function of adolescent female friendship is intimate sharing. These research findings demonstrate the strong relationship between language and social interaction, especially during adolescence.

HOME VERSUS SCHOOL LANGUAGE

The preschool child tends to talk about experiences in the immediate setting. Lack of specific vocabulary can be compensated with gesture and body expression. Conversation topics tend to be routine and familiar. Youngsters can initiate a conversation whenever they wish. They also produce monologues during play routines. Thinking aloud is considered to be another aspect of child talk. However, when children enter the school environment, expectations for conversation change considerably. The teacher determines what topics will be discussed, who will speak, when they will speak, and what language is appropriate to use when speaking.

Classroom Communication

Teachers, in general, have middle-class values and beliefs. They have language expectations for the students regarding how children address them and other individuals within the school. Each teacher also has assumptions concerning language manners and how verbal exchange is conducted in the classroom (Wallach and Miller, 1988). For example, most classroom discussion centers on questions posed by the teacher which often require children to produce narrow, predetermined responses. Children begin to realize that the questions posed are designed to test whether the child's answer corresponds with information already known by the teacher. This differs from home discourse where questions are posed to obtain unknown information such as, *What do you want to eat for lunch?*

In the classroom, the teacher decides who will speak by random selection. Children learn that if they would like to participate in the discussion, they must raise their hands. If they are chosen to provide a remark, their comment is acknowledged as being good, correct, or wrong. Blank and White (1986) note that this format for conversation takes place in few situations other than the classroom and runs contrary to the understanding of pragmatic rules of language. In fact, the researchers challenge this discourse format as being inconsistent with learning objectives which should include enhancement of thinking and cognition as well as fostering a free exchange of ideas.

Whereas home discourse is generally concerned with a shared situation between the conversational partners, classroom language tends to involve instructional material. That means the child in school cannot always depend on the immediate context like toys on the floor, food on the table, or clothes in the closet, to facilitate self-expression. Rather, the conversational topic may be **decontextualized,** or not related to the immediate situation. School discussions about community helpers or the definition of a word requires specific vocabulary and more abstract linguistic abilities (Silliman, 1984). As students move from lower to upper grades and from oral to written language contexts, they must apply more abstract and complex linguistic processing strategies to extract meaning (Nelson, 1986).

The culture, customs, experiences, and corresponding language framework that each youngster brings to the classroom is going to affect how well that child can cope with the language content, language manners, and teacher's expectations for classroom discourse (Hasan and Martin, 1989). Children who come from culturally different backgrounds or who have been exposed to limited experiences might have more difficulty participating in the formal instructional setting. Furthermore, students will vary in their ability to generate precise, abstract, and complex linguistic forms as they advance through school (Silliman, 1984).

Metalinguistics

As preschoolers, youngsters speak automatically to satisfy their wants and needs. They evaluate their utterances only in terms of obtaining the desired outcomes resulting from the communication effort. If particular words are not known, the child tries to substitute other words, use gestures, point, or modulate the tone of voice. The child's focus of attention is on what is being said and understood. Between the ages of four and eight, children begin to think about language. They begin to realize that the string of sounds emerging from a speaker's mouth are in fact divided into words. They also become aware of which sentences make sense, which words could only be uttered by a baby, and which words and sounds are alike. As discussed in Chapter 1, this conscious awareness of language which allows the child to control and make changes in utterances is known as metalinguistic awareness. Metalinguistic knowledge allows the child to observe, analyze, describe, and manipulate language.

After the age of seven or eight, children can concentrate on both linguistic correctness and the message meaning simultaneously (Owens, 1988). Children gradually learn to divide spoken sentences into words, words into segments or syllables, and syllables into their separate sounds. They become aware of which sounds correspond to specific letters or symbols. They also become conscious of the arbitrary nature of words. The English word *star* is called by other names in different languages. This word can also have more than one meaning such as an object in the sky or a person of celebrity status. Thus, children develop a greater knowledge of word meanings as well as structure (Estrin and Chaney, 1988).

Awareness of pragmatic characteristics of language also occurs. Children begin to repair communication breakdowns by requesting clarification or revising utterances. They adjust their language stylistically and make variations according to the age and status of the listener (Owens, 1988). Children also reflect on the words used to construct puns or figurative language. Van Kleeck (1984a) divides this metalinguistic development into three areas:

1. ***Awareness of language as an arbitrary conventional code.***
   Once youngsters realize that the sounds chosen by the community to denote a word are arbitrary, they understand that the actual object, event, or action is not related to the designated word. The letters *c*, *a*, and *t* have been selected to identify a furry animal that says *meow*. The animal could have also been named a *frugan*. The arbitrary selection of words has resulted in a short word (e.g., mile) which refers to a long distance and a longer word (e.g., centimeter) which refers to a shorter distance. At this stage, the child can begin to define words and tell whether a group of sounds constitutes a real word. A child can also identify synonymous words and foreign language words. Understanding language becomes less literal so that humor and figurative language can be interpreted. Extensions of word meanings can be created and understood.

2. ***Awareness of language as a system with specific rules to combine sounds and words.*** Children begin to understand that, when speaking, the stream of sounds can be divided into words. These words can be interchanged. For example, one can say *The weather is hot,* and then substitute other words in the statement such as *cold, warm,* or *temperate.* Being able to segment sentences into words and then words into sounds underlies reading proficiency. Children are expected to find words that contain the same initial sounds or rhyming words in early reading exercises. By understanding

the rules of the language system, they can perform these tasks.

3. *Awareness of language as a communication tool.* Youngsters become more sensitive to messages that communicate politeness or rudeness. They also begin to determine whether an utterance pertains to the conversational topic, to the listener, or to the particular setting. Youngsters will say, *Talk quietly, the teacher is coming!* This demonstrates their sensitivity to the appropriate loudness of an utterance in the classroom context.

Metalinguistic awareness is associated with success in early reading (Estrin and Chaney, 1988; van Kleeck, 1984b; Tunmer and Cole, 1991). Yet the development of metalinguistic knowledge can vary among normal children by several years (Kamhi and Koenig, 1985). Preschool children are sometimes taught by enthusiastic parents and teachers to try to match speech sounds with their corresponding written letter symbol. This can be problematic for those average youngsters who don't develop skill in segmenting words into their individual sounds until about age seven. In written language, there are spaces between words whereas in oral language three words can sound like one continuous word (e.g., *didjaeat?*). That is, oral utterances spoken at a normal rate have few words separated by pauses. There is often no physical basis for recognizing individual words in conversational speech. A child who cannot segment sentences into words will have an even more difficult time separating the various sounds within each word. Johnson (1985) argues that when a child has limited metalinguistic knowledge, reading and writing activities can actually accelerate these skills. Activities with words and sounds can promote greater awareness of their linguistic characteristics. In fact, the visual symbol system acts as a support to auditory language learning because the information can be reviewed. Unlike oral language which is spoken and disappears, written symbols are more permanent.

Continued cognitive growth is required for more advanced met-alinguistic skill. To consider how to convey a message effectively, the child has to attain a level of competence in language processing skills and cognitive reasoning abilities. There is considerable variability in both the overall development and cognitive development of children. Furthermore, metalinguistic skill requires basic linguistic skill. Because all of these factors affect a child's ability to succeed in academic and social environments, it is important to evaluate each child's language and cognitive development to determine the optimum period to teach various academic skills.

Developing Narratives: The Bridge to Literacy

Although children create narratives as preschoolers, the development of skill in generating well-organized oral stories that follow a logical series of events to a conclusion is important for literacy and school achievement (Westby, 1991). A *narrative* is an extended monologue rather than interactive dialogue. It retells an experience that has already occurred or predicts a future experience. Actual or imagined events must be observed, stored, recalled, and verbalized. Both the narrator and the listener are distanced from the actual event. To generate and comprehend meaning from the narration requires the ability to abstract. Therefore, the child must clearly identify who is speaking, the setting, and why the story is being told. All of these characteristics are related to literate style. Some children from culturally different environments have less exposure to aspects of narrative communication, such as the ability to generalize an experience by relating it to their experiences (Scollon and Scollon, 1981). Those youngsters who rely more on gestures, facial expression, and pointing to convey a narrative also will have a more difficult time with literacy. Because narratives reflect on past and future experiences, they combine features of both oral and literate language.

Klecan-Aker and Kelty (1990) view narratives as either written or spoken passages that form a unified whole. They can range in length from a sentence to a complete novel. These researchers have used Applebee's (1978) system for studying children's stories in their investigations of oral narratives. Their research indicates stories are well-developed by the fourth grade.

Applebee divides children's narrative development into progressively complex stages and has also identified stages of narrative skill during adolescence through adulthood. Table 4.2 summarizes Applebee's (1978) developmental hierarchy leading to true narrative skills and beyond.

Table 4.2

Developmental Stages of Narrative Ability

Approximate Age	Stage	Characteristics
2 years	Prenarratives: Heap Stories	• Children talk about whatever attracts their attention • Ideas are unrelated to one another and are usually expressed in present or present progressive (i.e., ing) tenses
2–3 years	Prenarratives: Sequence Stories	• Stories include characters, objects, and events but elements are "perceptually" related to one another rather than having a "logical" association • Stories lack a temporal sequence
3–4 years	Primitive Narratives	• Stories include a character, topic, or setting which complement each other logically • Events follow a central story core but may not be linked to each other. • First use of inferences in predicting and interpreting events though reciprocal causality between thoughts and events is not recognized

Continued

Table 4.2—*Continued*

Approximate Age	Stage	Characteristics
4–4½ years	Unfocused Chains	• Stories include a logical sequence of events but not a consistent theme (plot) or character • Conjunctions *and*, *but*, and *because* may be present
5 years	Focused Chains	• Stories contain a central character and a logical sequence of events • Listeners often need to interpret the ending • Plot is undeveloped
6–7 years	True Narratives	• Stories contain an initiating event, an attempt or action, and consequences • Cause-and-effect events are logically sequenced and integrated with other story elements • Story has strong well-developed plot, good character development • Characters' goals are dependent on their attributes and feelings • Story "problem" is resolved in the story ending
7–11 years	Categorization of Narratives	• Summarizes stories • Categorizes stories subjectively (e.g., funny, sad) and objectively (e.g., long, rhyming) • Considers story as a whole and places it in a general category
11–12 years	Complex Narratives	• Stories are complex because of multiple embedded elements
13–15 years	Narrative Analysis	When presented with stories, • Analyzes and evaluates stories or story components

Continued

Table 4.2—*Continued*

Approximate Age	Stage	Characteristics
		• Critiques stories from several perspectives
16 years–Adulthood	Sophisticated Analysis	When presented with stories,
		• Generalizes story meaning and how it applies to their own situation
		• Analyzes story message or theme to form abstract opinions and statements
		• Focuses on own reaction to the story

Narratives can be considered the bridge to literacy because the storyteller is generating a particular story after the experience has occurred. The entire story needs to be mentally constructed before telling it (Westby, 1984). Consequently, a narrative is distanced from the event itself and represents an interpretation of the experience. The narrative also contains an invented beginning and end to the event. People selectively attend to the ongoing flow of events in the world and highlight those that are meaningful to them. For example, a person may go to a movie and concentrate on the actions of the characters. Another person may attend the same movie but focus on the background music, perhaps recognizing it as a symphony heard at a recent concert. In subsequent narrations pertaining to the event, each moviegoer has a separate story to relate based on the aspects of the event that each has self-selected.

When presenting an oral story, the language used must be specific enough to provide a picture of the event without props in the immediate context. Therefore, explicit explanation of the event requires more precise linguistic usage. Oral conversation permits the speaker to use gestures, facial expressions, and pointing to elaborate a story. Written language, however, consists of the most precise language because these extralinguistic cues are not available.

Narrative skills embody interpretation of the world of events and feelings, as well as the use of specific linguistic forms to convey the story. They also organize information so that the listener can understand the meaning being presented. Developmentally, the oral narrative precedes the written story.

Language and Reading

When the child begins to read, communication and knowledge are now transmitted through the visual channel. Two reliable indicators for success in reading and writing are a child's oral language and metalinguistic skills (Owens, 1988). In the early stages of reading words, phonological segments and semantic features must be brought into conscious awareness. Those children who can discriminate between sounds presented orally, recognize and create rhymes, segment words into their sound components, and discuss aspects of language are best prepared to tackle the task of recognizing and decoding individual words. Children with a comprehensive experience base, large vocabulary, and the ability to analyze, integrate, and organize new information are best equipped to understand sentences and paragraphs. Thus, the complex process of reading is related to a variety of linguistic processes. Menyuk (1988) discusses the ability to segment words and the ability to comprehend sentences as predictive of later reading performance. She stresses that intuitive knowledge about various aspects of language must be brought to conscious awareness for success in reading.

A number of researchers (Menyuk, 1988; Nelson, 1988; Owens, 1988; Sorsby and Martlew, 1991) have associated reading and writing ability with language experienced in the home. Reading stories to children has been linked to language and literacy development as well as the more complex forms of language use. Reading promotes abstract thought which will help children deal with the decontextualized information found in school texts. Those youngsters with a limited symbolic system have difficulty organizing the events surrounding them. Parental speech during shared book reading tends to be more complex than during free play (Sorsby and Martlew, 1991). The more abstract the parent's speech, the more the child must rely on symbolic references that have been stored in the brain. Books, in contrast to other stimuli in the environment, also focus the child's attention to words and pictures which are symbolic representations. Dickinson and McCabe (1991) note that books that tell sustained stories are extremely important to read to preschool children.

As youngsters begin to decode words, teachers often select books with predictable rhyming texts in an effort to direct children's attention to print. This written style usually has weaker narrative style but students are able to decode greater portions of the text as compared to sustained story narratives. Some teachers have encouraged early readers to choose a linguistic pattern from a predictable rhyming text and then create their own version of the story to be read to other students.

As youngsters begin to read on their own, they shift their attention from an immediate audience that shares the child's experiences to less familiar speakers or listeners (Nelson, 1988). As writers, children have to gauge their material to a larger audience. This forces them to select those words which will convey a message to others who have not shared all of the same experiences. The written context becomes very important. That is, if a new word or experience is introduced in the passage, the words and ideas surrounding that word will help to provide understanding. This process is dependent not only on knowledge of more individual words but the way in which words combine to make meaning in sentences (i.e., syntax). Therefore, reading comprehension depends on shared experiences, word knowledge, and understanding of language structure. The printed symbol needs to be deciphered and put into the framework of the other words in the passage. The written information must then be related to the child's experience as well as the experience of the audience at large.

As students approach adolescence, literate forms of language assume a greater role in the development of linguistic knowledge as compared to children of younger ages who rely on oral language experiences.

Although most children acquire oral language without formal training, reading skills generally emerge only after direct instruction. One approach to early reading that emphasizes the similarities between oral language and the written text is *whole language.* Goodman (1986) believes that children should learn how to read in a format similar to the way they learn to speak. Providing an environment that is rich in materials that contain words and in writing tools like pens, crayons, and paper is emphasized. Whole language relates the written materials to the child's experience in a meaningful, purposeful, and functional way. That is, the youngster might read directions to play a game or devise a shopping list for a real party. Reading is taught from whole to part. Children learn by using reading and writing activities for specific purposes rather than by learning separate reading and writing subskills. This approach to reading and writing can be particularly beneficial to the child with language acquisition difficulties because it helps youngsters to understand the purposes of written language in concrete and meaningful contexts.

Another reading approach emphasizes teaching phonological awareness rather than functional literacy activities in kindergarten and first grade. Blachman (1991) stresses direct instructional activities in phoneme awareness and analysis to ensure early reading achievement. Some teachers have tried to use both whole language and discreet skills approaches by combining basal readers and workbooks with whole language reading and writing tasks during science or social studies lessons. Maria (1990) discusses both approaches and concludes that reading is a language process but more difficult to comprehend than speech because of its more formal syntax, organization, abstract concepts, and distancing between the author and reader. She states that because comprehension ability assumes greater importance as children achieve higher reading levels, those youngsters who have a strong language and experience base are able to engage in an interaction with the text more effectively. When students reach adolescence, proficient reading comprehension provides extensive opportunities for acquisition of world knowledge and linguistic growth.

SUMMARY

The examination of later language development demonstrates its impact on academic, social, and cultural growth. As youngsters acquire more mature language structure, expand their vocabulary, and learn to use language in conversation more effectively, their academic and social skills advance. Engaging in meaningful experiences, symbolic play, and shared book reading stimulates this development early on. However, the language used in the home environment is quite different from classroom language expectations. Children learn new rules at school for group discussion. As they enter elementary school, they also become more proficient in generating story narratives. This provides the bridge to literacy learning.

Reading and writing have been linked to language proficiency. Discussion regarding the most appropriate approaches to early reading has concluded that children need metalinguistic skill for early success. However, those teachers who use relevant and meaningful reading tools with a solid storyline are teaching most closely to the way oral language is acquired. Academic language becomes more abstract and decontextualized as the child progresses through school. As each student matures, conceptual, linguistic, and pragmatic knowledge expands. The child comes to understand and know people, things, and ideas; what oral and visual symbols represent this knowledge; and when to use them in the correct context. This complex process actually continues through adulthood.

SUGGESTED READINGS

Goodman, K. (1986). *What's Whole in Whole Language?* Portsmouth, NH: Heinemann.

Nippold, M. (Ed.). (1988). *Later Language Development: Ages Nine Through Nineteen.* Boston, MA: College-Hill Press.

Wallach, G., and Miller, L. (1988). *Language Intervention and Academic Success.* Boston, MA: College-Hill Press.

5 LOOKING AT CULTURAL AND LINGUISTIC DIVERSITY

One educational challenge in the United States today concerns meeting the needs of increasing numbers of bilingual and multi-cultural children. Estimates from the 1990 U.S. census are that the minority population exceeds 25% and are projected to be more than 30% by the year 2000 (Carey, 1992). Some school systems in California, Texas, New York, and elsewhere have a majority of culturally and linguistically different children. Of the 25 largest public school systems in the U.S., all but two have a majority of minority students (Willig and Greenberg, 1986). Children with language differences stemming from a language background other than English or from a culture that varies from the "majority" culture are often (erroneously) labeled as language disordered.

The speech-language specialist determines which children in fact do require special intervention for language disorder and provides input concerning specific intervention strategies. Cole (1992) states that in the American Speech-Language-Hearing Association (ASHA), only 3.7% of its members have identified themselves as Black, Hispanic, Asian, or Native American. This suggests that the majority of the members of the profession may not have personal knowledge or empathy for the needs of an increasingly multicultural society.

This chapter seeks to examine these seven issues related to cultural and linguistic diversity:

1. define terminology pertinent to understanding linguistic and cultural differences;

2. provide an historical perspective of cultural diversity within the United States, from "melting pot" ideology to the current recognition of "cultural pluralism";

3. contrast bilingualism with English dialect variation and present expectations of language acquisition within each group;

4. examine issues in assessment including the determination of a communication disorder for children who are culturally and linguistically different;

5. discuss meaningful intervention for language acquisition including home and school language models;

6. acknowledge the critical role of parents in the intervention process; and

7. examine cultural diversity issues in teacher training programs.

TERMINOLOGY

When discussing linguistic and cultural differences, an understanding of the pertinent terminology is essential. Children are often described as "bilingual" when they live in an area where the dominant language is different from their own. In fact, some children are **monolingual.** They speak only one language. In discussions of linguistic diversity in the U.S., that language is any language other than English.

Some children can speak two languages. They are then considered **bilingual**. Children who can speak more than two languages are **multilingual.** Some youngsters have only moderate proficiency in two languages. Initially, they may have learned the language of their family and before they are competent language users, they begin using another language. Under these circumstances, neither the original language nor the new language is acquired satisfactorily and these children are called **semilingual** (Duncan, 1989). Professionals in the field of bilingual education refer to children who lack proficiency in the English language as **limited-English proficient (LEP)** and **non-English proficient (NEP)**. In the United States, the majority of the population speaks English. The linguistic minority are those people who speak languages other than Standard American English.

People living in specific communities may speak a "dialect" of a language. **Dialects** are variations of a specific language. In the United States, Black English (also known as Black dialect or Ebonics) is such a dialect. Vocabulary, sentence structure, phrasing, word meanings, pronunciation, and language use can account for the variations (Hegde, 1991). **Regional dialects** sometimes occur when a group of people has remained socially isolated with limited exposure to the dominant language over a long period of time. Language variety also is affected by gender (e.g., girls are expected to speak in more polite forms) and age group. For example, adolescent youngsters use words, gestures, and phrases that constantly change and often represent different meanings from adult expectations. *That's cool, chill out*, or *go bananas* are expressions of teen dialect from various times.

A discussion of language difference due to cultural diversity requires a review of the interdependence of language and culture. **Ethnography** is the investigation and study used to understand the culture of a group of people. The use of communication and language of the group can be analyzed through ethnographic approaches.

Culture constitutes the way a specific group of people collectively work, behave, think, and believe at a certain time. The experiences and environment encountered by a group of people will affect behavior and beliefs. They also will affect language, especially choice of words, word meanings, and concepts (Patton and Westby,

1992). Thus, the culture and the language of a group of people are affected by the same experiences and environment. For example, the language of Eskimos has multiple words for *snow* whereas the English language just uses *snow* whether or not it is wet, has large flakes, is just falling, or lies glistening in the sunshine. Even among people who speak the English language, various "cultures" can have different vocabulary and word meanings depending on their experiences. In the computer culture, the words "virus" and "mouse" have meanings that elude a person who has never been exposed to computers. The more that is known about a person's culture, the better one can determine the proficiency of an individual's language use. Furthermore, when shared experiences are similar, communicators of a language are more likely to select similar vocabulary and word meanings.

HISTORICAL PERSPECTIVE

Many countries in the world are multicultural and multilingual. Each language has dialects. However, the United States has one official language, English. Zangwill (1910) introduced the term *melting pot* to describe the blending of immigrant groups from Europe to America early in the twentieth century. At that time, when immigrant children attended school, they were to learn English as quickly as possible and blend their diverse cultural patterns together into the dominant one. This ideology excluded Latin Americans, Asians, Africans, Middle Easterners, and others who were not of European descent. Yet, immigrants from these areas were part of the American fabric. Some groups were not "melting" and retained their cultural practices and ethnic backgrounds.

More recently the ideology of cultural pluralism has been embraced. **Cultural pluralism** (Payne, 1986; Poplin and Wright, 1983) recognizes the distinct variety of races and cultures which retain group identity. Cooperation, mutual appreciation, and understanding of diversity are assumed. In this "salad bowl" of cultures, individuals do not shed their heritage or identity. Rather than eradicating the ethnic origins, the American language and culture are added to the person's original background.

Educational models are still imbued with "melting pot" ideology, although legislation (The Bilingual Education Acts) has attempted to rectify this. Some American teachers note that their parents and grandparents arrived from Europe with no English and were able to attend school without support services, learn the English language and the American customs, and succeed. They can't comprehend why bilingual education is necessary. Yet, not all ethnic groups aspire to the dominant culture. Members of certain groups recognize the value of their own language and customs. The dominant culture's language will be learned in addition to their own. Cultural pluralism as an educational model requires teachers to empathize with linguistic and cultural differences, to familiarize themselves with the culture and customs, and to value and respect all cultures equally. The child has the right to maintain his or her identity.

Currently, Americans are expected to know English. Diversity, especially linguistic difference, is seen as an obstacle to national unity. Government policy continues to stress cultural conformity, as in the 1940 Nationality Act requiring English literacy to become a naturalized citizen (Erickson and Iglesias, 1986). Yet cultural pluralism is tolerated. The Bilingual Education Acts of 1968 and 1974 assist children who have been labeled "educationally disadvantaged" because they don't speak English. This includes teaching in a language other than English. The Education for All Handicapped Children Act of 1975 (PL 94-142) states that educational evaluations should be conducted in the child's primary language and provision of services should not be racially or culturally discriminatory.

THE BILINGUAL CHILD

There are three primary ways in which a bilingual child acquires dual language exposure (Schiff-Myers, 1992). First is **infant bilinguality** where two languages are spoken to the child from early infancy. Sometimes a specific individual speaks only in one language while another language is spoken by others. The baby associates the individual with the language spoken and usually can acquire two languages most easily under these circumstances. Other infants hear the same speakers changing their choice of language depending on the context.

A second way children acquire two languages is by early **childhood bilinguality**. Typically, the child hears one language at home and as a preschooler is exposed to a second language in community settings such as daycare. Languages are learned consecutively and the children are designated sequential language learners.

The third type of dual language acquisition is **school-age bilinguality**. Usually the child has developed proficiency in the family language and sometime during the school years (after age five or six) learns another language. The child who takes "foreign language" as a school subject is not included in this group because exposure to the second language tends to be limited and the child is not using that language to learn in other subject areas. School-age bilinguality is also sequential language learning.

Bilingualism and Language Disorders

For the child with a language disorder, developing minimum proficiency in a first or primary language (L1) may take more than the typical first five years. Depending on the degree of severity, an individual may never become a competent language user. Cummins (1989) points out that the level of proficiency a child has in L1 when initially exposed to L2 (the dominant language of the community) will affect future development in both languages. This even applies to children without language disorder. That is, normal children who are exposed to another language before the primary language is fully developed can be delayed in both languages for a period of time. Cummins urges competence in L1 before exposure to L2 to avoid problems. In fact, regression in the primary language (L1) may result from exposure to L2 at an unsuitable time.

The normal child developing early childhood bilinguality might demonstrate arrested or regressive language development in L1 or semilingualism. This causes confusion for teachers and language specialists when trying to separate language and cultural differences from true deficiencies and disabilities. Those children who are clearly identified as having disability need intervention that is appropriate to the disability and also to their dominant language and culture. Many teachers are from the majority culture and perceive minority cultural differences as problems. They might mistake language dialect or accent with a speech and language disability. Determining when a child will learn most efficiently in his or her dominant language and when English is most appropriate requires thorough evaluation in a variety of settings and tasks. Because language and culture develop from one's own unique experiences within a specific ethnic group, using typical school materials which were developed for middle-class America can be deleterious.

The American Speech-Language-Hearing Association (ASHA), in their 1985 position paper on communicatively handicapped minority language populations, states that LEP children are considered **communicatively handicapped** when there is limited competence in both the minority language and the English language. ASHA goes on to say that assessment of LEP children should be conducted in the client's primary (L1) language with a proficient bilingual examiner. If the normal but semilingual child is in a state of language regression, even a skilled bilingual evaluator will have to interpret language behaviors cautiously.

Bilingualism and Academic Language Use

School-age bilinguality poses further complications. The experiences that a child encounters at home develop corresponding language forms and uses. Home language tends to be informal and based on activities occurring in the "here and now." Therefore, a child's primary language tends to have distinctly everyday informal characteristics imbued with the home culture. The language taught in school tends to be more formal and more polite because the communicators aren't family members with whom the child feels at ease. The subject matter also begins to change. Topics are no longer centered on everyday occurrences but on curricular subject matter. Therefore, the language learned in school tends to be academic in nature. For the school-age bilingual child, this means that L2 has very different vocabulary, structure, and use from L1. When a school-age youngster is evaluated, the child could still be acquiring L2 and appear language deficient. The bilingual evaluator now conducts the testing in the primary language (L1) of the child. The test format and subject matter is academically oriented but the child's expertise in L1 is everyday, informal and home-centered. Results of the test can be very misleading due to these circumstances.

Bilingual children often switch from one language to another during conversations. Known as **code switching**, this linguistic device is most noticeable when complete mastery has not been achieved. However, sometimes code switching occurs because one language expresses a concept better than another. Other times children switch from one language to another during a conversation because they do not have the label for a particular concept in the language they are speaking.

Language Acquisition Time Lines

Normal time requirements for second language acquisition vary depending on the length of time the child has been exposed to the language, the age of the child, and the types of language acquisition techniques that are provided (Langdon, 1989). One should account for a child's cognitive development (concepts, memory, attention, sequencing, associations, etc.) in determining language proficiency time lines as well. The school-age child without cognitive or sensory deficits usually can use the new language in 18–36 months for social interpersonal functions (Duncan, 1989).

Wong-Fillmore (1991) points out that the length of time required to learn the "academic" forms of a second language depends on the structure of the classroom environment, the characteristics of the individual students in the class, and the kinds of language used in the academic setting. Other factors facilitating second language acquisition by the school-age youngster include more extensive first language experience, heightened awareness of how language is structured, and awareness of its meaning and use (metalinguistic awareness). Often the school-age child has encountered literacy, reading, and writing experiences as well. Despite these positive elements, Cummins (1984) argues that children who begin to learn another language in school must not only learn language for social communication but also academic language proficiency. He reports that academic language competence in a new language can take up to seven years to develop for normal children beginning to learn L2 after the age of six. Therefore, these children may achieve inadequate test scores in L2 for an extended time.

It can be argued that because linguistic proficiency equal to monolingual native speakers is so time-consuming, children should begin to learn L2 before the elementary school years. Pacheco (1983) cites several studies that take issue with this notion. Cummins's hypothesis proposes that a child must reach a threshold of competence in the primary home language before a second language (L2) can be mastered. Otherwise both languages lag in development (i.e., semilingualism).

The UNESCO Study

A classic study of children placed in a new cultural and linguistic environment is discussed in the findings of the Finnish National Commission Report to UNESCO (Skutnabb-Kangas and Toukomaa, 1976). This study supports the notion that the first language of a child should be developed to proficiency before another language is introduced to expect most efficient learning of both languages. The study is particularly important for decisions in the United States because Finland, the country from which the immigrants came, and Sweden, the host country, are highly developed, modern societies. Issues of health care, diet, and unemployment were not variables which could contribute to lack of school achievement for the immigrant children. Results indicated that those children who moved to Sweden from Finland at about the age of ten, when the Finnish language was firmly established, could most quickly develop proficiency in the Swedish language equivalent to children born in Sweden. Those children who came to Sweden before the age of six did not do as well. Children who moved to Sweden after the age of 12 could develop language skills comparable to Swedes but not as quickly as the ten year olds.

THE CHILD WITH ENGLISH DIALECT VARIATIONS

The child from a different culture who speaks a dialect of the English language is expected to learn the customs, behaviors, and language of the dominant language community at school. Some members of the African American and Native American communities fall under this category. To separate the child with a dialect and cultural difference from one with a language disorder is complex. One problem involves the lack of an adequate empirical definition of normal language behavior for nonmainstream speakers. The inadequate definition results in inaccurate language assessment (Stockman, 1986).

There are many ways to speak the English language. In England, Ireland, Australia, the south and midwest United States, English has many variations. Yet, perception in the dominant culture as to which of these dialects is acceptable is rooted in historical, political, and social bias.

Historically, Standard American English was the language that people in the U.S. aspired to learn and most languages and dialects were characterized as the speech of the oppressed and ghetto minorities. The dialects associated with oppressed people tended to be regarded as inferior to Standard American English. Because standardized tests were developed within the dominant white culture, assessment scores proved this thesis. For example, African American people have been socially isolated for centuries in the U.S. and it is not surprising that they developed English dialects. For many years, teachers have devoted themselves to "correcting" Black English features to their Standard English equivalents. Linguists, however, stress that nonstandard dialects of English are highly structured systems with specific rules as to form and use. English dialects are not "primitive" forms of the language. Rather, they reflect the same cognitive skill and cultural expression that any language system does. ASHA's position paper on social dialects stated that no English dialect can be considered a language disorder; each social dialect in English is considered effective and functional, serving communication and social solidarity needs of the dialectic community (American Speech-Language-Hearing Association, 1987).

When one views a dialect as a distinct and highly structured language with a specific rule system which relates to the culture of the community of speakers, the children speaking this language should be treated in a manner similar to the linguistically different and bilingual youngsters. Their home language should be fully developed. Teachers must study, respect, and value the child and the child's community, culture, and language dialect. Culturally different children have the right to maintain their identity and pride. Standard American English is considered a second language and theories of bilingual language acquisition apply to culturally diverse children. The youngsters learn Standard American English in addition to their original dialect. It is not meant to replace their dialect (Light, 1972).

ASSESSMENT

When assessing children who may be language disordered but who are culturally and/or linguistically different, one must carefully examine the testing instruments, the culture and customs of the child, the tester's expertise and familiarity with the child's culture and language, and, of course, the child's family and community (Crago, 1992). If the child has no language disability in the primary language, the child cannot be considered language disordered.

Test Limitations

Assessment instrumentation continues to create barriers to effective determination of a child's difficulties. Some state laws require at least one standardized testing instrument in any assessment. Most speech and language tests have only a selected population from which their standardized norms are derived. The population could be a group of inner-city children from Detroit, suburban children from New Jersey, and rural children from Iowa. Yet, none of those groups may compare to the particular child referred for evaluation in terms of culture and custom. Furthermore, few assessment instruments are specifically designed for non-English speaking youngsters.

Language competence is affected by cognitive ability, culture, sensory adeptness, and meaningful experiences. Language can be viewed in various ways including understanding, expression, and use in various contexts. No one language test can account for all of these factors. Even if there were one test that encompassed these critical considerations, that test would not be standardized with children using every dialect of every language from every culture that exists in the United States. Thus, standardized testing instruments are extremely limited as to what aspects of language they can effectively test and on whom. Even when tests are translated accurately into a child's language and dialect, the test cannot account for cultural differences.

IQ Testing and Language Differences

State laws differ with regard to standardized IQ testing to determine a child's level of intellectual functioning when making a special education placement. For those youngsters who have apparent linguistic and cultural differences, standard IQ tests are often invalid. Furthermore, intelligence and language are sometimes difficult to separate. Poor language skills can be confused with lowered intellectual ability. In fact, disproportionate numbers of linguistically and culturally different children have been placed in classes for children with mental retardation (Cummins, 1983a; Pacheco, 1983).

IQ tests, even nonverbal portions of IQ tests such as block design, object manipulation, and form boards are geared to middle class English culture children (Samuda, 1975). As Willig and Greenberg (1986) point out, attempts to devise "culture free" IQ tests are unsatisfactory because a child's view of the world is based on his or her experience. Even adeptness at puzzle assembly relies on experience. Many specialists (Cummins, 1989; Erickson and Iglesias, 1986; Langdon, 1983, 1989; Maldonado-Colon, 1986; Zavola and Mims, 1983) regard using standardized testing for culturally and linguistically different children with extreme caution and only when such tests are used in combination with other criteria.

Assessment Guidelines

When assessing children from a culturally or linguistically different background, Kayser (1989) considers the following:

- the language used by the family
- the child's length of stay in this country
- the educational level and work experiences of the parents
- the use of language outside the home by the family in situations such as church
- the language used in newspapers and other media by the family
- the attitude of the family toward the primary and dominant language and culture
- the attitude of the community towards the dominant culture

Other factors affecting test scores of culturally diverse children, in addition to the use of language in the home and community, include child-rearing practices, exposure to various schooling practices, self-concept (including previous failures), prior experience in testing situations, and the cultural conventions of the family. The physical appearance of a test environment may also affect a child's test scores. The child's reaction to an examiner who may not fully understand cultural differences can influence test outcomes as well. Evaluators need training in cultural variability. For example, white middle class children have been taught to be competitive, individualistic, and hard working as a means to a future end. Other cultures teach collective decision making, respect for the wisdom of the elders, mutual support, and goals through common effort (Miller, 1984).

Table 5.1 contrasts several cultures in their use of English language components. The examples depict differences in the use of syntactic and morphological structures and pragmatic conventions and exemplify the need to fully understand the child's culture and its conventions to accurately differentiate language difference from language disorder. The reader is referred to the sources listed for extended examples which contrast several cultures and their use of English.

Table 5.1

Contrasting Cultural Conventions in the Use of English

	Black English	Asian Speakers of English	Standard American English	Hispanic English
Morphological and Syntactical Components				
Plural *s* Marker	Nonobligatory use of marker *s* with numerical quantifier. *I see two dog playing. I need ten dollar. Look at the dogs.*	Omission of plural marker *s* or overregulation. *I see two dog. I need ten dollar. I have two sheeps.*	Obligatory use of marker *s* with a few exceptions. *I see two dogs. I need ten dollars. I have two sheep.*	Nonobligatory use of marker *s*. *I see two dog playing. I have two sheep.*
Past Tense	Nonobligatory use of *ed* marker. *Yesterday, I talk to her.*	Omission of *ed* marker or overregulation. *I talk to her yesterday. I sawed her yesterday*	Obligatory use of *ed* marker. *I talked to her yesterday.*	Nonobligatory use of marker *ed*. *I talk to her yesterday.*
Pragmatic Components				
Rules of Conversation	Interruption is tolerated. The most assertive person has the floor.	Children are expected to be passive; are discouraged from interrupting teachers; are considered impolite if they talk during dinner.	Appropriate to interrupt in certain circumstances. One person has the floor until point is made.	Official or business conversations may be preceded by lengthy introductions.
Eye Contact	Indirect eye contact during listening. Direct eye contact during speaking denotes attentiveness and respect.	May not maintain eye contact with authority figure but may make eye contact with strangers. May avert direct eye contact and giggle to express embarrassment.	Indirect eye contact during speaking. Direct eye contact during listening denotes attentiveness and respect.	Avoidance of direct eye contact is sometimes a sign of respect and attentiveness. Maintaining eye contact may be considered a challenge to authority.

Adapted from *Language Disorders: A Functional Approach to Assessment and Intervention* by R. Owens, 1991, New York: Charles E. Merrill; and from "Cross-Cultural and Linguistic Considerations in Working with Asian Populations" by L. Cheng, 1987, *ASHA, 29*(6), 33–38.

An ethnographic approach can be extended to children by observing them in a variety of settings to determine what languages are used in which contexts and the effectiveness of the use. This might include observing children at home, in the classroom, in the lunchroom, and on the playground interacting with a variety of people including members of the family and community.

Erickson and Iglesias (1986) have suggested using standardized tests in a nonstandardized manner. The purpose is to account for the academic, cultural, and linguistic competencies of the minority child. The examiner would first determine that the child has had exposure to the material examined in the test. Among other considerations, the researchers discuss rewording instructions, allowing additional test time, comparing answers from the dominant language to the child's dialect or primary language, practicing test taking, having the child explain an "incorrect" response, or using real examples instead of the pictures used in the test.

Tests are used to determine what the child *can do* and not to trick the child. Look at the child as an individual with learning potential. Respect the child's differences. Children from culturally different environments are not necessarily deprived. Sometimes teachers impose their own cultural values and make such assumptions. The tester must listen most carefully to *what* a child says rather than *how* he or she says it. Expression of ideas by linguistically and culturally different children should carry more weight than grammar and pronunciation or accent. Take into account how the child learns, the rate the child learns, and those areas the child learns most easily.

Careful assessment must be stressed. There are data (Dew, 1984) from one hundred school districts which note that in sixteen of these districts, 100% of the LEP (limited English proficient) students have been placed in special education. More than forty of these districts had placed between 50 and 100% of their LEP students in special education. In proportion to their general population, Hispanic students were underrepresented in all special education categories except learning disability where they were over-represented by 300%. Improper assessment or outright discrimination must account for such imbalanced numbers.

INTERVENTION

Children with cultural and linguistic differences further complicated by language disorders have been placed in a variety of settings. In many instances, the programs have been well-meaning but largely unsuccessful. Statistics concerning graduation of these youngsters from high school are disappointing. In some large school systems, regulations ensuring appropriate bilingual services for these children are in place. Unfortunately, certain schools don't have available personnel to comply with the regulations and the children in need are left unserved. Parents who are unaware of the educational rights of their children don't know how to access the programs their children are entitled to receive. Some parents are overwhelmed with their everyday survival and find school meetings adversarial. School personnel sometimes use technical language when discussing a child or when answering parents' questions. This is perceived as threatening and intimidating. Therefore, the first steps to effective intervention must include knowledge and respect for the child's culture and language. The program can be designed more suitably when pertinent information is known about a child and the child's family.

The Immersion Question

When teaching children who speak a language other than English, a central question is when to introduce English into the curriculum. **Immersion programs** have been interpreted as being an approach where the minority student is "immersed" in English-only programs. Children with moderate language disorders are frequently taught using English immersion techniques. It is argued that only one language should be used for school instruction although it may differ from the home language (Carrow-Woolfolk and Lynch, 1982). The rationale is that children with moderate language disability have difficulty learning even in one language and bilingual instruction creates confusion.

Cummins (1983a) states that immersion should be an "additive" process where English is added without sacrificing competence in the first language (L1). This is accomplished by promoting proficiency in L1 so that it can be transferred to English (L2) learning and literacy most effectively. This requires emphasizing L1 through the mid-elementary grades. Even after English is introduced as the language of instruction, the L1 continues to be a subject for the student.

When the child has language disability, difficulty in learning L1 can delay proficiency drastically. The concept that L1 would then facilitate acquisition of English is questionable. In fact, by mid-elementary school, the language of a child with language disability could be equivalent to a preschooler. Research has shown that preschool bilingual acquisition can interfere with language development and even cause it to regress (Miller, 1984; Pacheco, 1983). Children can become confused and frustrated. Therefore, careful assessment of each child's abilities and thorough discussions with the parents are critical in developing any program for the youngster with language disability. Sometimes too a particular child doesn't fit the educational program devised for linguistically different children with language disorders in a particular school district and accommodations need to be made.

Using Meaningful Curricula

A major group of theorists view the appropriate way to instruct language minority students is to establish a process of meaningful input that is interesting and relevant to the child (Cummins, 1983a; Miller, 1984; Omark and Erickson, 1983; Ruiz, 1989). Miller differentiates language acquisition from language learning. Acquisition focuses on communication and meaning. The child acquires language in natural situations as opposed to language learning which stresses structured lessons reinforcing specific language forms or skills that are practiced out of their real situation. Thus, the emphasis is on meaningful communication in concrete contexts and not grammatical usage drills. This allows the students to observe and use paralinguistic cues (gestures, facial expressions, and other nonverbal cues) to infer intended meanings of the communication. Bruck's (1982) research in Canada with children in French immersion programs illustrates that children with language disability in true immersion programs, with a meaningful and relevant curriculum, develop linguistic and academic skills equivalent to similar children taught only in English, the primary language.

Students should be actively involved in the learning process. For culturally and linguistically different children, the subject content must relate to their prior background and experience to ensure comprehension. This also reinforces the child's sense of cultural identity and pride. Incorporating the language and customs of the minority student into the school program as well as increasing the participation of members of the minority community at school extends cultural identity. Specific suggestions for sharing rather than suppressing the minority languages include these (Cummins, 1989; Ruiz, 1989):

1. placing signs in the school written in the minority languages;

2. recruiting people to tutor in the minority languages;

3. providing books in the minority languages;

4. displaying pictures of various cultures represented at the school;

5. encouraging students to write newspaper articles in their primary language (L1);

6. integrating the minority language into content areas; and,

7. incorporating collaborative learning whenever possible, which provides opportunities for natural language practice.

Home and School Language Models

When children from another linguistic background begin learning English at school, teachers sometimes advise parents who have some bilingual proficiency to use English in the home environment as much as possible. The intent is to reinforce language development in the natural home setting. Before making such advisements, analyze carefully the English language competency of the parent. Young children, in particular, who are still developing proficiency in their primary language (L1), should be exposed to the most developed language models possible. It is better not to communicate with a child in English at home if it is limited and broken English or English dominated by code switching with L1. This could result in fewer interactions between parent and child or qualitatively weaker language experiences for the child (Cummins, 1983a).

The child with a language disorder needs exposure to accurate models of language geared to his or her level of comprehension. If parents have equal proficiency in both English and the child's primary language, then an evaluation of the language needs of the youngster at that time can determine how the parents can best help the child. Literate parents can be encouraged to read appropriate books with the child. The teacher can discuss book selection and how best to read and discuss books. Parents from other cultures are not always aware of public libraries in their neighborhood. Assistance in obtaining a library card can provide the family with access to various media to enrich the child's experience.

Studies in Intervention

A study (Ruiz, 1989) was undertaken of an 11-year-old Mexican-American child named Rosemary who was identified as mildly disabled and placed in special education. Her story represents the education of many Hispanic youngsters who come from large families that are poor, struggling, and isolated. Yet, with proper intervention, this child became a successful learner. Rosemary was born in Mexico and moved to California at age 2. The family only spoke Spanish. She entered school for the first time at age 7½ and was placed in an English speaking multigrade classroom. Rosemary displayed learning problems, was provided with special help, and continued to progress slowly. An intelligence test (*WISC-R*) was administered in English, with resulting scores in the midseventies in both verbal and performance areas. The speech-language pathologist evaluated the youngster in both English and Spanish and determined that she had a four-year language delay although scores on the *Language Assessment Scales* were in the near-proficient range. This score convinced the bilingual teacher providing special help to continue teaching reading and writing in English.

Rosemary's next placement was a bilingual special education class for students with communication disabilities. Dual language instruction was provided in an alternate day method. She continued to lag until a special consultant-researcher began to work with the school. Two pictures of Rosemary emerged. In the classroom, she was a child struggling with language-related academic tasks. In other contexts, the researcher found Rosemary's communication in both oral and written form to be quite competent. When writing in Spanish on self-selected topics, the content was clear and interesting with few grammatical errors. When participating in sociodramatic play, Rosemary was a leader who could generate specific and detailed language for descriptions and instructions. Thus, depending on how the task was organized, the student could display either competence or incompetence in reading and writing tasks. When educational contexts and activities indicate discrepancies in language ability, the educator must consider these factors in providing appropriate educational intervention.

Another study emphasizes the need for culturally sensitive professionals to work with diverse populations. Cheng (1989) discusses Asian/Pacific children and the extreme variability in this population whose influx into the U.S. has swelled in recent years. Cultural traditions, religion, history, language background, and discourse styles are very different among the many children from Malaysia, China, India, Hong Kong, Taiwan, Japan, Korea, Thailand, Vietnam, Laos, and elsewhere. Within any one of these countries, multiple languages abound. Southeast Asian groups, like the Hmong, did not have a written language until the 1950s and many Hmong adults cannot read. Religions such as Buddhism, Confucianism, Taoism, Animism, and Shintoism are not well known by many Americans. For example, Taoism promotes passivity. When initiative is needed to obtain appropriate help for youngsters with disability and the family practices Taoism, they may experience a sense of fatalism and resignation which could be an obstacle to service. Cultural traditions dictate that children be quiet, less active, cautious, and observant in some groups, and exploration and competitiveness are deplored. The Asian/Pacific population exemplifies the diversity of cultures and language that any one country can possess. Familiarity with the culture, language, and community of a particular child is critical for effective assessment and intervention to be achieved. Duncan (1989) studied Punjabi and Bengali students living in England with language disabilities by working closely with the family and community, teaching with a team of bilingual personnel familiar with the language and culture, and teaching in English and the child's primary language concurrently. Duncan's data indicated that even children with language disorders can learn bilingually.

A research project on the language of Navajo children (Saville-Troike, 1986) illustrates how basic American educational concepts can be misconstrued by children reared in "minority" cultures. When meeting unfamiliar people in new situations, it is the Navajo custom to remain silent for a period of time. On the first day of school, a teacher immediately talks to the children. Children are asked to give their name but traditional Navajos, by religious taboo, don't reveal their names. Colors and shapes also are viewed differently. In Navajo, certain colors are grouped under the same name and others, like black, have two distinct names depending on the hue or tint. Most Navajo preschoolers can identify a hexagon but triangles are not learned early in their culture. Because language development depends so much on a child's culture, teachers must be careful not to misinterpret lack of knowledge or experience with disability. Furthermore, segments of the Navajo population have a high frequency of untreated hearing loss in children which could create a predisposition for true language disability.

In examining the education of the "disadvantaged" or "culturally deprived" children, Fantini (1972) stresses that when referring to minority populations, these terms reflect a "colonial" perspective. They also imply that it is the learner who has difficulties and not the school or the educational process. Programs such as Project Head Start were developed by white professionals as compensatory education programs to rehabilitate children so that they could join regular learners in the standard educational system. It is suggested that the established educational system might need to be changed to fit the individual learners. Early education is deemed essential but shaping a minority child into the middle American mold sometimes leads to failure in school or misdiagnosis of learning disability. This can be seen in the number of minority children labeled as language and learning disabled as services for children with disabilities have grown (Erickson and Walker, 1983; Ochoa, Pacheco, and Omark, 1983).

THE ROLE OF PARENTS

Parents are critical members of the educational team. Because language continues to be used when the child leaves school, the parent and educator should collaborate to help the child with language difficulty. The parent is also an important informant to the school concerning family and community customs and culture when the school is working with linguistically and culturally diverse children. The Individuals with Disabilities Education Act requires school districts to involve parents in planning educational programs for their children with disabilities. However, parents may choose not to be involved. In reality, parent involvement varies greatly from community to community. Race, culture, and language variation also seem to be factors affecting parent participation. Stein (1983) found that Hispanics and African Americans participate less than whites in assessment and program conferences for their children with disability. African American parents are more involved and aware of services than Hispanic parents. The study suggests that cultural differences, parent trust, awareness of parental rights, and language barriers influence parent involvement. The concept of "participation" varies in different cultures. Parent involvement is also affected by cultural trust of the schools as institutions.

Knowledge of parental and cultural views of disabilities, their causes, and treatment is extremely important for school personnel interacting with parents. In some Asian cultures, parents do not perceive their children as having a disability unless there are physical manifestations. Recommending intervention or a special class for a child with a language disorder can be difficult for the parents to understand. In some countries, there are no services or recognition of certain disabilities. Other cultures view disability as the will of some spiritual force that can't be corrected by secular means. To communicate with parents effectively, school personnel must consider not only the family culture but also their own cultural biases.

Researchers have outlined specific guidelines when communicating with parents (Carrasquillo, 1986; Matsuda, 1989; Stein, 1983). Consideration of status, authority, compromise, silence, nonverbal clues, and avoidance of direct personal questions are among the issues examined. Schools are encouraged to do the following:

- Conduct meetings and home communications in the language of the family.

- Learn about and respect the customs of the child's family so parents will be in a more conducive environment for expressing their views and insights.

- Provide parent training on the educational rights, responsibilities, and services for their child.

- Discuss instructional strategies and demonstrate how the parent can reinforce school learning at home.

- Promote collaboration between the home and school.

TEACHER TRAINING

Currently there are many children from culturally and linguistically different backgrounds who have language disability and are not being taught with any of the aforementioned models (Bernal, 1983). Most frequently, there are no bilingual-trained staff members to properly evaluate and provide instruction. Taylor (1992) describes the issue as "alarming" and stresses teaching about cultural diversity issues in teacher training programs at the universities and in continuing education settings. Recruiting culturally diverse speech-language pathologists is a priority of the American Speech-Language-Hearing Association (Cole, 1992). Teachers need to learn effective pedagogic principles, special education issues, and knowledge of various cultures. Those educators working with minority language children who have language disabilities should be familiar with normal first and second language development, appropriate instructional approaches for children with language disorders, and characteristics of language impairment. A teacher's cultural background similar to the student being served does not guarantee expertise in educating that youngster. Bilingual special education as a specialty within special education will require expanded coordination and collaboration among bilingual, special, and general educators. A collective problem-solving process among teachers can prevent and resolve identified problems (Harris, 1991). Educators need to understand their own perspectives, attitudes, and values. Research into the most accurate and appropriate assessment and instructional strategies also must continue. Knowledge should be obtained concerning what language behaviors can be expected in a child's cultural peer group at specific ages. All these critical competencies must be developed for effective education of culturally and linguistically diverse children.

Unfortunately, the number of bilingual special education teacher training programs has decreased by about 50% to just 16 in 1988. Of these 16 programs, 9 were single-faculty member programs (Hoover and Collier, 1991).

SUMMARY

Cultural and linguistic diversity affects increasing numbers of children in the United States. Some children enter school without having developed a rich primary language. Some immigrant and minority families have had inadequate health care and nutrition. Overburdened parents sometimes haven't engaged in special activities and quality interaction with their children due to issues of housing, work, substance abuse, and community disintegration. These factors impact on educational decisions concerning the linguistically and culturally different child who may have special education needs. Assessments using traditional instruments can provide inaccurate information about the child's true language and learning abilities. This has resulted in inappropriate class placement and services for many youngsters who are not members of the mainstream culture. Educational programs and services should determine when to introduce English into the curriculum using criteria such as the age and first language proficiency of the child, language learning abilities, English proficiency of the youngster's family, the child's culture, and the resources of the educational system. Experience-based learning using meaningful, relevant activities promotes functional language and improves conceptual understanding. Subject content must relate to the child's cultural identity. For some students, school might be the only opportunity to learn that they can communicate with others, that wonders exist in the world, and that hope for the future is possible.

Parents can have unrealistic expectations about their child, the school, and the language disorder. This is especially true for families who are not familiar with American education. Some parents make no attempt to learn English. Others desire their child to learn in the minority language only. Effective education for each youngster requires careful consideration of all issues. The challenge is to teach students to be literate and fluent in Standard American English without sacrificing their primary culture and positive self-image. Bilingual students need to understand that knowing more than one language is a special achievement to be valued and preserved. Children with language disability must be carefully examined so that they can achieve their potential in either the language of the majority or bilingually. Under either condition, children with language impairment should maintain pride in their culture and heritage.

SUGGESTED READINGS

Cummins, J. (1984). *Bilingualism and Special Education: Issues in Assessment and Pedagogy.* Austin, TX: Pro-Ed.

Omark, D., and Erickson, J. (Eds.). (1983). *The Bilingual Exceptional Child.* San Diego, CA: College-Hill Press.

Taylor, O. (Ed). (1986). *The Nature of Communication Disorders in Culturally and Linguistically Diverse Populations.* San Diego, CA: College-Hill Press.

6 UNDERSTANDING LANGUAGE ASSESSMENT

The process of child language assessment has undergone modifications which reflect the various ways that researchers view language. Over the last fifty years, researchers have studied "normal" language of children, causes of language disorder, descriptions of the characteristics of each child's language, and how various situations affect children's language (Lund and Duchan, 1988).

Experience in assessment has taught speech-language pathologists that language is not an isolated entity. Assessment must reflect the communicative function of language which involves a community of people, a culture, and shared events. Observing individual children out of their everyday environment in isolated testing rooms can create a different or atypical picture of their language ability. Furthermore, assessment must account for language as the medium for learning. Children use language to listen, speak, read, and write. They also use language to obtain, synthesize, and express information about their world. The relationship among language, academic, and cognitive functions impacts on assessment results. Tools of assessment currently do not encompass the spectrum of social, cultural, and academic forces affecting the language ability of a youngster.

The complex and variable nature of language itself also challenges accurate assessment. The sounds, syllables, words, and sentences in language interface with word meanings and use. Meanings change in both linguistic and situational contexts. Language varies when used in conversation, mediation, narration, and classroom lessons.

No single test can evaluate all facets of language comprehension and production for all children from all cultures. Selection of assessment tools and procedures is affected by the evaluator's approach to language, the evaluator's perception of the child, the purpose of the assessment, the availability of assessment tools, and the time available to the evaluator.

In recent years, real communication contexts, such as a play situation or conversation with peers and familiar adults, have been more valuable for assessment of expressive language than formal or standardized tests (Klee, 1992). Children often exhibit more developed interaction skills with their classroom teachers and other familiar individuals during an assessment. When they are attuned to their conversational partner, youngsters tend to converse with more complex linguistic forms and with more detailed and elaborated linguistic output. They can concentrate on language and not be distracted by unfamiliar surroundings and people as might be found in a formal testing situation.

The role of the communication context has resulted in a reappraisal of standardized tests. If the goal of assessment is to determine the most effective intervention strategies, then the selection of testing instruments, whether formal or informal, will impact on that intervention. Yet, some government agencies and education systems have mandated approved lists of tests when determining language intervention. Uniform testing is presumed to promote greater reliability in determining eligibility for intervention services. This requirement usually promotes use of norm-referenced formal tests which cannot thoroughly assess the complexity and variability of a child's language and can exclude youngsters that don't meet pre-specified eligibility criteria (ASHA, 1989).

This chapter discusses several critical aspects of assessment:

1. the purposes of various assessment measures and their ability to reflect an accurate and comprehensive picture of a particular child's language and communication skill; and

2. advantages and disadvantages of standardized and informal assessment procedures. Comprehensive assessment measures require considerable time to administer and interpret. Accurate determinations regarding a child's language abilities and appropriate educational programs are derived from a person's knowledge about the child, interpretation of evaluation data, and the collective knowledge of those individuals who interact with the child.

THE CHANGING FOCUS OF ASSESSMENT

The approach to language disorders taken by speech-language pathologists affects the assessment process. In the 1950s, when the medical model of intervention was utilized in schools and clinics, assessments determined probable cause or etiology for language difficulty. Once diagnosed, it was assumed that the "condition" could be improved by employing specific intervention plans. For example, an influential researcher of the period, Helmer Myklebust (1954, 1971) used the term *childhood aphasia* to diagnose those youngsters with seemingly normal intelligence but language deficits. He suspected neurological irregularities and recommended interdisciplinary diagnostic measures including pediatric, neurologic, and psychiatric consults as well as an evaluation by the speech-language pathologist. The intensive evaluation was designed to reveal the underlying deficits affecting the youngster's ability to manipulate oral language. The condition *childhood aphasia* could then be differentiated from other disorders such as mental retardation, hearing impairment, and emotional disturbance. This "medical" approach introduced collaboration in determining a diagnosis, but it provided few guidelines for the "speech therapist" on how to further examine and control the presenting symptoms of the disorder.

By the 1970s, the implementation of the Education for All Handicapped Children Act (PL 94-142) (revised as the Individuals with Disabilities Education Act) required designation of a specific handicapping condition for a child to receive service. Programs were established for children with different etiologic categories such as mental retardation or autism. Expected language outcomes varied, however, within these groups. For example, one child with autism might speak in sentences and another child might not speak at all. Children might exhibit ranges of severity for various behaviors associated with the disorder, or be diagnosed with multiple conditions such as autism and hearing impairment.

Public law specifies that assessment instruments reflect the child's aptitude or achievement level rather than impaired sensory, manual, or speaking skills (Federal Register, September 29, 1992, p. 44822). This approach to assessment describes the language of the child rather than to emphasize etiology. Known as the **descriptive approach**, the purpose is to outline specific linguistic characteristics such as language comprehension variables and the production of linguistic forms (Miller, 1983).

Standardized tests examine particular dimensions of language and compare the child's performance to a group of "normal" children selected by the test creator. The descriptive approach provides more specific guidelines for intervention strategies because individual areas of the child's linguistic system have been analyzed. However, by focusing on specific linguistic functions and deficits, the functioning of the whole child within the environment, and how that impacts on the ability to understand and use language, is not given full attention.

During the 1980s, pragmatics research led speech-language pathologists to interact with youngsters in natural settings and to engage in realistic activities rather than in drills to improve specific language deficits. Researchers became aware of children's linguistic competencies and deficiencies in multiple situations. Another focus to assessment emerged that examined children's communicative competence in different contexts (Brinton and Fujiki, 1989; Lund and Duchan, 1988). Language was assessed in relation to a listener and to a particular environment (Roth and Spekman, 1984a; 1984b). Assessment stressed the factors affecting a child's ability to communicate successfully. Formal testing tools were replaced by guided observational protocols.

In summary, the focus of assessment shifted from a medical orientation emphasizing causal factors and underlying deficits affecting a child's language to a model which described the child's language ability. The most recent approach to assessment has attempted to explore children's communicative competence and how well their language serves them in everyday contexts. Each successive approach to assessment does not necessarily override the preceding orientation. Rather, each approach should extend the evaluator's vision of children, their language, and how they interact with environmental factors.

CHALLENGES TO ACCURATE LANGUAGE ASSESSMENT

Language difficulties are associated with educational, emotional, and social problems (Corcoran, 1989; Wiig, 1990). Federal legislation mandates appropriate educational services for children between the ages of 3 and 21 with disorders. Many states have enacted legislation which provides assessment and intervention for children with disabilities from birth. Programs from infancy have been organized to meet the needs of these youngsters. However, deciding what constitutes a language disorder challenges even the experienced speech-language pathologist.

Each child has individual abilities and a unique environment which serve as the framework for language acquisition. This results in considerable variation in normal language development (Bishop and Edmundson, 1987). In hindsight, a given set of abilities in language for one child might constitute a delay, whereas for another child the same set of abilities is within the realm of normality. That is, at a particular time, youngsters who are the same chronological age may exhibit similar language delay. Yet, over time, a positive physical and social environment may stimulate more rapid language development in one of them. It may be determined that this child has normal language whereas the other child may continue to demonstrate language delay.

The range of "normal" in the communication skills of children is considerable. Corcoran (1989) discusses studies demonstrating a variation of 30–36 months in "normal" four year olds. This situation contributes to a "wait-and-see" attitude among some professionals to determine genuine language deficits. When the diagnosis of language delay has finally been specified, valuable and often irretrievable intervention time has been lost.

Another barrier to accurate language assessment concerns the many complexities of language as well as the interrelationship of language with social, linguistic, and cognitive factors. Disorder may involve one aspect of language such as grammatic development or multiple facets of language such as using language appropriately in different contexts, or understanding abstract concepts. The complex nature of language is further complicated by the fact that disorder has a range of magnitude. A youngster may demonstrate a mild deficit in language understanding and a severe inability in combining words. These inherent difficulties must all be considered when making an assessment of children's linguistic skills. Yet a definitive framework for stages of normal language development, the unique language abilities of individual children, and the range of severity in language disorders continues to be debated.

Assessment of Infants

Infants who are prelingual present challenges in assessment. Coggins (1991) suggests looking at an infant's communicative intentions. The child may gesture, gaze, or change posture to indicate needs and wants. Sparks (1989) emphasizes observation over time to determine an infant's developmental patterns. Because language is used in contexts, assessment includes interactions between the infant and caregiver. The infant's family strengths and needs are also considered (Ensher, 1989; MacDonald and Carroll, 1992).

Because of natural variation among infants, many are seen by speech-language pathologists because they are "high-risk" or "at-risk" youngsters. Early assessment and intervention are promoted because research suggests that these infants have a higher incidence of later speech and language difficulties (Proctor, 1989). Yet many newborns with overwhelming birth complications cannot be assessed accurately with current instruments and identified definitively as language impaired (Sparks, 1989).

Assessment of the Older Child

When youngsters begin to verbalize, new challenges to assessment emerge. Because both normal and language disordered children exhibit such variation in language ability, criteria for identifying disability might be inaccurate when applied to a particular youngster. Conceptual definitions for disabilities lack professional and scientific consensus (Silliman and Wilkinson, 1991). In addition, each youngster matures at an individual rate so that quantifying the severity of each aspect of language is difficult. Compounding this difficulty is the fact that a child's language competence appears to change when viewed in different contexts. Depending upon who the child speaks with, what the topic is, and where the linguistic exchange occurs, the quality and quantity of language understood and used can vary.

In summary, accurate assessment must account for the professional who administers the tests as well as the child. Any two people interacting together will create a language climate that differs from any other. The amount of time spent on the assessment also should be considered. Oftentimes a school schedule allows a limited period of time such as 60–90 minutes for a tester to evaluate a youngster. Important placement and intervention decisions are based on this single meeting. Most researchers concur that several encounters with the youngster in various situations will provide more accurate data on language ability (Brinton and Fujiki, 1989; Duchan, 1988; Silliman and Wilkinson, 1991). Lastly, the selection of assessment tools and procedures will influence the outcome of the evaluation. Any test will focus only on certain aspects of a child's language. Even a broad selection of tests cannot analyze all linguistic behavior. Assessment instruments cannot be adjusted to account for differences in social, cultural, emotional, cognitive, and academic forces affecting each child. Therefore, results of assessment must be viewed cautiously with an expectation for diagnostic refinement and modification over time.

Collaborative Evaluation Teams

IDEA specifies that a team of at least two or a group of persons, including at least one teacher or other specialist with knowledge of the suspected disability, evaluate each child. However, youngsters with speech or language impairment as the primary disability are not required to complete psychological, physical, or adaptive assessments. The qualified speech-language pathologist who administers the evaluation may be responsible for referrals for additional assessments that might be needed to make appropriate placement decisions. This mandate has been interpreted in individual states in varying ways. Some only require that the language evaluation be comprised of multiple assessment tools rather than a team of evaluators. Interpretation of evaluation data to determine service options for certain communication disorders also can be instituted without educational team collaboration.

Nevertheless, because language ability relies on particular physical settings as well as conversational partners, extensive evaluation results provided by several sources ensures more accurate information.

Classroom teachers contribute their observations of the child's use of language in academic and social domains. Parents provide insight on the youngster's language function in the home community. The school psychologist presents information on the child's ability to integrate linguistic and cognitive ability. Referrals to an educational evaluator, learning disabilities specialist, or reading specialist may also be indicated for those youngsters whose language difficulties are affecting academic areas. Observations of the child's interactions with peers can be included as well. By analyzing and comparing a child's understanding and use of language in a variety of contexts, more accurate decisions regarding educational placement options and services can be made. Furthermore, team collaboration informs more individuals on the linguistic abilities of the child as well as expected outcomes from specific interventions.

PURPOSES OF ASSESSMENT

The language assessment process assumes different purposes during various stages. Initially, tests are used to identify children with language difficulties. Further testing to determine the degree and types of language problems is then conducted. Based on this assessment, appropriate intervention strategies can be developed. Finally, the effects of intervention are monitored consistently.

The Screening Test

When determining whether or not a child has a language problem, a **screening test** is generally used. This instrument differentiates those youngsters with suspected problems from children who appear to be functioning normally. Often the individual administering the screening is not well known to the youngster.

Language screening tools tend to require children to respond in artificial circumstances. They might be required to point to pictures or shapes in an arbitrary manner or repeat unfamiliar sentences that aren't related to one another. Sometimes the child performs these tasks in unknown surroundings. These test conditions can affect linguistic production and can lead to inaccurate results (Duchan, 1988). Therefore, language screening tests generally do not require a long time (i.e., more than a few minutes) to administer. Still, they tend to cover only a few aspects of language. Screening tests only identify the possibility of a language problem and the need for further assessment. To determine effectively whether a youngster has a language problem requires more comprehensive information on the linguistic abilities of the child.

Comprehensive Language Assessment

Once the possibility of having a language problem has been identified, the examiner needs to determine whether the child has a language disorder and the characteristics of the child's linguistic ability. To determine whether a child has a language problem, information regarding the child's communicative abilities is compared to the abilities of normal children. Formal tests that have been standardized on a group of children are generally used as a comparison. If the performance on the test of the child who is being assessed deviates significantly from the average of the test scores of "normal" children, the youngster is diagnosed as having a language disorder.

Descriptive language tests designate linguistic components which are used to analyze a child's language. These tests may be standardized or informal assessment instruments. For example, one examiner may look at language comprehension and expression. Within the realm of comprehension, the child's ability to understand vocabulary, directions, concepts, paragraph narratives, questions, and abstract language might be evaluated. Language expression might be examined to determine the child's lexicon or breadth of vocabulary, grammar, narrative competence, pronunciation, as well as the ability to generate categories, opposites, and word definitions. Other diagnosticians may analyze the child's capacity to understand and use language structures (syntax, morphology, and phonology), language meaning (semantics), and language contexts (pragmatics). Still other testers might focus on the child's social interactive skills in various situations. The activities which stimulate the most complex language might be examined as well as the people and environments which promote linguistic competence.

Ongoing Assessment

Once the language assessment test has determined the presence of a language deficit and descriptive tests have specified the range and severity of the deficits, a determination regarding the need and type of intervention is made. Specific goals and objectives are formulated. As intervention procedures evolve, continued assessment is necessary to determine their effectiveness. **Ongoing assessment** monitors change in the child's language behaviors. Standardized tests may be used. Most frequently, informal protocols are administered. Language behaviors are examined in various contexts to determine whether the child has a complete understanding of when and how the behaviors are used. This generalization of a language behavior usually indicates successful learning. Ongoing assessment provides a rationale for modification and refinement of intervention strategies as well as a gauge of changes in the child's linguistic abilities.

TYPES OF ASSESSMENT MEASURES

A comprehensive language assessment usually combines standardized and informal test instruments. The Individuals with Disabilities Education Act specifies the use of evaluation materials which "have been validated for the specific purpose for which they are used" (Federal Register, September 29, 1992, p. 44822). In some states, "valid" has been interpreted to mean "standardized" and results from formal tests have been required to place youngsters in language intervention programs (Wilson, Blackmon, Hall, and Elcholtz, 1991). However, IDEA requires that a qualified speech-language pathologist evaluate "using procedures that are appropriate for the diagnosis and appraisal of speech and language impairments" and that "no single procedure is used as the sole criterion for determining an appropriate educational program for a child." Standardized tests are used to determine the degree of language strengths and weaknesses and to identify some language deficits of a child in comparison to a group of other children. However, an in-depth description of a child's language ability must also include informal assessment measures and direct observation (Lahey, 1988, 1990; Leonard, 1990).

Standardized Assessment Measures

Standardized tests are developed as one means of obtaining reliable and valid results. A test has **reliability** if various examiners obtain consistent results. To obtain reliability, conditions under which the original test is administered must be replicated. Test **validity** refers to the ability of the test to measure what it was intended to measure. One way researchers ensure test validity is to compare the assessment tool to other standardized tests purported to test the same set of skills. Language can be generated in infinite combinations. Any test will have a circumscribed set of tasks that it will assess. Therefore, validity for many tests is valuable only for the specific items provided in the actual test. Whether the child can apply the skills in other nontest language contexts is not determined. Consequently, judgments of validity sometimes require experienced evaluators.

For example, a test of language concepts does not include every concept in the language used in all multiple contexts. Any test selects a group of representative concepts and uses one manner of presentation such as pictures to demonstrate each concept. Each child has an individual framework of conceptual ability. Perhaps the items selected on the test are not those most familiar to the child. Furthermore, the child may understand the concept in certain circumstances but not in the picture format chosen by the test creator. Thus, the test may not be a valid instrument for this youngster. It does not accurately predict the child's nontest performance (Lund and Duchan, 1988; McCauley and Swisher, 1984a, 1984b).

As stated earlier, formal tests have been standardized based on the average of test results of a group of youngsters selected by the test creator. The typical behavior of these youngsters is the norm with which the child being assessed is compared. The youngsters comprising the norm sample may or may not have similar cultural, social, or linguistic parameters with the youngster completing the test. For example, members of different cultures or localities may call the shoes worn in cold or inclement weather *boots, overshoes,* or *galoshes.* A standardized test, which must be uniform and objective, cannot always accommodate response variations or a lack of response due to differences in English usage. Therefore, it is extremely important to determine which children comprise the group from which the norm was derived. If there are regional, cultural, or social differences, the test may not assess accurately the child being evaluated (McCauley and Swisher, 1984a). It may be necessary, then, to re-norm the standardized test with members of the same linguistic community as the child taking the test.

A further concern is the number of youngsters actually used as subjects when obtaining normative data for a test. Because tests often are designed to evaluate youngsters over a wide age range, norms within each chronological category must be derived. For example, a test may be designed for children from the ages of 5–12 years. Standardization requires a sample of youngsters whose average score has been computed for a specific developmental period. Some tests have been standardized using perhaps 50–100 children for each age designation. With the complexity and variability of language, examiners question whether just 50 other youngsters are a fair comparison with the child being assessed.

Standardized tests are helpful in determining some strengths and weaknesses in a child but are unable to develop a complete language profile. They do suggest language deficits which can then be explored in greater detail. For evaluators with limited experience, standardized tests provide objective criteria for comparing the language skills of a particular youngster to another group of children of comparable age or grade. Yet standardized tests cannot be used exclusively as descriptors of a child's language strengths and weaknesses.

Standardized Expectations in Comprehension Tasks

There are dozens of standardized tests on the market today. Many require the child to engage in one or a series of comparable tasks in order to complete the test. Leonard (1990) discusses some of the expected response modes used in standardized tests. When tests evaluate language comprehension, the child may be asked to "identify" or select a picture or object which best relates to something the examiner says. For example, a group of three pictures might be displayed. The child is requested to point to the picture that depicts a word or phrase (e.g., *Show me, "The girl is sitting"* or *"Point to the large red circle"*). A variation of this task is to actually manipulate objects and to put the doll into a sitting position at the request of the evaluator. Another type of comprehension task is to judge an utterance provided by the examiner by responding with yes or no (e.g., *a dog says meow*).

Standardized Expectations in Production Tasks

Traditionally, tests of language expression have required the youngster to repeat sentences. This **elicited imitation** task directs the child to repeat a sentence exactly the way the evaluator stated it. It is assumed that grammatical differences exhibited by the child reflect a lack of mastery of that feature (e.g., *The boy is sitting down*). When the youngster repeats this sentence by saying *The boy sit down*, the examiner assumes that the present progressive verb tense has not been mastered. This assumption has now been severely questioned and elicited imitation is no longer a recommended assessment task (Bloom, Hood, and Lightbown, 1974; Fujiki and Brinton, 1987; Prutting and Connolly, 1976).

Another task used in expressive language tests is **word definitions.** A stimulus word is provided and the child tries to explain what the word means. **Cloze tasks** are also frequently used. A sentence is stated by the examiner and a word or phrase is omitted. The child completes the sentence with the appropriate word (e.g., *Mary has a dress and Joan has a dress. They have two* _____). These completion tasks sometimes are accompanied by a picture. Expressive language is also evaluated by providing a stimulus word and requesting that the child generate a sentence using the word.

These tasks that are used repeatedly in standardized language tests explore very circumscribed aspects of children's language. They are of limited use in understanding children's natural language and the communication competencies needed in conversation, narration, and classroom discourse. In addition, skills needed by adolescents for communicative and educational success require more comprehensive procedures. Narrative organization and conversational skill as well as assessments based on the student's curriculum requirements can be analyzed to provide a more balanced assessment of adolescent language ability (Damico, 1993).

Informal Assessment Measures

In-depth examinations of the child's understanding and use of language can be obtained using informal assessment measures. Unlike standardized testing, the examiner organizes the informal test based on each child's individual needs. An examiner can begin by selecting the specific components of language to be described, the methods and materials to be used to analyze the child's language behaviors, and the interpretation of the information obtained. This is more conducive to accurate descriptions of the child's language abilities and to formulating individualized intervention strategies. In certain instances, parts of standardized tests are administered. The intent is to observe the child's language behaviors, the child's approach to the task, and how the child's language abilities change in different contexts.

Language Samples

One type of informal testing measure frequently used is the **language sample**. In its basic form, the examiner provides a comfortable communicative environment for the child and either conversational or narrative discourse is evaluated. Youngsters are encouraged to choose and talk about a topic of interest and the examiner facilitates the communication. The atmosphere should be relaxed and natural so that the linguistic output will be a true representation of the child's language ability. Language samples can be derived from various formats. Some are conversations, others are story or script narratives, and another is the classroom lesson (Lund and Duchan, 1988). These everyday types of communication allow examination of language use in naturalistic discourse.

Conversational Exchanges

A **conversation** involves two or more individuals and requires the participants to understand the needs of the listener. Explanations must be complete and focused so that the listener can identify the important objects, events, and people of the verbal exchange. Therefore, the speaker must know the extent of the listener's world knowledge. Once a topic is established, it is maintained and elaborated during conversation. The conversational partners are required to change or modify topics during a conversational exchange. For example, two students could be deciding what game to play at recess and one says, "Let's play John's game." This statement assumes the listener knows who John is as well as John's "game." If the listener's world knowledge does not include John or his game, this statement cannot be acknowledged. The listener must then inform the speaker that clarification of the remark is needed. Thus, a simple conversation involves the ability to initiate a topic that contains appropriate information for the listener, the ability to understand the needs of the conversational partner, and the ability to maintain, elaborate, and end the conversation.

Narrative Contexts

Narratives defined earlier such as stories or scripts are generally monologues told to one or more listeners. They are an organized sequence of ideas that describe an event or the outcome of an episode. Stories generally have a scene and characters that need to be described. **Scripts** are descriptions of common, everyday experiences. These routine events could be preparation for school or how to make a peanut butter sandwich. Ross and Berg (1990) have found that linguistic proficiency as well as individual experience and knowledge affect the quality of scripts youngsters generate.

Classroom Lessons

Classroom lessons differ from conversations and narratives because one individual, usually the teacher, controls what will be discussed and also evaluates the child's utterances. For example, if the child is asked a question, the response is judged for its correctness (e.g., *that's right*). If more than one student is involved, taking turns to speak and waiting to be recognized to speak comprise the communication format (Silliman and Wilkinson, 1991).

Variation and Length

Language samples obtained from each of these communication contexts provide varying perspectives on the child's ability to manipulate language for different purposes. Roth and Spekman (1984a, 1984b) emphasize the importance of variation in language tasks. They also suggest that the language samples involve different partners and settings because the quality of language output is determined by the context. However, the settings should be familiar to the child, such as lunchtime, recess, group projects, or classroom presentations, so that the sample obtained represents the child's actual communication abilities.

The language sample has no correct length in terms of time or number of utterances. However, 30 minutes has been suggested (Reed, 1986) or between 50–100 utterances generated by the child (Miller, 1991). The language sample can be recorded by audiotape or videotape. If audiotape is used, notations by the examiner as to the activities and contexts of the utterances are recommended.

Language Sample Analysis

When analyzing the child's language, examiners should consider the comments of the conversational partner, the context, and the nonverbal behaviors of the participants (Reed, 1986). Once the language sample is obtained, the examiner can use it to analyze various types of linguistic output. One area to examine might be language form such as grammar or sentence length. Another analysis might include the child's range of vocabulary. Pragmatic ability can also be evaluated using the language sample. For example, the examiner might analyze whether the child takes appropriate conversational turns or responds to questions. The approach in evaluating the language sample depends on the examiner's initial observations of the child's abilities.

The language sample became almost a standard component of a language evaluation in the 1970s when the importance of pragmatic elements of child language was recognized. No standardized tests examined pragmatic aspects of language at that time. Even today, standardized tests do not include all aspects of pragmatic skill and the language sample continues to partially close that gap. The significant drawback to its use in the educational setting is that proper administration and analysis are extremely time consuming, often beyond the assessment time allotments of the most generous school schedules.

Researchers (Brinton and Fujiki, 1989; Klee, 1992; Miller, 1991) have attempted to simplify and quantify the language sample so that inclusion in a school evaluation is feasible. Miller (1991) has found three significant identification measures of expressive language in differentiating specific language deficit from normal children:

1. the mean length of the child's utterances (MLU);

2. the total number of words the child generates during a fixed period of time (TNW);

3. the number of different words produced by the child during the specific timeframe (NDW).

Prutting and Kirchner (1987) have developed a pragmatic protocol to analyze language behaviors obtained during a 15-minute interaction. Thirty pragmatic features are analyzed and rated as either appropriate, inappropriate, or not observed. They include verbal production such as the child's ability to maintain the topic of conversation or the ability to take turns during a conversational exchange. They also review paralingual aspects of the language sample which include the fluency or flow of the child's utterances and whether the child speaks with the proper loudness for the conversational situation. Finally, nonverbal elements of the interaction are examined. These include the child's eye contact, use of gestures, body posture, and appropriate physical proximity to the conversational partner. This type of protocol lends itself to descriptive analysis but can't be quantified so that any particular characteristic exemplifies a particular age group or type of language disorder.

Direct Observation

Another important informal test procedure is direct observation of the child's language behaviors. These behaviors can be compared to those of similarly aged youngsters. Lahey (1988) states that information derived from observation depends on the abilities of the observer. Effective observation depends on the observer's understanding of the behavior under scrutiny and how that behavior relates to the purpose of the observation. If untrained observers such as parents and teachers are a part of the assessment, specific questions regarding language behavior should be provided so that relevant information about the child is obtained. This will provide the evaluator with information concerning what the child knows about language so that a determination regarding intervention can be made. Rather than requesting general reports from other professionals, particular information should be sought that enhances the evaluator's understanding of the child. For example, the teacher might be asked to describe the child's language output in small group projects and in classroom presentations.

Silliman and Wilkinson (1991) stress that assessment should relate directly to the requirements for interaction within the classroom. Observation by the speech-language pathologist of children in actual school contexts provides information on the causes of communication difficulties that create academic problems and affect motivation. Variations in teaching approaches and the communication styles of teachers affect learning. Classroom observation documents teacher-child interactions and which strategies promote communication. It also allows the examiner to assess the impact of the child's language deficits on written communication and other content areas. Furthermore, observation in natural contexts such as the classroom provides confirmation of results from standardized tests. For example, the child who was unable to demonstrate knowledge of basic concepts in the test format may be observed understanding these concepts in the natural context of the classroom. Varying contexts can reveal changes in the child's communicative competence.

Dollaghan and Miller (1986) examined the observational process and have attempted to provide a reliable and valid framework so that observation can be used for clinical and research purposes. They suggest that specific behaviors of the child be delineated before the observation, with a clear intent on how the information concerning these behaviors will be used. Thus, all observations should have objectives. By selecting defined behaviors for the observation, the observational process becomes a focused assessment with measurable results. This research begins to bridge the gap between standardized and informal assessment procedures.

THE EFFECTS OF ASSESSMENT TOOL SELECTION ON INTERVENTION

Assessment tools, whether they are standardized or informal, are selected to answer questions about the language function of a particular child. The instruments that are chosen determine strengths and weaknesses of the child as well as the direction of the intervention. Goals are generally based on the results of the assessment. Therefore, assessment must be focused on the most important needs of an individual child. For example, a specific child might be referred to a speech-language clinician in a school because he doesn't understand the teacher's directions and has difficulty expressing himself. The evaluator may administer a test of language comprehension and a vocabulary test. A language sample might be obtained as well.

Based on the results of the selected testing instruments, possible goals are determined. If the vocabulary test administered indicates deficient vocabulary, vocabulary enrichment may be recommended. If the child did not understand questions and complex sentences in the test of language comprehension, intervention is indicated to improve these aspects of language comprehension. The language sample may be analyzed for grammatical errors and inadequate sentence structure which are both judged to be areas needing remediation. If the child's pragmatic skills were evaluated, the results may have indicated that this area affected the child's classroom functioning more than vocabulary skill and question comprehension. Thus, whatever assessment information is gathered tends to form the basis and focus of intervention.

Language is extremely complex. Yet evaluators have time constraints which limit the evaluation process. No assessment can provide a complete profile of language ability. Therefore, before any evaluation begins, the clinician should have definitive and appropriate areas to explore. Otherwise, intervention strategies, if warranted, may not include those goals which provide the child with the most expedient means for language and communication development, and for improved academic performance and social functioning.

TEACHER GUIDELINES FOR REFERRALS

Classroom teachers and other individuals who know a particular child well are often the most accurate referral sources for language assessments (Snyder and Godley, 1992). They observe youngsters engaged in a variety of language contexts such as class presentations and peer conversations. Teachers are also familiar with the range of behaviors exhibited by groups of children of a specific age. Finally, teachers have linguistic expectations for academic achievement. Classroom material is taught using language in both oral and written form.

Teachers who have been provided with specific referral guidelines often can identify children with language deficits accurately. Damico and Oller (1980) provided two groups of teachers with inservice training for language referrals of youngsters in their classes. One group of teachers was taught to observe only surface characteristics of language such as verb tenses, noun-verb agreement, irregular plurals, and pronoun case or gender. This corresponds to the focus of some standardized language assessment measures. The other group was trained to observe pragmatic aspects of language as criteria for referral. Each group of teachers referred a number of youngsters for evaluation, but those teachers examining pragmatic criteria referred approximately 50% more children. After in-depth assessments, it was found that the pragmatic protocol more accurately identified children with language difficulties. Those teachers observing surface criteria overlooked youngsters who, in fact, should have been identified. Seven pragmatic behaviors were introduced to the classroom teachers as the basis for referral criteria:

1. ***Nonspecific vocabulary.*** This refers to generic words such as *thing* or *those* when a more specific word is preferable. The listener is placed in the situation of not knowing exactly what the speaker is referring to. Nonspecific vocabulary also refers to the use of pronouns, proper nouns, and other words that are not explained or elaborated so that the listener has no reference and must ask the speaker for clarification.

2. ***Need for repetition.*** The child does not respond in conversational contexts when a response is expected. Additional information or message repetition is necessary for the child to take a conversational turn.

3. ***Poor topic maintenance.*** During conversational exchanges, the child changes the topic without explanation. The listener is under the impression that the remarks of the child don't correspond with the topic under discussion.

4. ***Inappropriate responses.*** The child does not respond during conversations in predictable ways. Answers to questions are not topic-related, as if the child has been inattentive to the conversation or misunderstands.

5. ***Linguistic nonfluency.*** This is not to be confused with true stuttering although words, sounds, and phrases are repeated. The child may also use filler words such as *um* or *ah*, have pauses, and generate jerky spurts of words as well.

6. ***Revisions.*** The child seems to have difficulty getting an utterance started and developing it. Like a car that keeps

stalling out, the child says a few words, stalls, sometimes can keep moving for another couple of words and sometimes completely stalls and starts from the beginning. Oftentimes roadblocks cause the youngster to start again using a different set of words.

7. *Delays before responding.* The child disrupts the conversation by pausing so long before responding that the conversational partner can assume that the child has become disengaged from the conversation. At times, the child might respond appropriately just when the partner has determined that the interaction is terminated.

These guidelines have been elaborated and used in research with bilingual and adolescent children in determining language difficulty (Damico, Oller, and Storey, 1983; Damico, 1993). Complete criteria descriptions have also been outlined for in-depth functional language assessment (Damico, 1991). Dollaghan and Campbell (1992) acknowledge that pragmatic criteria such as those outlined above constitute disruptions in conversation which interfere with communicative proficiency. However, they find little research supporting spontaneous language disruptions as confirmed indicators of language difficulties. They look to the impact on the listener and suggest using a child's social community to validate communicative performance (Campbell and Dollaghan, 1992). Teachers, peers, and family members are important sources for confirmation of a child's communicative success in real contexts as well as for changes during intervention.

SUMMARY

The complexity and variability of language resist assessment. Its interrelationship with social, academic, emotional, cultural, cognitive, and physiological forces make assessment time-consuming. The individual framework from which each child's language was developed defies standardized tests which look at normal and average skill.

Over the last few decades, language assessment has shifted from a medical model, which sought etiologies for a child's language difficulty and outlined the youngster's underlying deficits, to a descriptive model which tended to fragment language and subdivide it into separate components to be analyzed. Both standardized and informal assessment instruments were used to examine discreet skills and behaviors. More recently, child language has been regarded as a total system. Children are assessed in natural contexts using real activities to determine communicative competence. Each assessment model has advantages and disadvantages. Whereas formal tests can quantify results, their scope of language is limited. Natural context or pragmatic assessment depends on the expertise of the examiner.

Natural variability in language behavior among children challenges even experienced evaluators. Researchers continue to debate the stages of normal development and ranges of severity in language disorder. Children mature at variable rates and show strengths and weaknesses in differing linguistic areas. These factors challenge effective assessment.

Testing protocols can be used to screen youngsters to determine who has a suspected language problem. Once further assessment is determined, both standardized and informal instruments are used in the process to identify and describe the characteristics of the language difficulty. Judicious selection of assessment tools is imperative so that the results can be translated into effective intervention strategies, if warranted.

Classroom teachers and other individuals familiar with a particular youngster are important contributors to the assessment process. They are often the first to recognize the effect of language disorder on the child's ability to complete classroom activities. Specific observational guidelines for referral to professional language evaluators can be an efficient means for helping to identify youngsters with language impairments. Collaboration and respect for the differences and needs of each child help to accurately focus language assessment.

SUGGESTED READINGS

Damico, J. (1991). Clinical Discourse Analysis: A Functional Approach to Language Assessment. In C. Simon (Ed.), *Communication Skills and Classroom Success: Assessment and Therapy Methodologies for Language and Learning Disabled Students* (pp. 125–150). Eau Claire, WI: Thinking Publications.

Dollaghan, C., and Miller, J. (1986). Observational Methods in the Study of Communicative Competence. In R. Schiefelbusch, (Ed.), *Language Competence: Assessment and Intervention* (pp. 99–130). San Diego, CA: College-Hill Press.

Duchan, J. (1988). Assessment Principles and Procedures. In N. Lass, L. McReynolds, J. Northern, and D. Yoder (Eds.), *Handbook of Speech-Language Pathology and Audiology* (pp. 356–376). Philadelphia, PA: B.C. Decker.

Lund, N., and Duchan, J. (1988). *Assessing Children's Language in Naturalistic Contexts* (2nd ed.). Englewood Cliffs, NJ: Prentice-Hall.

Silliman, E., and Wilkinson, L. (1991). *Communicating for Learning: Classroom Observation and Collaboration.* Gaithersburg, MD: Aspen.

7 SPECIFIC LANGUAGE DEFICIT

Language proficiency is reflected in each child's success in academic activities, peer acceptance, and basic interaction and communication skills. In learning about normal language development, the complex and multidimensional nature of language becomes evident. Language can include understanding, production, and appropriate use. Narrative skill, classroom discourse, metalinguistic knowledge, and literate language use also reflect language proficiency.

Furthermore, selective aspects of language skill are always in a state of flux. For example, a child may develop adeptness in following directions at a particular stage of development but make no progress in combining a series of related ideas to form narrative discourse. Therefore, when studying children's language proficiency, there are aspects of the total language system that can fall at various points on the "normal" to "disordered" continuum. Children can display an uneven pattern of abilities.

When making a determination of language disorder, the American Speech-Language-Hearing Association (ASHA Reports, 1989) reports that some education agencies make comparisons to youngsters who are the same age or to children who have an equivalent mental age. However, using chronological age or mental age criteria exclusively to document a language deficit clashes with the complex issues of language and cognition as well as consensus concerning the range of deviation that defines language disorder. It is recognized that there are youngsters who demonstrate language disability which is secondary to more pervasive disorders. These disorders include hearing loss, mental retardation, autism, emotional disability, learning disability, vision loss, and physical disability. However, when evaluations separate these youngsters from the general population, there remains a group of children exhibiting language difficulties with no known etiology. Their disability has been given terms such as *clinical language disorder* (Carrow-Woolfolk and Lynch, 1982), *specific language disorder* (Johnston, 1988); *developmental language disorder* (Prather, 1984; Snyder, 1984), *specific language impairment* (Dale and Cole, 1991; Leonard, 1991) and *specific language deficit* (Stark and Tallal, 1981). Each label denotes different semantic interpretations. The word *deficit* implies a shortage or lack of language. Yet it does not imply physical irregularities as *disorder* or *impairment* could.

The purpose of Chapter 7 is as follows:

1. define specific language deficit;

2. present theories which suggest possible causes of specific language deficits;

3. clearly differentiate language disorders and language delays;

4. describe typical behaviors associated with language disorders as they impact on the child's linguistic, academic, social, and emotional development; and

5. suggest general underlying principles for consideration in providing proper educational intervention.

WHAT IS SPECIFIC LANGUAGE DEFICIT?

The vast majority of children with language difficulties that are not associated with sensory disorders such as hearing loss, or other serious developmental and neurological disorders, usually are described as exhibiting a **specific language deficit**. It is a primary language disorder that is not secondary to some other condition and is determined through the process of elimination (Craig, 1993). Children with a lack of opportunity to learn language are excluded from the group. With intensive and appropriate intervention, these children could develop adequate language skills. The capacity to learn efficiently is present but the exposure to language has been denied.

No standardized criteria have been developed to define youngsters with specific language deficits. Studies of these children describe a variety of language and learning characteristics. Aram, Morris, and Hall (1993) state that typical definitions of specific language deficit employ either discrepancy and/or exclusionary criteria. A discrepancy definition identifies a disparity between cognition and language ability. That is, the child's "normal" cognitive skills cannot explain the impaired language. Exclusionary criteria differentiate children with language deficits from youngsters with known handicapping conditions (e.g., mental retardation or autism).

State education agencies have developed separate definitions of specific language deficit by comparing language performance with grade level, chronological age, mental age expectations, or standardized nonverbal intelligence tests (Nye and Montgomery, 1989). The combinations of formal and informal assessment measures that are used also vary among states, schools, and individual evaluators. These factors, in combination with the multiple aspects of language which can be impaired, have created barriers to identification criteria for specific language deficit.

The issue of standardized criteria for defining and identifying the disorder known as *specific language deficit* has also created controversy in separating it from language disorders associated with specific learning disabilities (see Chapter 8). That is, learning disabilities usually affect the child's ability to read, write, listen, and express language effectively. Language also impacts on these skills. In fact, a majority of youngsters who have language deficits as toddlers and preschoolers are diagnosed as having language-based learning disabilities during their school years (Simon, 1991; Wallach and Miller, 1988).

Generally, youngsters with specific language deficits reach physical milestones within normal limits and they can complete nonverbal tasks age-appropriately. The parents and pediatricians caring for these children initially tend to reassure themselves that although the youngsters show delay in verbal ability, they demonstrate normal development in other areas.

Young children with specific language deficits seem to say words but their utterances are "vague" and "difficult to follow." Still others don't seem to understand directions, forget family routines from one day to the next, or appear not to "listen." The parents of these youngsters sometimes question their child's ability to hear. Sometimes a young child with a specific language deficit will be described as "just lazy" or "pampered, with no incentive to learn to talk."

Leonard (1991) characterizes many children in this diverse group as falling within the low end of a random distribution of normal youngsters. Rather than regarding them as disordered, he describes them as limited in language ability. He compares the children with other youngsters who may have little musical ability or who lack physical coordination. Leonard's point of view has been challenged by a number of researchers who suggest that by placing youngsters with specific language deficit in the normal development arena, no explanation can be provided to parents and professionals as to the cause of the child's difficulty. Frequently, it is helpful to know why a child is having particular problems. Parents can be frustrated with the commonly provided interpretation that children have varying aptitudes for the wide range of skills needed by human beings. They are told that, unfortunately, language skill, which is critically important in our society for school and social success, happens to be impaired.

Such a view also stymies research efforts (Johnston, 1991). If the language deficit is considered to be in the normal range, it is difficult to engage in scientific inquiry which would need to differentiate deficient language behaviors from normal ones (Tomblin, 1991). In fact, Dale and Cole (1991) have demonstrated that morphology is the component of language most tied to general language learning ability. Yet, their initial research was unable to show that this aspect of language can separate disordered language from predictable language development variability.

Aram (1991) suggests that specific language deficit is an umbrella characterization for several subtypes of developmental language disorders. She states that there are language strengths and weaknesses in separate components of language among children with this diagnosis which may result from variable causal factors. Thus, some aspects of language ability may be related to causes that are unrelated to other language skills. Specific language deficit takes many forms and to attempt to attribute all of them to one cause may be erroneous.

POSSIBLE CAUSES

Although minimal brain dysfunction was an early theory to account for specific language deficit (Barry, 1961), researchers have been unable to document this belief with consistent positive findings. In the 1940s and 1950s, children with poor language skills were compared to adult stroke victims and the term *aphasia* was used (Barry and McGinnis, 1988; Eisenson, 1972). However, unlike the adult counterparts, most of the youngsters have no known indications of brain dysfunction. Neurologists usually do not detect positive signs such as abnormal reflexes and irregular brain waves. Thus, children with specific language deficit show a discrepancy between expected and actual achievement in language skill. Yet there is usually no substantiated physical, organic, or environmental explanation for the language problem. Some authorities continue to presume that very subtle central nervous system irregularities do exist that cannot be detected with traditional technology. Aram (1991) projects that with sophisticated nuclear neuro-imaging techniques such as MRI (Magnetic Resonance Imaging), these subtle irregularities in brain activity will be substantiated.

Curtiss and Tallal (1991) propose the notion that specific language deficit is a processing impairment. They state that processing deficits cause youngsters to struggle with language comprehension and production. Carrow-Woolfolk and Lynch (1982) have outlined research that suggests three auditory processing areas that may affect specific language disability. They propose that language impairment may be the result of deficits in one or more of these three areas.

Auditory Processing Deficit

Children with specific language deficit are believed to exhibit difficulty processing incoming auditory messages. One example can be seen in children who confuse sounds or syllables in words. Expressively, they might say *efelant* for *elephant*. These mistakes are known as errors in **temporal ordering**. Sound confusion can be exacerbated by a rapid rate of presentation. If sounds are heard at a slower pace, many children with language deficits are better able to discriminate and process them.

Auditory processing difficulties that involve background noise also have been shown to interfere with the ability to perceive sounds by children with language difficulty. This means that when the speech message is competing with other sounds at the same level of loudness, the children with specific language deficit frequently cannot extract auditorially the important speech message and are described as "only hearing what they want to hear" or "just not paying attention." Researchers call this deficient **auditory figure-ground discrimination**.

Additionally, difficulty in auditory memory has been indicated as being related to specific language deficit. Short-term memory difficulties have been documented, especially if the material has little meaning to the youngster, as in the task of repeating a group of arbitrary numbers in a test situation. Some children have even struggled to repeat sentences that they had generated themselves at an earlier time.

The correlation between auditory processing deficits and specific language deficit can be readily observed in many children. Further research is needed to study what casual relationships between the two might exist.

Symbolic Deficit

Children with specific language deficit are known to engage less in symbolic play. (Symbolic play is discussed in detail within Chapter 3.) Whereas other youngsters are reenacting common routines of their daily life, the child with language problems can be seen pushing or arranging toys without any sense of make-believe. Children with language difficulty are less likely to pretend one object represents another such as a pot placed upside down on the child's head designating a hat. Deficiency in visual imagery and conceptual development has been associated with delayed symbolic play. As these youngsters undergo assessment for intelligence, the *verbal* portions of the tests reveal significant deficits.

Children with language disorder who score somewhat lower than expected on *nonverbal* portions of intelligence tests are suspected of deficits in representational or symbolic ability. This too has been associated with visual imagery difficulty and concept development.

Stark and Tallal (1981) found that some children who had been identified by speech-language clinicians as exhibiting specific language deficits, but were in the normal range of intelligence, scored unusually low on the nonverbal or performance portions of IQ tests as well as the verbal subtests. At first, the researchers concluded that the verbal directions of the tests might have accounted for the low scores. Nonverbal intelligence tests were administered to some of the youngsters. Even using these instruments, the children scored in the retarded range.

Many education departments require a 15 point discrepancy between the verbal and performance abilities of the youngster on an intelligence test to determine the presence of a specific language deficit. Children with problems in visual imagery may score poorly on both sections of IQ tests and be inaccurately labeled as mentally retarded. Because cognition and language are so interrelated, the subtests of language and intelligence measures are often evaluating the same behaviors (ASHA, 1989).

Attentional Difficulties

Attention is critical for language development. A child must notice and observe when and how to use language in specific situations, what words signify specific events and objects, and the correlation between spoken and written texts (Carrow-Woolfolk and Lynch, 1982). The interrelationship between language deficits and attentional problems should not be confused with ADHD (attention deficit hyperactivity disorder) which is discussed in Chapter 9. Any individual who listens to incomprehensible sounds and words (e.g., a radio program in an unknown foreign language) or who reads a difficult written text (e.g., a book which describes a highly technical operation which is unfamiliar to the reader) will not sustain attention. Poor comprehension of a linguistic context causes the individual to switch to another activity or daydream about other matters.

Children who have limited understanding of their environment due to specific language deficits may also display attentional problems. Some children are impulsive, some lack proper inhibition, some are easily frustrated, and others are extremely active and fidgety. Although attentional deficit is associated with language difficulties, the impulsive and overactive child with language impairment is usually calm and focused for certain tasks that the child understands and enjoys. Therefore, these youngsters are described as having problems in **selective attention**. The interplay between attentional difficulties and language ability reduces the child's potential for interpersonal relationships and all learning.

Genetic Factors

Some studies have looked to genetic factors to explain specific language deficit (Aram, 1991; Pembrey, 1992; Tomblin, 1989). Tallal, Ross, and Curtiss (1989) discuss several studies of families of children with specific language deficit. Data indicate that statistically significant numbers of the parents and siblings of these youngsters exhibit language difficulty. The results of the study are presumed to be an underestimate of familial language difficulty because many siblings were still too young to demonstrate symptoms. Tallal et al. (1989) found that when both parents reported a history of specific language deficit, 52.6% of the siblings of the children with language difficulty also were affected.

Tomblin (1989) also studied the families of youngsters with specific language deficit. He concluded that some of the factors that produce language difficulties are associated with the family. In that study, 53% of the children with language deficits had one or more affected family members. The question of genetic transmission of language disability still remains. Perhaps variation in child-rearing practices which could influence language development has affected the results. Thus, the possibility exists that environmental factors can skew the results of these genetic studies.

When examining the research on possible causes of specific language deficits, many theories emerge. A relationship to brain function can be found in the most well-known explanations. Yet language deficit cannot be attributed conclusively to cerebral irregularities, because in many instances no positive clinical evidence has been uncovered. Perhaps there are several causes for this complex and multifaceted disorder which can occur in isolation or in combination with one another. Lahey (1990) states that inferences about the nature of the underlying system of language disorder are less important than understanding the differences in language behaviors.

LANGUAGE DISORDER VERSUS LANGUAGE DELAY

Children learn various aspects of language at different rates and in a variety of ways due to the complex nature of language itself and the diverse environmental and cultural influences affecting language. In the past, a specific language deficit has been called a *language disorder, language delay,* or, by some, a *language deviancy* or a *language-learning disability* (Craig, 1993). In differentiating language disorder from language delay, Reed (1986) explains delay as slower than normal acquisition of all aspects of language.

This contrasts with children having language disorders who exhibit uneven progress in attaining various aspects of language. Language delay can be viewed as a condition that is correctable with intensive, appropriate intervention. There are no interfering variables, whether organic or environmental, that will impede language improvement with proper therapy. Young children are often given the label *language delay* when language development is not progressing as expected and when no known etiology or causal factors are evident. In some instances, as the child matures, that label may be removed or changed depending upon the acquisition of more accurate information about the child.

Researchers have been concerned about whether a child with language difficulties is exhibiting a delay in the development of language or whether there is some fundamental deviation both in the manner of language acquisition and the content of the language acquired. The language of every child can be observed to determine how it is being learned and whether the language-learning style differs from the way most children acquire language.

Additionally, the language forms and meanings that the child is developing may be deviant as well as the way the child is using language in communicative situations.

The way children with language problems acquire the structural components of language has been studied in great detail since the 1960s (Johnston, 1988). The overall sequence of development of language structures (phonology, morphology, and syntax) generally is similar for all children, but the rate of development is much slower. Lee's (1974) study of children with language disorders found them to have particular difficulty with the copula verb *to be*. She also found that children with language difficulties used simpler grammatic rules.

Damico (1991) examined pragmatic issues and found his subjects with language disorders to be less fluent, to fail to provide significant information to the listener, to respond inappropriately to questions, to need statements regularly repeated to comprehend them, and to have difficulty staying on the topic when carrying on a conversation. Carrow-Woolfolk and Lynch (1982) have characterized youngsters with language disorders as exhibiting different structural or semantic language. Their language may appear to resemble that of younger children, but on closer analysis, it is atypical.

Whereas most children learn to speak without intervention, the child with a language disorder needs intensive special instruction. Curtiss and Tallal (1991) attribute the need for intensive instruction to deficits in specific aspects of information processing, cognition, and memory, which produce adverse consequences to language learning.

A young child who has experienced a serious illness requiring hospitalization may have setbacks in some areas of language development. Once the illness is treated and proper language intervention is provided, the child should demonstrate more normal language proficiency. This example of language delay assumes that the child's innate abilities to learn are adequate, that appropriate language stimulation is provided upon recovery from the illness, and that the illness has not produced a severe emotional overlay which could interfere with learning. It also presupposes that the duration of the illness was short enough to permit realistic and adequate language improvement.

This situation can be contrasted with language disorder, which seems to defy the notion of "catching up." Wallach and Liebergott (1984) suggest that young children with language disorders experience some sort of language difficulty throughout life. During the school years, reading and other academic problems can arise. As adolescents, social and pragmatic growth may be affected. Thus, there is a change over time of the symptoms of language disorder but it generally does not totally disappear, even with appropriate intervention.

BEHAVIORS ASSOCIATED WITH SPECIFIC LANGUAGE DEFICIT

Because language difficulties can be mild or severe, can affect language comprehension and production, can involve language structure, meaning, or use, and can fluctuate and change over time and in varying environments, the behaviors associated with the disorder also vary. No child exhibits all characteristics associated with language disorder. Each child's unique language capabilities and culture will determine which of the concomitant behaviors will appear. Characteristics associated with specific language deficit can be separated into linguistic, academic, emotional, and social attributes. These divisions sometimes blur because of the underlying interconnections between language, learning, and social development. Table 7.1 outlines problem behaviors exhibited by youngsters with specific language deficit.

Table 7.1

Problems Related to Specific Language Deficit

LINGUISTIC PROBLEMS
Difficulty with Understanding and/or Expression

LANGUAGE STRUCTURE:

- Omissions and distortions of speech sounds
- Omissions of parts of words
- Sounds or syllables of words out of sequence
- Omissions of morphological endings of words
- Immature syntax
- Limited ability with complex sentences
- Undeveloped age-appropriate grammar
- Unintelligibility: can't be understood

LANGUAGE MEANING:

- Difficulty with directions
- Confusion with concepts and ideas
- Difficulty with questions
- Paucity of vocabulary
- Literal interpretation of words and concepts
- Difficulty with figurative language, humor, slang, and double meanings of words
- Poor word classification and association skill

LANGUAGE USE:

- Difficulty initiating, maintaining, and terminating conversational exchanges
- Immature turn-taking strategies
- Inadequate code-switching—change of language to suit specific person or situation
- Pauses, word fillers, word repetitions, and circumlocutions
- Difficulty assuming listener's point of view

Continued

Table 7.1–*Continued*

METALINGUISTICS:

- Difficulty expressing ideas about language
- Poor syllabication skills
- Poor phonics skills
- Poor rhyming skills

SOCIAL PROBLEMS:
Difficulty Interacting Appropriately

CONVERSATIONAL DEFICITS:

- Poor eye contact
- Inappropriate comments and responses to questions
- Excessive pauses before responding
- Inappropriate voice quality: intonation
- Poor social language (e.g., please, thank you)
- Insufficient information for listener
- Redundancy

SOCIAL-INTERACTION ISSUES:

- Poor sense of fair play (e.g., sharing, win/lose rules)
- Inadequate setting of limits or boundaries
- Inconsistent responses and actions in social encounters
- Difficulty with new situations
- Inappropriate clinging, touching, and kissing
- Excessive demands for attention
- Inappropriate laughing and crying
- Difficulty expressing wants, needs, and ideas
- Inappropriate clowning

Continued

Table 7.1–*Continued*

EMOTIONAL PROBLEMS
Difficulty Monitoring Behavior

PERSONAL ISSUES:

- Egocentric
- Poor self-concept
- Limited repertoire of emotions
- Rigidity of routine
- Low frustration level
- Need for immediate gratification
- Impulsive
- Perseverative and repetitious
- Poor differentiation of fantasy and reality

EMOTIONAL-INTERACTION ISSUES:

- Inability to accept responsibility
- Dependency (i.e., on parent, teacher)
- Gullible; easily led
- Sensitive to criticism
- Withdrawn or acting out
- Poor coping strategies
- Unpredictable

CLASSROOM ISSUES:

- Poor retention of material; need for constant repetition
- Problems in organization and planning
- Difficulty problem solving
- Left/Right confusion
- Symbol reversals: numbers and letters
- Difficulty expressing known information
- Poor generalization of information to novel situations
- Difficulty with inferences and deductions

Continued

Table 7.1–*Continued*

- Poor judgment and understanding of cause and effect
- Inability to self-monitor and self-correct
- Poor integration of information
- Poor short- and/or long-term memory

METACOGNITION:

- Inability to verbalize about academic tasks
- Inability to self-regulate behaviors

ACADEMIC PROBLEMS

Difficulty Learning and/or Retaining Information

SENSORY DEFICITS:

- Hyper- or hypo-sensitivity to smell, touch, or taste
- Immature body image
- Underdeveloped sense of one's position in space
- Distractions by visual and auditory stimuli
- Over- or under-reactions to sight and sound
- Attentional deficits
- Auditory and visual perception, discrimination, and memory deficits, including figure-ground and sequence problems

ASSOCIATED PHYSIOLOGICAL ISSUES:

- Awkward gait
- Excessive eye blinking
- Hyper- or hypo-activity
- Poor motor coordination: fine and gross
- Allergies and asthma
- Poor posture
- Restlessness
- Slow processing and response time

Linguistic Problems

When linguistic problems are translated into children's behaviors, we observe youngsters who are difficult to understand. Often the individual words are intelligible, but ideas are vague, disconnected, and not quite related to the topic at hand. Some children use simple sentences and imprecise vocabulary. They lack understanding of the multiple meanings of words. Concepts are only understood in their most literal sense. For example, the exclamation, *I can't stand to wash the dishes,* could be interpreted by the child with language difficulties as meaning that the person can only wash dishes sitting down. Youngsters tend to lose the humorous meaning of language and fail to understand jokes, puns, and gags. Current slang expressions are either overused or confused. Evidence of difficulty in language meaning can be seen when the child is groping for words to express an idea. Often the child has the conceptual notion but does not express it linguistically. Directions may be difficult for the youngster to follow. Frequently, directions have to be presented individually for comprehension. Forming and comprehending questions may also be difficult for these children. Sometimes there are long pauses before the child responds to a question, or the child may generate an inappropriate question or response to a question.

Linguistic problems are most noticeable in pragmatic contexts. During conversational exchanges, the child may not provide enough basic information to the listener, causing ideas to become confused. Children with language deficits may have poor turn-taking strategies. They might interrupt or fail to respond during conversational exchanges. Topic maintenance may be difficult. Sometimes they may stand too close to the listener or use voice volume and pitch inappropriately. These children need to be reminded to use their "inside voice" or to "give others a chance to speak." Children with language problems have been called *socially tone deaf.* Body language may be poorly understood. For example, if a person was standing with hands on the hips, knit eyebrows, and pursed lips, the child with a language deficit may start to laugh because the posture is misinterpreted. Sarcasm and subtle nuances often pass by the child with language deficits.

Language structure difficulties are also observed in these children. When speech sounds are distorted or words are omitted or misused, the listener has concrete evidence of linguistic problems. As children with language deficit begin to become consciously aware of language and how it is formed and used, they may have difficulty in analyzing its components. The child may not make associations between sounds and letters, identify rhyming words, or judge whether a series of sounds constitutes a word. Difficulty understanding and expressing language structure, meaning, and use, as well as being able to verbalize information about language has an impact on academic achievement.

Academic Problems

The child with specific language deficit also exhibits some learning difficulties. Table 7.1 summarizes typical academic problems manifested in the child with a language deficit. Information is poorly perceived, organized, and retained. Even when it is learned, the child does not always express known knowledge. A poor knowledge base causes a low level of interest in new information. Children are most interested in knowledge that relates to ideas that are already integrated into their knowledge repertoire. With a general paucity of information comes poor retention and the need for constant reinforcement. For example, when a student is trying to learn a new child's name, it may be easier if the name is the same as a sister's name. There is a familiar association between the old information (i.e., the sister's name) and the name of the new child. As discussed earlier, attentional and perceptual difficulties are believed to be related to these information processing problems.

Concepts may be particularly confusing to these children. Notions of time, space, quantity, and emotion must be presented with concrete examples. Yet the child with language deficits does not typically generalize examples of a concept to new situations. This results in rote understanding and poor integration of isolated bits of information. Ineffective use of known knowledge makes it difficult for the child to make decisions, predict outcomes, and understand cause and effect relationships. Disconnected information is more difficult to remember. Consequently, academic tasks become overwhelming and result in the child becoming distracted and working slowly. These youngsters may have difficulty pacing themselves as they complete their tasks. Often they shift from one activity to another or become confused with the various words, pictures, or examples on a single work page. Strategies to help the children regulate their activities independently are not self-generated and must be taught. For instance, the child may not consciously realize that the directions to an assignment must be read and understood before approaching the actual examples.

Social Problems

From a general lack of understanding about the world, social problems emerge and intensify. Very young children with language deficits do not automatically integrate knowledge about human interaction. Whereas most children learn to tap an individual to attract attention, the youngster with a language deficit might bite or shriek to obtain the same goal. These undesirable behaviors might generate a desired response but the child has not learned intuitively by observing and internalizing what other individuals do to attract attention. Therefore, interactional skills are extremely inconsistent and often inappropriate. Children are seen laughing during serious occasions and getting angry when there seems to be no cause.

As the child matures, assuming the role of the listener may become difficult. Sometimes adequate information is lacking for comprehension of verbal statements. Other times the child becomes redundant, repeating information that has already been given.

Appropriate use of social communication is difficult for the child with a language deficit. A child might say "excuse me" when a gift is presented rather than "thank you." Often the child omits these social words. Difficulty verbalizing pleasure in a social interaction may cause the child to act overly friendly to an unknown authority figure. Excessive clinging, touching, and kissing have been reported by teachers.

Youngsters with language problems often experience frustration playing games. The rules might be poorly understood so that winning and losing are not anticipated. The child who does not win is disappointed. Sharing toys and personal belongings may also be difficult. The child sometimes assumes that by playing with another person's toy, it becomes one's own. Because expression of feelings and needs is generally difficult, group situations are problematic. The child then looks for ways to camouflage language misunderstandings. Many of these youngsters become the class clown. This role permits the use of gestures which are easier to produce than words. The child assumes that being the clown satisfies the strong desire to be included in the group.

Emotional Problems

The inability to understand one's environment and express one's needs and ideas leads to emotional issues for many children with language deficits. Academic and social failure leads to poor self-concept. Once youngsters believe that they are less worthy, they have difficulty accepting responsibility and making independent decisions. Typically, the child becomes very dependent upon parents and teachers. This is viewed as immaturity. The child can be very sensitive to criticism and generally exhibits a low frustration level. Coping strategies are typically poor and behavior can be extremely unpredictable. The child may have periods of positive performance and, for no apparent reason, periods of regression.

Poor language comprehension creates an image of naivety for children with language deficits. They are described as gullible and easily deceived. Often they are the brunt of gags and tricks at school. Children erroneously believe that the peer group is including them rather than setting them up for trouble or ridicule. They tend to be egocentric and oriented to the immediate present. This results in momentary gratification without being able to project the consequences for their behavior. As the child enters adolescence, many of these behaviors become less apparent. Yet difficulty in school, feelings of self-doubt, and inadequate interpersonal skills often persist.

In conclusion, although no one child exhibits all of the problems related to specific language deficit at any one time, the difficulties described and outlined in Table 7.1 frequently are observed in these youngsters. Each child will change over time, encounter new environments, and exhibit varying behaviors.

Many children will be labeled learning disabled as they enter school and their language difficulties impact on academics. (Chapter 8 discusses learning disabilities in detail.) Snyder (1984) reports that in those states that have no designation of "language disorder" as a legal handicapping condition, the prevalence of language disorders in school-age children declines substantially and the incidence of "learning disability" increases proportionately. In states like Colorado, where the term *perceptual and communicative disorder* is used, the incidence of language disorder remains constant across the school years. Indeed, many of these children will be labeled learning disabled and language disordered and will receive the services of a learning disabilities teacher and a speech-language pathologist. The child described in this chapter may be one and the same as the child described as having a learning disability in Chapter 8.

EDUCATIONAL ISSUES

The complexity and variability of language problems precludes utilization of one approach or method in dealing with children diagnosed with a specific language deficit. Each child must be carefully observed and evaluated in diverse environments and situations. Varying materials, techniques, and groupings should be considered. However, several general underlying principles are important. Because children's language behavior can be affected by different people and settings, interdisciplinary decision-making is imperative. Any school personnel who interact with the youngster should be apprised of the child's behaviors. Many adults confuse "naughty" actions with inappropriate responses due to confusion or lack of understanding of the circumstances by the child. Shrieking, hitting, and tantrums can be a child's attempt to communicate rather than intentional belligerent behavior. Teaching strategies need to be coordinated so that concepts can be generalized to novel situations. Parents are a source of important information, feedback, and reinforcement. They need to be informed and updated continually. A language deficit is not just the child's problem. Families need training as well so that improvement can progress expediently.

Children with language deficits learn language and world knowledge best when their lessons are related to functional situations (Duchan and Weitzner-Lin, 1987; Shafer, Staab, and Smith, 1983). Experiences that are meaningful to the particular child, with much language interaction and feedback, provide the most positive environment for language learning. For example, if the child is expected to learn about food groups, sorting, tasting, and preparing specific foods provides real opportunity to explore the topic. Selecting an apple for the "fruit" category, talking about it, and distinguishing it from other fruits can confirm the child's hypotheses about fruits. Furthermore, the language associated with the lesson provides immediate feedback to the child regarding the communication of the messages pertaining to the topic.

Particular subjects are internalized more readily when they are related to and integrated with other subject areas. Information can be generalized in new situations which refines and broadens conceptual knowledge. That is, a discussion of food groups can expand to include writing and spelling assignments such as creating a shopping list. It can also incorporate math knowledge. A child can scan supermarket advertisements and compare the price of apples at different food outlets. These activities are experience-based and real. They discourage learning isolated bits of information which the child has difficulty associating with any prior experience or knowledge.

Johnston (1988) recommends activities that are **child-centered**, those which are chosen because they have special significance for the child. This encourages optimum attention to the task and promotes more rapid learning. Language forms are modeled for the child which express the ideas related to the activity that the child should internalize. Carrow-Woolfolk and Lynch (1982) suggest modifying each child's learning environment to help the youngster compensate for language deficits. For example, one child may need linguistic information presented at a rate that is slower than normal. Another may need directions simplified and/or separated into smaller units. Another may need quiet surroundings without competing background noise. This approach contrasts with those who believe that specific deficits identified for each child should receive direct instruction (Barry and McGinnis, 1988). In that style of intervention, a child who has difficulty sequencing auditory signals would be given drills to practice skills. One activity might be the presentation of arbitrary numbers which would be recited back to the teacher in order by the child. Still other approaches (Alley and Deshler 1979; Larson and McKinley, 1987; Schwartz and McKinley, 1984) suggest helping the youngster develop "strategies" to compensate for the language deficit. Additional educational issues are reviewed in Chapter 15.

SUMMARY

The term *specific language deficit* is one of several labels that describe those youngsters who most often appear to score within normal limits in measures of nonverbal intelligence, perceptual acuity, emotional stability, and physical development, but who are exhibiting difficulty with language learning. One or many of the dimensions of language could be affected. Deficits can fluctuate in severity and change over time. The cause for this disorder is often unsubstantiated but minimal brain damage resulting in perceptual, symbolic, and/or attentional deficits is surmised. Recent research suggests genetic factors affecting multiple family members.

Language delay can be contrasted with language disorder by characterizing delay as a condition which is correctable with appropriate intervention. Behaviors associated with language deficit vary considerably. However, the disorder impacts on linguistic, academic, emotional, and social development of the child. These pervasive characteristics result in the need for proper educational intervention. Interdisciplinary planning and collaboration to bring consistency to the child's education program are critical. Meaningful language experiences developed specifically for the child's individual needs provide the groundwork for effective language learning.

SUGGESTED READINGS

Curtiss, S., and Tallal, P. (1991). On the Nature of the Impairment in Language-impaired Children. In J. Miller (Ed.), *Research on Child Language Disorders: A Decade of Progress* (pp. 189–210). Austin, TX: Pro-Ed.

Fletcher, P., and Hall, D. (Eds.). (1992). *Specific Speech and Language Disorders in Children.* San Diego, CA: Singular Publishing Group.

Johnston, J. (1988). Specific Language Disorders in the Child. In N. Lass, L. McReynolds, J. Northern, and D. Yoder (Eds.), *Handbook of Speech-Language Pathology and Audiology* (pp. 685–715). Philadelphia, PA: B.C. Decker.

8 THE NATURE OF LANGUAGE DISORDERS AMONG CHILDREN WITH LEARNING DISABILITIES

Learning disabilities are usually considered when children have difficulty in school. To provide professional help to children who are having considerable difficulty learning, the disorder contributing to their difficulties must be clearly defined. A number of outstanding individuals in the field of education have put their minds to this task, yet a clear definition of learning disabilities remains elusive. There is consensus, however, in the observation that these children are intelligent and capable, but are not achieving academically.

Federal guidelines for defining **learning disabilities** (U.S. Office of Education, 1977) emphasize that there must be a "significant" discrepancy between measurements of ability (i.e., intelligence tests) and performance in one or more areas of academic achievement. What constitutes a significant discrepancy varies from state to state. In other words, to be classified as learning disabled, the child's achievement must lag behind expectations to the degree determined by the state in which the child lives.

In some states, a significant discrepancy is reached when a child of normal intelligence scores one year below grade level on achievement tests. Other states consider a lag of one year significant for a second grader, but require scores on achievement tests of at least two years below grade level for a fifth grader to meet the criteria (Smith, 1983). And still other states define significant as a 20–25% discrepancy between expected achievement based on intelligence and actual achievement. Keep in mind that students with learning disabilities have at least normal intelligence, and that they have many strengths among the disabilities.

Learning disabilities are usually not identified until the primary grades. Assessment protocols are not sensitive enough to conclusively identify learning disabilities in three- to five-year-old children. Practically speaking, by the time school-age children are identified, tested, and classified as having learning disabilities, they have had to struggle for a considerable period of time. Most likely, they exhibit severe difficulties reading with comprehension, writing with clarity, and listening with understanding. Under these conditions, the child's emotional stability and social development probably have been compromised, with serious ramifications.

Too often, children with learning disabilities are not identified at all. They continue to struggle, often until the junior high school grades where they falter under greater linguistic demands and the need to rely on basic skills they never learned. Ironically, the factors contributing to academic failure were evident long before the children entered school and long before they could communicate using a symbolic linguistic code.

Specific language deficit as described in Chapter 7 and the language deficits directly related to neurological factors as described in this chapter represent two different points of view or perspectives. The learning disabilities specialist and also specialists in neuropsychology are concerned with how humans receive, organize, and store information and use language to think about, analyze, and utilize the information received. All the current definitions of learning disabilities indicate that the disorder is reflected in language deficits and academic difficulties due to central nervous system dysfunction (i.e., related to abnormal cortical functioning). Through the use of noninvasive technology and postmortem anatomical studies of the brain tissue of individuals with known learning disabilities, the correlation between specific functions in the cortex of the brain that involve language processing and their relation to reading, writing, and problem solving is becoming better understood. Some of these devices include: electroencephalogram

[EEG], evoked potential [EP], computer-assisted tomography [CAT], magnetic resonance imaging [MRI], positron emission tomography [PET], superconducting quantum interference device [SQUID], and single-photon emission computerized tomography [SPECT]).

Whether sophisticated technology actually documents central nervous system dysfunction or not, classroom teachers are faced with children with significant learning problems. The teachers' focus is on how to help those students learn despite their CNS dysfunction, or suspected dysfunctioning. The cause of the learning disability is not as crucial as the services provided by the teacher.

In discussing the nature of language disorders among individuals with learning disabilities, this chapter

1. presents several definitions of learning disabilities;

2. considers the various factors that contribute to learning disabilities;

3. examines the relationship of language deficits and learning disabilities; and

4. suggests intervention strategies for students with learning disabilities.

DEFINITIONS OF LEARNING DISABILITIES

Three "official" definitions have been proposed to describe children with learning disabilities. They are summarized in the next three sections.

PL 94-142, Education for All Handicapped Children Act

In its definition, PL 94-142, now known as IDEA, attempts to differentiate learning disabilities from other disorders and also from the effects of environmental, cultural, or economic deprivation:

Specific learning disability means a disorder in one or more of the basic psychological processes involved in understanding or in using language, spoken or written, which may manifest itself in an imperfect ability to listen, think, speak, read, write, spell, or to do mathematical calculations. The term includes such conditions as perceptual handicaps, brain injury, minimal brain dysfunction, dyslexia, and developmental aphasia. The term does not include children who have learning problems which are primarily the result of visual, hearing, or motor handicaps, of mental retardation, of emotional disturbance, or of environmental, cultural, or economic disadvantage. (U.S. Office of Education, 1977, p. 42478)

Statement by National Joint Committee on Learning Disabilities, 1988

The following definition is the "most widely accepted definition in use today" (Hammill, 1990, p. 78).

Learning Disabilities is a general term that refers to a heterogeneous group of disorders manifested by significant difficulties in the acquisition and use of listening, speaking, reading, writing, reasoning, or mathematical abilities. These disorders are intrinsic to the individual, presumed to be due to central nervous system dysfunction, and may occur across the life span. Problems in self-regulatory behavior, social perception, and social interaction may exist with learning disabilities but do not by themselves constitute a learning disability. Although learning disabilities may occur concomitantly with other handicapping conditions (for example, sensory impairment, mental retardation, serious emotional disturbance) or with extrinsic influences (such as cultural differences, insufficient or inappropriate instruction), they are not the result of those conditions or influences. (NJCLD Memorandum, 1988, p. 1)

The member organizations of the NJCLD include: the American Speech-Language-Hearing Association (ASHA), the Council for Learning Disabilities (CLD), the Division for Children with Communication Disorders (DCCD), the Division for Learning Disabilities (DLD), the International Reading Association (IRA), the Learning Disabilities Association of America (LDA), the National Association for School Psychologists (NASP), and the Orton Dyslexia Society (ODS).

Unlike PL 94-142, the National Joint Committee's definition emphasizes

1. the intrinsic nature of learning disabilities (i.e., caused by physiological factors and not by external factors);

2. the fact that learning disabilities is a problem not only of school years, but also of early childhood and adult life; and

3. the idea that the disorder may occur "concomitantly with" other handicapping conditions and in individuals from different cultural and socioeconomic environments.

Definition Adopted by the U.S. Interagency Committee on Learning Disabilities, 1988

The members of the U.S. Interagency Committee on Learning Disabilities are the National Institute of Child Health and Human Development, National Institute of Neurological and Communicative Disorders and Stroke, National Institute of Allergy and Infectious Diseases, National Eye Institute, National Institute of Environmental Health Sciences, Division of Research Resources of the National Institutes of Health, Food and Drug Administration, National Institute of Mental Health, Centers for Disease Control, Environmental Protection Agency, Office of Human Development Services, and Department of Education. Together they drafted this definition:

Learning disabilities is a generic term that refers to a heterogeneous group of disorders manifested by significant difficulties in the acquisition and use of listening, speaking, reading, writing, reasoning, or mathematical abilities, or of social skills. These disorders are intrinsic to the individual and presumed to be due to central nervous system dysfunction. Even though learning disability may occur concomitantly with other handicapping conditions (e.g., sensory impairment, mental retardation, social and emotional disturbance), with socioenvironmental influences (e.g., cultural differences, insufficient or inappropriate instruction, psychogenic factors), and especially with attention deficit disorder, all of which may cause learning problems, a learning disability is not the direct result of those conditions or influences (Kavanagh and Truss, 1988, pp. 550-551).

ETIOLOGIES

In each definition above, learning disabilities have been attributed to presumed central nervous system dysfunction. Evidence relates the various types of cortical dysfunction to biochemical and genetic factors, viral infections of a pregnant mother (e.g., rubella, herpes simplex, syphilis, tuberculosis), drug and alcohol ingestion and smoking during pregnancy, oxygen deprivation due to prematurity or birth trauma, low birth weight, trauma by accident or physical abuse, poor nutrition during pregnancy, and viral infection of the child postnatally (e.g., encephalitis, meningitis, Reye's syndrome, otitis media) (Eimas and Clarkson, 1986; Feagans, 1986; Johnson, 1988; Lerner, 1985; Sever, 1986; Smith, 1983; Streissguth, 1983, 1986a; Streissguth, Clarren, and Jones, 1985; Tallal, 1988).

Symptoms of central nervous system dysfunction in a child are quite different from the symptoms of central nervous system dysfunction acquired as an adult. "Central nervous system dysfunction in the child is typically reflected in deficient development of cognitive, perceptual, linguistic, academic, and behavioral skills, whereas insult to the adult brain generally results in the loss of previously acquired skills" (Lyon, Newby, Recht, and Caldwell, 1991, p. 377).

LANGUAGE DEFICITS AMONG STUDENTS WITH LEARNING DISABILITIES

There appears to be general agreement between educators and investigators that students with learning disabilities have difficulty using and comprehending language. They often have particular difficulty processing new linguistic information. Their serious language deficits contribute to the difficulties they encounter when attempting to read with comprehension (Catts and Kamhi, 1986; Liberman, 1983; Mann, 1991; Vellutino and Denkla, 1990; Vellutino and Scanlon, 1986; Wallach and Butler, 1984; Wiig and Semel, 1984).

Deficits in Metalinguistic Awareness

Before children can learn to read, they must acquire metalinguistic awareness. As discussed in Chapter 4, metalinguistics refers to how the child thinks about language, talks about language, and manipulates language (Gleason, 1989). Long before children speak in complete sentences, they learn the purposes of print and become interested in labels, letters, magazines, books, and signs. When stories are read to them, children become aware that the pictures and words provide knowledge.

At about four years of age, the child begins to break down language into linguistic units. The child recognizes that written language is comprised of words we speak (Tunmer and Bowey, 1983). Before children understand that sounds match written letters, they must be able to delineate words in continuous discourse, and then segment words into their component syllables. Unlike printed sentences, spoken utterances do not always have perceptible spaces, or pauses between each word. The child learns that sentences are made up of words. Children who are exposed to nursery rhymes and play with words learn that words are made up of sounds.

Young children in preschool and kindergarten who do not enjoy nursery rhymes, sound games, songs, and storytelling time are indicating a lack of metalinguistic awareness and are revealing behaviors that are often referred to as "soft signs" of potential learning problems. Obviously, there are many reasons why children are not willing to participate in games and act out during storytelling time. They may have come to school without having eaten breakfast or they may be in physical discomfort. When the undesirable behaviors are consistently present during auditory activities, but otherwise absent, then they are legitimate causes for concern. Children who have not grasped basic metalinguistic awareness are not ready to comprehend sound/symbol relationships (Liberman and Liberman, 1990).

Deficits in Information Processing

The brain must make sense of the speech or manual code used to convey information, as well as the nonverbal clues and visual and auditory stimuli in the environment. It must process (i.e., identify, discriminate, and categorize) the myriad sensory stimuli carried to the cortex by complex neurological connections and pathways. These stimuli are temporarily held in short-term memory while the individual components are routed to specific areas of the cortex for further processing. The brain must recognize the relevancy and relationships of these new incoming data to the ever-expanding store of related information in long-term memory. The new information, now combined with related, already learned information, must be organized in such a fashion that it is readily accessible for still further processing.

Higher-level language processing depends upon the integrity, or reliability, of the sensory and perceptual systems. In addition, effective information processing relies heavily on the following abilities:

- the ability to focus attention on the topic and the specific details of the incoming message;

- the ability to deliberately attend to selected, relevant information and disregard the irrelevant details; and

- the ability to sustain attention for the time required to obtain from the utterance all the information necessary for comprehension.

The final stage of this processing procedure requires using inner language to think about, make decisions about, and formulate ideas about what has been learned (i.e., metacognition). Students with learning disabilities often do not have integrity of their perceptual, attentional, or memory systems to process the stream of linguistic information to which they are exposed during the school day. One or more of these systems is not functioning adequately and, therefore, they cannot process information without strategies to organize and systematize this information. These deficits manifest themselves in severe difficulties listening to and learning from oral instructions, learning to read with comprehension, applying logical reasoning and higher-level analytic skills, and using language as a tool to process information more efficiently.

Deficits in Oral Language Processing

When children are in school, they are immersed in a linguistic environment where they are required to communicate with others to solve problems, to share space and materials, and to complete the tasks that the teacher has assigned. Students are continuously exposed to conversational interactions, oral and written instructions, questions, discussions, lectures, stories, textbook assignments, and narrative writing assignments. Students with learning disabilities often flounder in such an intensive linguistic environment.

Instruction presented orally often causes particular problems for students with learning disabilities (Bloome and Knott, 1985;

Norton, 1989; Valletutti and Dummett, 1992). The beginning of a new lesson is important, and the teacher often introduces new information by defining and explaining the topic carefully. Students with learning disabilities may spend a number of frantic moments trying to identify the topic. By the time they focus on the relevant details of the new lesson and perceive what the lesson is all about, the teacher has progressed far ahead, and many of the important facts are missed.

Students with learning disabilities also may have difficulty sustaining attention to important details. If they are momentarily distracted, they do not easily pick up the trend of the teacher's oral commentary nor do they readily visualize the concepts being presented. They have organized their experiences and their knowledge in long-term memory inadequately, incompletely, or in a distorted fashion, and do not have easy access to this information. They cannot quickly retrieve related facts from memory and they have difficulty integrating previously learned ideas with new material presented orally by the teacher.

Deficits in Listening Comprehension

Studies indicate that students with learning disabilities reveal deficits in listening comprehension, particularly the complex syntactic structures in spoken language (Byrne, 1981; Donahue, Pearl, and Bryan, 1983; Hallahan and Bryan, 1981; Menyuk and Flood, 1981; Perfetti and Roth, 1981; Siegel and Ryan, 1984; Wiig and Semel, 1984).

Students with spatial perceptual learning disabilities, for example, may experience particular problems comprehending pronouns. Their specific type of disability is manifested in their inaccurate perception of the changes in location of objects and people as they move in space.

Demonstrative pronouns *this* and *these* (close to the speaker) and *that* and *those* (remote from the speaker) cause confusion for children with spatial perceptual learning disabilities. Children with this deficit are not certain how far or near the object or other person is in relation to themselves. In addition, the speaker and the listener may move in space during their conversation, and the object that is remote from the speaker at one moment may be near to the speaker the next.

Difficulty comprehending the use of personal pronouns, *I, you, they,* and *we,* also may involve orientation in space while conversing. During personal interactions, the terms *I* or *we* are used by speakers to refer to themselves alone or in combination with specific others, and *you* or *they* to refer to the listener or to other people or objects. During these interactions, speakers and listeners constantly change roles, and the personal pronoun *I* is interchanged between speakers, while the personal pronoun *you* is interchanged between listeners. The pronoun *it* or *they* may refer to persons other than the speaker or listener, or to animals, objects, or ideas (Wiig and Semel, 1984). Students with spatial perceptual learning disabilities who reveal deficits in the comprehension of pronouns are often observed to be confused during personal interactions. Their confusion will also be evident when attempting to comprehend written dialogue.

Deficits in Comprehension Monitoring

Many students with learning disabilities have **comprehension monitoring deficits,** that is difficulty recognizing that they have not comprehended a portion of the teacher's oral message (Brinton and Fujiki, 1982; Dollaghan, 1987). If students are aware, they often do not know how to obtain the teacher's attention to indicate that they are confused. They have difficulty formulating a question or a request for clarification. When the teacher has rephrased the confusing statement, they often are not certain whether the rephrasing is sufficient or whether they need further clarification.

Deficits in Processing Questions

Students are required to answer a great many questions, both oral and written, in the course of an average school day. Students with learning disabilities often have particular difficulty answering questions (Parnell, Amerman, and Harting, 1986). They are often not aware when a speaker's question is poorly phrased and not entirely comprehensible. To respond to questions asked by the teacher, students must determine whether they clearly understand the question or whether more information or clarification is needed. If more information is required, students must express an appropriately phrased question to request clarification. As mentioned earlier, this is often particularly difficult for students with learning disabilities.

When the teacher has revised the question, it has to be analyzed to determine how to respond to it. Moreover, students have to consider whether their personal knowledge is adequate or whether they need more information to answer the question adequately (Gavelek and Raphael, 1982). Based on clinical observations, Wiig and Semel (1984) ranked *wh-question* terms in the following order of increasing complexity with respect to interpretation by students with learning disabilities: *what, who, which, where, when, why, how, whose.*

Deficits in Note-Taking Skills

The process of taking notes is considerably more complex than listening to and processing the teacher's instructions alone. Although both skills include receptive language comprehension, adequate short-term memory capacity, attention capacity, selective attentional ability, and semantic and syntactic knowledge, note taking also requires intact intersensory integration (i.e., simultaneous writing, seeing, listening, motor planning and kinesthetic integrity). When a student engages in note taking, the additional skills of writing, spelling, and reading are involved. Students with learning disabilities tend to write down everything that the teacher has said and everything that has been written on the chalkboard or overhead transparency.

Furthermore, students with learning disabilities often have difficulty copying from a chalkboard or overhead transparency. Glancing back and forth may cause them to lose their place and return to an incorrect sentence. They may omit large portions of information and then may not be aware that their notes are incomplete or do not make sense. Long after the notations are erased, they realize their notes are valueless.

The note-taking difficulties described appear overwhelming unless they are considered individually in a task analysis addressing the question, "Which skills are necessary to take adequate notes?" Table 8.1 analyzes the various skills required to take notes during a classroom lecture. Students may have problems with some, but rarely with all of the required skills. When individual skills are identified as deficient, compensatory strategies can be taught to the student.

Table 8.1

Skills Required to Take Adequate Notes

- Adequate attention span
- Ability to focus on material being discussed
- Adequate short-term sequential memory
- Ability to process complex verbal sentences that contain embedded clauses
- Adequate vocabulary
- Ability to perceive relationships among objects, events, and situations presented both visually and auditorially
- Ability to grasp inference and figurative language
- Ability to follow 3–4 step directions
- Ability to differentiate the main idea, relevant details, and information that illustrates that idea
- Ability to hold words in mind while writing them down, at the same time listening to additional words
- Ability to process simultaneous visual and auditory stimuli
- Ability to copy from a chalkboard or overhead transparency and simultaneously listen while the teacher explains notations
- Ability to switch between sensory tracts: auditory (listening), visual (seeing), and motor-kinesthetic (writing)
- Auditory discrimination ability
- Auditory closure ability to "fill in" when information spoken has not quite been distinguished
- Auditory figure-ground ability

Deficits in Written Expression

The same problems that interfere with learning disabled children's ability to express their thoughts orally and to comprehend spoken language are apparent when they attempt to express their thoughts in written form. Written language is a symbolic, graphic representation of oral language. However, written expression requires more precise syntactic structure and less redundancy than spoken language.

By the age of seven years, most children are telling fictional stories with a centered plot and one or more episodes involving a character or characters (Brown, Day, and Jones, 1983; Stein, 1983; Sutton-Smith, 1986). The structure of the plots continues to increase in complexity through early adolescence (Roth and Spekman, 1986; Sutton-Smith, 1986). Students with learning disabilities often reveal serious expressive writing problems that persist over time (Graham and Harris, 1989a; 1989b). Their plot structures appear to be poorly organized, and they have problems sequencing events (Montague, Maddux, and Dereshiwsky, 1990). They often pay little attention to characters' attitudes, feelings, goals, and motives (Moran, 1988). When writing a descriptive narrative, their imagery is often distorted or disconnected and missing many important facts and details. Such omissions cause the reader to envision a different scene, person, or event than the one envisioned by the writer. After writing a first draft, these students often do not know how to make the necessary revisions.

Deficits in Reading

One of the most complex learning tasks required of school-age children is reading. An important question to be considered when students are having exceptional difficulty acquiring the necessary reading skills is, "Specifically, which aspects of the task cause the most problems?" The classroom teacher must identify the problem areas quickly and often informally to teach children remedial strategies. A good technique for analyzing the component skills of a complex process such as reading is a task analysis that will address the questions, "What skills are necessary to be able to decode unknown words?" and "What skills are necessary to be able to read with comprehension?" These skills are summarized in Table 8.2 .

Table 8.2

Task Analysis of Reading Skills

Skills Required to Decode Unknown Printed Words

Phonological Skills

- Awareness of differences and similarities between phonemes
- Knowledge of phonological rules of the language
- Ability to blend individual phonemes into a meaningful word
- Knowledge of sound-letter association

Synthesis

- Ability to combine sounds into larger units

Attentional Skills

- Ability to focus attention on a specific sound or task
- Ability to sustain attention for the length of time it requires to complete a specific task
- Enough attentional capacity to simultaneously decode and comprehend the text

Auditory Perceptual Skills

- Ability to isolate a sound within a word in initial, medial, and final position
- Ability to perceive relationships between words that rhyme (i.e., to perceive the sounds of parts of two or more words that sound the same)
- Ability to perceive the double sound of consonant blends in words, such as *play* and *table* (*bl, br, cl, cr, dr, dw, fl,tr, gr, pl, gl, pr, sc, sk, sl, sm, sn, sp, st, ng*)
- Ability to perceive the consonant combinations that represent one sound (*sh, th, wh, ch, ph, ng, gh*)
- Ability to perceive differences between the sounds of short vowels in words, such as *fan, fin, fun, tan, tin,* and *ten.*

Continued

Table 8.2—*Continued*

- Ability to perceive the sounds of vowel combinations (e.g., *ie, ea, oo, oi, ou, oa, ai*)

Knowledge of Morphological Rules

- Ability to divide perceived words into their smallest grammatical units, or morphemes (e.g., *unanswerable* contains *un, answer,* and *able*)

Sequential Memory

- Rapid recognition and retrieval of the letters and words

- Ability to remember the order of phonemes that when combined comprise a word

- Ability to recall the sounds within a word and words within a phrase or sentence

- Ability to recall from memory the syntactical, phonological, and morphological rules that govern the arrangement of words in a phrase or sentence

Visual Perceptual Ability

- Ability to distinguish different letter shapes

- Ability to discriminate letters of varying size

- Ability to perceive the differences between the amount of space separating letters within words and that which separates words in a phrase or sentence

- Ability to distinguish the direction and orientation of different letters

- Ability to perceive any angle, slant, or other deviation from the horizontal or vertical

- Understanding that the letters have permanent shapes despite the fact that we view them vertically on a chalkboard, horizontally on a desk, and from a variety of orientations, and that we often move while we are viewing them (shape constancy)

- The ability to separate the letters from the lined paper on which they are written and/or separate the printed letters from illustrations on the same page (figure-ground discrimination)

- Ability to recognize or identify the letters despite distortion, illegibility, partial erasure, or overlap (closure)

Continued

Table 8.2—*Continued*

Skills Required to Read with Comprehension
Attention

- Enough attentional capacity to simultaneously decode and comprehend the text
- Ability to focus attention on the relevant and most important aspects of written text
- Ability to withhold attention from irrelevant and incidental information in the text to be read

Syntax

- Ability to understand complex spoken sentences with embedded clauses
- Ability to understand relationships between sentences and across sentence boundaries (paragraph)

Semantics

- Ability to understand the multiple meanings and subtle nuances of spoken language
- Appropriate and adequate vocabulary
- Ability to associate and generalize concepts
- Ability to interpret idiomatic, figurative, and colloquial speech

Memory

- Ability to access stored lexical knowledge
- Ability to hold the sentences in working memory long enough to establish relationships among the concepts expressed by the sentences being read and related concepts stored in memory
- An adequate sequential auditory memory to enable child to hold the words of a relatively long and complex sentence in short-term memory long enough to extract the most pertinent and important components
- Ability to tap past experiences and previously stored information that relate to the topic, the problem, and the meaning of the material to be read
- Ability to draw from long-term memory lexical information pertaining to words and word meanings
- Appropriate and adequate general information stored in long-term memory, based upon past personal experiences with objects, situations, and events

Continued

Table 8.2—*Continued*

- Ability to draw from long-term memory information that enhances and supplements what is read (i.e., analogous reasoning ability)

- Ability to hold in working memory the correct sequence of events in a story

Imagery

- Ability to envision the scene described by the author, not only the visual details, but also the smells, the sounds, the entire physical and emotional environment

Pragmatics

- Ability to quickly identify the topic of the paragraph or chapter to be read

- Ability to perceive the relationships between experiences of a character in the story and one's own

- Appropriate and adequate social skills with peers and adults in real life

- Ability to understand affect denoting emotions when communicating with another person

- Ability to understand motivation that causes individuals to react and respond to another person, event, or situation in a particular way

- Knowledge of cause-effect relationships and ability to identify consequences of fictional characters' actions

- Ability to predict what will happen in a story or how the character will react

- Ability to role play

- Ability to empathize with people who are unhappy, embarrassed, or frightened in real life

- Ability to understand the emotional reactions of a character in a story

- Ability to predict the character's response in a given situation, and also to envision the character's affect indicating the emotions that are felt

- Ability to determine just from the description of the dialogue the tone of voice, the stress of words, the sarcasm, and the inflection in the voices of the characters as they speak

Continued

Table 8.2—*Continued*

Higher-Level Cognitive Skills

- Ability to find evidence in a passage to support logical generalizations and conclusions

- Ability to differentiate between the main idea of the story and supporting details

- Ability to infer concepts that are not explicitly stated

- Ability to perceive the author's purpose or intention

- Ability to distinguish among facts, opinions, hypotheses, and assumptions

- Ability to differentiate conclusions from supporting statements, facts from opinions, and explicit from implied statements

- Ability to determine how details relate to main ideas, whether sufficient information is provided by the author, and whether the author's ideas are coherent

- Ability to apply criteria or standards with which to make judgments on content, ideas, methods, products, and people that are presented by the author

- Ability to combine components of information into a coherent and connected whole

- Ability to apply ideas learned in one situation to new or related situations

Students with learning disabilities do not have difficulties in all of the skills cited in Table 8.2. The global picture of a poor reader erroneously gives the impression of an individual who is struggling with "all aspects" of written language. In fact, the students have deficits in very specific skills related to reading, and these deficits affect the students' overall ability to decode with ease and comprehend the text. Students with decoding deficits and those with reading comprehension deficits should be considered separately because each task requires different cognitive and linguistic skills.

Decoding

Specific problem areas for young students with learning disabilities who are having exceptional difficulty acquiring decoding skills include these:

- *Phonological processing*—The ability to discriminate sounds in songs and nursery rhymes and to relate sounds of spoken language (phonemes) to specific letters of the alphabet are good predictors of reading success; deficient phoneme awareness is a consistent predictor of reading problems (Bradley and Bryant, 1985; Brady and Shankweiler, 1991; Mann, 1993; Perfetti, 1985; Stanovich, Cunningham, and Freeman, 1984). Children with phonological processing deficits have difficulty learning to decode because they cannot discriminate vowels and consonants and cannot blend the sounds together until a familiar word is "recognized."

  Among the factors contributing to problems of phonological processing are auditory perceptual deficits. Children with this particular type of learning disability have serious problems when trying to discriminate the sounds of speech, delineate and separate words in continuous discourse, perceive similarities between sounds that rhyme, and separate particular speech sounds from background ambient noise.

- *Phonological memory*—In addition, the child with phonological processing deficits often has poor memory with regard to verbal information, both spoken and written (Mann, Cowin, and Schoenheimer, 1989) and cannot hold sentences in memory long enough to obtain meaning from them (Baddeley, 1986; Hulme, 1981; Katz, Shankweiler, and Liberman, 1981; Mann and Brady, 1988; Pratt and Brady, 1988; Swanson, 1983; Torgesen, 1985, 1988).

- *Visual perception*—Visual perceptual ability is required to discriminate the shapes, sizes, and orientation of individual letters. Learning disabled children with visual perceptual deficits may have no difficulty with phoneme discrimination when trying to decode a word, but may not be able to differentiate letter shapes or separate the printed letter or word from the lines on which they are written.

Spatial perceptual learning disabilities can contribute to decoding difficulty. In reading, groups of letters are recognized as words because there is space surrounding them that separates them from other words in the sentence (Lerner, 1985). There is also more space between words in a sentence than between letters in a word. Students with spatial perceptual deficits frequently are unable to distinguish the amount of space between words and letters and read a sentence as one long word.

- *Attention*—Learning disabled children who have decoding difficulties expend so much energy focusing on the decoding task that there is not sufficient attentional capacity available to comprehend the text.

- *Word recognition*—The child painfully decodes individual words instead of rapidly and efficiently recognizing them. This puts heavy demands on memory, thus making comprehension a frustrating process (Ackerman and Dykman, 1982; Lorsbach, 1982; Samuels, 1987; Samuels and Peterson, 1986; Shiffrin and Schneider, 1984; Spear and Sternberg, 1986; Sternberg, 1984, 1985; Sternberg and Wagner, 1982).

- *Word knowledge*—If the student has a poor vocabulary, or if the word is not in the child's lexicon, it will not be recognized even after the struggle to decode it phonetically.

Comprehension

Specific problem areas for older students with learning disabilities, who are expected to comprehend the language of the printed passage and to glean the necessary information, include these:

- *Knowledge base*—Insufficient knowledge due to lack of meaningful experiences or to inaccurate storage of information related to an experience may account for some comprehension difficulties by students with learning disabilities (Gerber, 1991; Kolligian and Sternberg, 1987).

- *Visual processing*—The visual scene at any given moment is a complex picture consisting of lines oriented in a variety of angles, contours, shapes, and perspectives, as well as colors, shading, highlights, textures, and patterns. The human brain receives these minute details through the retinas of the eyes and then, by way of complex neural systems, they are brought to the processing areas of the cortex where understanding and storing of all of these details take place. There are many opportunities along this pathway where problems can cause interference and distortions of the image being processed. When this occurs, perceptions of the visual scene are inaccurate, and resulting images and concepts that are stored in long-term memory are inaccurate as well. This particular kind of learning disability can interfere with reading comprehension.

- *Visualization*—The ability to recall the visual details of a scene or event and compare one's own experiences to one described in a written passage is essential for reading comprehension. Quite often, the response to a visual experience also awakens memories of the smells, sounds, and tastes of the experience, making it richer and more vivid (Lorch, 1982; Shaw, 1982). If the visual experiences that have been stored in memory are either distorted or missing some essential details due to visual perceptual learning disabilities, the individual retrieves inaccurate images. In many instances, this perceptual deficit will distort the memory of the entire event. The student will then draw inaccurate conclusions and will have difficulty when having to interpret, infer, analyze, compare, and thus comprehend narratives, essays, and descriptive texts.

- *Linguistic concepts*—Adverbs (e.g., *quickly, slowly, timidly, boldly*), adjectives (e.g., *round, enormous, pliable*), and prepositions (e.g., *near, above, close to*) are examples of concepts expressed in words or phrases. Linguistic conceptual development contributes to comprehension of written narratives. When learning disabilities interfere with normal concept development, linguistic terms expressing these concepts may not be understood. For example, spatial perceptual learning disabilities will affect the development of concepts expressed by linguistic terms, such as *depth, length, width, size, slope, curvature, tilt, slant, to the left, to the right, in front of, and toward the center.* A reader who cannot envision depth, height, width, and circumference cannot comprehend a story of a rescue attempt of a man who has fallen down a narrow gorge: *The walls on either side of the gorge press against the lone, slender rescuer as he lowers himself by ropes to the victim.* The restrictions forced upon the entire rescue team by the terrain, and the distance that the victim must be raised to level ground are important details for comprehension. A reader with a visual perceptual deficit in space perception and spatial orientation will not be able to envision or comprehend what is happening or predict what will happen.

Deficits in Nonverbal Communication

Paralinguistic information, such as tone of voice, inflection, intensity of voice, and attitudes and emotions that are embedded within the voice itself, is frequently misinterpreted by children with nonverbal learning disabilities (also referred to as right hemispheric learning disabilities). When interacting with other people, they derive little or no meaning from emotions apparent in facial expressions or gestures. They may not respect personal space between themselves and other people with whom they are conversing. These children reveal serious pragmatic deficits.

If students do not empathize, do not perceive the emotions revealed by a person's facial expressions, and do not perceive paralinguistic cues in personal interrelationships, they will not perceive these subtle, essential bits of information during conversations or in stories they are reading. They will not understand the motives and reactions of their conversational partners or of the characters portrayed by an author.

INTERVENTION WITH STUDENTS WITH LEARNING DISABILITIES AND CONCOMITANT LANGUAGE DEFICITS

Metacognitive strategies are helpful to students with learning disabilities. Metacognition requires that the students step back and

- consider the skills, strategies, and resources needed to perform a task,

- implement the steps necessary,

- monitor the activities, and

- evaluate the effectiveness of their efforts (Brown, 1982).

Inner Language

An effective tool for metacognition is inner language. As defined in Chapter 1, inner language is the language with which one thinks. It is not used as language is ordinarily used, to communicate with other human beings; it is the process by which speech is internalized into thought; it is the means by which one communicates with oneself.

Functions of inner language include the following:

- planning actions before undertaking a problem-solving task

- "trying out" possible approaches to the solutions of problems

- deciding how well the materials have been understood, whether the ongoing strategies are effective, or whether some modifications of these strategies should be considered

- evaluating the progress and the outcome of the strategies used to solve a problem

Evaluating the task itself and the effectiveness of the strategies used to solve problems involves comprehension monitoring or analysis of how well the information in the text is understood. Students with learning disabilities have the ability to evaluate their comprehension of text, but they often fail to do so without prodding and supervision. They can evaluate their comprehension if taught appropriate strategies (Bos and Filip, 1982; Ryan, Ledger, Short, and Weed, 1982).

When students are given very specific instructions as to the procedures they should use to evaluate their understanding of spoken or written information, they are much better at monitoring their comprehension (Baker, 1982; Markman and Gorin, 1981). Even kindergartners are quite capable of noticing more obvious irregularities if they are specifically alerted to watch for them (Pace, 1980). These findings suggest that an essential component of metacognition is selective attention.

Self-Impressions

Children's self-impressions of capabilities and limitations are important forms of metacognition (Brown, 1982). Studies of students with learning disabilities indicate that many of them have the following self-perceptions (Butkowsky and Willows, 1980; Diener and Dweck, 1980; Dweck and Licht, 1980; Grimes, 1981; Pearl, Bryan, and Donahue, 1980):

- They have very little control over academic success or failure.

- Their failures are due to their lack of ability.

- Their successes are due to luck, to their teacher's explicit help, and other external factors to which they do not contribute.

- Their chances of success in learning situations are poor.

These self-perceptions have been referred to as **learned helplessness**, or the perceived inability to overcome failure. Research on students' attributions for causes of their own successes or failures has revealed important differences between good and poor readers. Skilled readers tend to attribute successes to their ability and their failures to lack of effort. Poor readers tend to attribute success to external circumstances and failures to their lack of ability. The poor readers exhibit the symptoms of "learned helplessness" in that they expect to fail and feel there is nothing they can do about it (Borkowski, Weyhing, and Carr, 1988; Borkowski, Johnston, and Reid, 1987; Butkowsky and Willows, 1980; Dweck and Licht, 1980).

Metacognitive Training

Metacognitive training, sometimes called **cognitive behavior modification**, provides explicit guidance in self-monitoring skills, and the use of "self-talk" (Billingsley and Wildman, 1990; Wong, 1991). When given metacognitive training, the student is taught to

1. consider the goal of the task and define it in concrete terms;

2. select a strategy from among several possible strategies to accomplish this goal;

3. monitor the effectiveness of the strategy selected;

4. make modifications and alterations if necessary;

5. evaluate results;

6. praise oneself for success; and

7. cope with problems encountered during the process.

The teacher initially directs the sequence of the steps required to complete the task and models the questions the children must ask themselves. Next, the children perform each step of the task asking themselves the questions "aloud" or, if deaf, signing in view of the teacher. Finally, the children perform the task alone, proceeding through each step and asking the questions using inner language (Chan, 1991). Self-instructional, metacognitive training, with its emphasis on self-regulation through the use of inner language, is particularly appropriate for teaching students with learning disabilities (Chan, 1991).

Self-instructional, metacognitive training programs have also been successful for developing higher-order thinking abilities, such as comparing and contrasting, categorizing, analyzing, summarizing, making inferences, interpreting information, problem solving, reasoning logically, drawing conclusions, making judgments, visualizing, reflecting on various considerations, organizing, prioritizing, and generalizing (Chan, 1991; Grossen, 1991; Valletutti and Dummett, 1992).

"Patting oneself on the back" is an important component of the sequence. The student must recognize when something has been accomplished by self-effort. Too often, the student with learning disabilities waits for the teacher to offer words of encouragement. The process of self-monitoring requires the awareness that motivation needs a boost occasionally, and that accomplishment deserves recognition.

The following is an example of metacognitive self-talk, or self-instruction, for a mathematical computation:

Step 1. "What is it I have to do?"

Step 2. "I have to find the sign."

Step 3. "This sign means *add*. I start with the 3 and add it to the 9. That adds up to 12. I write the 2 at the bottom of the ones column. Then I write the 1 above the 4 in the tens column."

Step 4. "Good! I'm doing a great job."

Step 5. "Now I have to start on the next column. Go back, you skipped a column. That's okay. Just erase and start again."

Step 6. "Now I have to check my work for mistakes."

Step 7. "Uh, uh, I added wrong. Adding 7 and 4 equals 11 not 12. Correct the mistake. It's okay! Now it's fine!"

Step 8. "You did a good job!"

Although it is generally agreed that metacognitive training has been successful, and has value in teaching specific strategies to students with learning disabilities that will enhance their performance on school-related tasks, many studies have failed to demonstrate generalization of the training over time and across situations (Torgesen, 1980; Wong, 1991).

Attempts to analyze the problems interfering with transfer and later use of strategies acquired by metacognitive training produced some valuable and constructive conclusions. Transfer and later use of problem-solving strategies appear more likely when problems used in instruction are like those that will be often encountered later on (Niedelman, 1991). It is necessary to recognize the sameness between the learning situation, one's own past experiences, and the new or transferred situation. It is necessary to experience a wide range of examples in different, but related contexts in order to perceive the common characteristics encountered (Grossen, 1991; Niedelman, 1991; Salomon and Perkins, 1987). Also, teachers must understand students' unique abilities and disabilities so that compensatory strategies can be taught to further ensure the effectiveness of the training (Stone, 1989).

A more accurate estimate of analytic and inferential abilities may result from teachers' understanding of the impact of basic cognitive deficits on the students' impressions and interpretations of events. When students with learning disabilities are observed or tested on their interpretations, inferences, or conclusions regarding specific information, teachers are frequently alarmed at what appears to be confusion, or gross misinterpretation of the information presented. Teachers should keep in mind that there may be different ways of interpreting the students' "misinterpretations." For example, students with perceptual deficits may have stored information in memory in a form very different from that of their teachers. While teachers may think the students have misinterpreted the information, they may be drawing reasonable inferences considering their perceptions. This mismatch of student and teacher interpretations can result in the implementation of inappropriate remediation and also in serious emotional ramifications for the student—feelings of frustration, confusion, and anxiety.

SUMMARY

The emphasis in this chapter was on the ramifications of learning disabilities upon language and concept development and usage. Students with learning disabilities are a heterogeneous, complex population. Classroom teachers often do not know where to begin to help them. Certain conclusions and inferences can be drawn from the vast amount of research available regarding learning disabilities.

There are many different contributing factors that cloud the difficulties encountered by students with learning disabilities. When considering specific disabilities, such as those encountered in reading acquisition and reading comprehension, professionals cannot just focus on language alone. The student must have integrity of neurological systems controlling memory, attention, and visual and auditory perception. Teachers must anticipate problems. To do so, they must have a thorough understanding of the abilities that are necessary to do the tasks they are asking their students to perform. When evaluating students' abilities and their completed assignments, teachers must keep in mind that the students' impressions are often based upon distorted perceptions. Their conclusions and thought processes are not illogical when considered in light of the distorted concepts they have stored in long-term memory. Their "basic" cognitive skills are often deficient, not their higher-level cognitive abilities. Compensatory strategies can be very helpful.

Children with learning disabilities have at least normal intelligence and can benefit from skilled, well-constructed remedial methods/procedures. The vast majority of students with learning disabilities have serious language deficits, no matter what their specific learning disability. These language deficits are manifested in difficulties with reading comprehension, expressive writing, information processing, vocabulary development, long-term memory accessibility, selective attention, study skills, and pragmatic skills.

Students are further debilitated by learned helplessness. They are convinced that their failure is due to their inability and their successes are due not to their ability, but to luck, to their teacher's assistance, or to some other extraneous source. Students with learning disabilities benefit from cognitive training techniques that teach them how to use inner language as a tool to think about the task, to consider the problems involved, and to plan and develop solutions to the problems.

SUGGESTED READINGS

Johnson, D., and Myklebust, H. (1967). *Learning Disabilities: Educational Principles and Practices*. New York: Grune and Stratton.

Lerner, T. (1985). *Learning Disabilities: Theories, Diagnosis, and Teaching Strategies* (4th ed.). Dallas, TX: Houghton Mifflin.

Wong, B. (Ed.). (1991). *Learning about Learning Disabilities*. San Diego, CA: Academic Press.

THE NATURE OF LANGUAGE DISORDERS AMONG CHILDREN WITH UNIQUE LEARNING DIFFICULTIES

9

Dyslexia, attention deficit/hyperactivity disorder (ADHD), and nonverbal information processing disorder share common characteristics with learning disabilities in that they are neurologically based and they each contribute to severe learning problems. Indeed, many students with learning disabilities have severe reading deficits, symptoms of hyperactivity or impulsivity, and/or difficulty processing nonverbal information. However, the above disorders are each unique, and they differ substantially from other forms of learning disabilities. Hence, information regarding these disorders is being discussed in a separate chapter.

The most debilitating problem of individuals with dyslexia is learning to read. However, dyslexia differs from other types of severe reading disabilities not only in its severity, but also its resistance to conventional remediation, its persistence throughout adulthood, and its intrinsic association with linguistic deficits. Too often the term is used indiscriminately when referring to individuals who have difficulty learning to read. All individuals with dyslexia have difficulty learning to read, but not all individuals with severe reading problems are dyslexic. The problem is made more confusing by the fact that dyslexia is included as a specific learning disability by definition in federal legislation (IDEA). Nevertheless, the special needs of students with dyslexia warrant discussion of the disorder apart from other reading and learning disabilities.

Attention deficit/hyperactivity disorder has also been classified by federal law as a specific disorder that warrants special educational services. Until 1991, ADHD had not been included among the disorders considered as learning disabilities. Having at least normal intelligence, children with ADHD often did not receive special services until they began to fail in school and were subsequently designated as being learning disabled, or became so disruptive in school that they were designated as having a behavioral or emotional disorder. Attentional deficits are often observed among the behaviors of children with learning disabilities, and all children with attentional deficits have problems learning. However, all children with learning disabilities do not have an attention deficit/hyperactivity disorder. The effects of the attentional problems of children with ADHD are pervasive in that they interfere with learning across activities and environments. In many cases, severe impulsivity compounds the learning problems of these children. ADHD also can be considered a pragmatic disorder with serious social and emotional ramifications. For these reasons, ADHD will be considered separately from other attentional learning disabilities.

Children with nonverbal information processing disorder have severe pragmatic deficits. The ramifications of this disorder are pervasive in that it not only affects pragmatic and social development, but causes serious academic problems in all content areas. Another distinguishing characteristic is **dyscalculia** which is a severe deficit in mathematical concepts and difficulty acquiring arithmetic computation skills. The disorder is also referred to as right hemispheric dysfunction and social imperception disorder. These students' difficulties are exacerbated in regular classrooms because of the linguistic demands in content areas.

Language disorders underlie all three unique learning difficulties. These difficulties can be addressed appropriately when they are anticipated and understood. Chapter 9 seeks to describe the nature of language disorders associated with these unique learning difficulties:

1. dyslexia;

2. attention deficit/hyperactivity disorder; and

3. nonverbal information processing disorder.

DYSLEXIA

Dyslexia is characterized by extreme difficulty in learning to read and spell words despite continuous and specially designed instruction. This disorder is not attributable to intellectual deficit. Individuals with dyslexia are often extraordinarily gifted and highly intelligent. Dyslexia is associated with brain dysfunction and neurological anomalies. The disorder is considered to be congenital and also persists through adulthood (Aaron and Phillips, 1986; Forrell and Hood, 1985; Frauenheim and Heckerl, 1983; Read and Ruyter, 1985).

Language Processing Deficits Underlying Dyslexia

Although language deficits are associated with all reading disabilities, the degree and specificity of language processing deficits characterize dyslexia. The deficits are pervasive in that they affect all activities and all areas of development—academic, social, and emotional. The difficulties that individuals with dyslexia experience are manifested in several distinct levels of language processing: auditory perception, phonological awareness, word recognition, phonetic short-term memory, listening comprehension, general information base, reading comprehension, and written expression.

Auditory Perception

Dyslexia is most often characterized by severe deficits in auditory perception, specifically in the individual's ability to analyze the sounds of speech for these purposes:

1. to discriminate sounds within words;

2. to isolate a sound or sound combination from others;

3. to detect the similarities between sounds in words that rhyme; and

4. to determine which of the specific sounds in words such as "mat" and "bat" differ and which are the same.

All of the above are auditory perceptual abilities, specifically related to discrimination of speech sounds in oral language.

Phonological Awareness

The term *phonological awareness*, as described previously with regard to preschoolers, is quite different from the term as it is used to describe a reader who is attempting to decode the written word. In this context , the term refers to the skills of analyzing, manipulating, blending, synthesizing, and segmenting the phonological elements of spoken language in a written form.

Individuals with dyslexia have been observed to be lacking sensitivity or awareness of speech sounds of the language. They have difficulty perceiving similarities or differences between speech sounds and have difficulty separating the sounds within words (Aaron, Kuchta, and Grapethin, 1988; Brady and Fowler, 1988; Catts, 1989a, 1989b; Doehring, Trites, Patel, and Fiederowicz, 1981; Fox and Routh, 1983; Mann, 1991; Vellutino and Scanlon, 1988). No differences have been found between children with dyslexia and those without dyslexia in perception of nonverbal, environmental sounds (Brady, Shankweiler, and Mann, 1983; Godfrey, Syrdal-Lasky, Millaj, and Knox, 1981). Only verbal stimuli seem to be problematic.

Children with dyslexia are often identified when they begin to learn to read and are being taught how to decode words phonetically. They must recognize individual phonemes that comprise spoken words before they can assign a phoneme to a corresponding graphic symbol or letter. Written words are symbols that represent the phonemes of spoken language (i.e., the vowels and the consonants).

Children with dyslexia reveal extreme difficulty breaking down words into their component parts and blending these parts together to pronounce them and to form recognizable words.

Some children and adults with dyslexia tend to reverse and transpose letters and words. Spelling is a source of frustration throughout their lives. Dyslexic spellers have problems that either reflect deficits in sound-symbol association, short-term memory deficits regarding the sequence of letters and the visual configuration of words with irregular, nonphonetic spelling patterns, or a combination of both (Boder and Jarrico, 1982). Spelling problems of individuals with dyslexia persist into adulthood (Aaron and Phillips, 1986; Cone, Wilson, Bradley, and Reese, 1985; Ganschow, 1984; Kitz and Tarver, 1989).

Word Recognition

Children with dyslexia have difficulty acquiring word-recognition skills. When attempting to decode words that have irregular spelling patterns or to recognize familiar sight words (e.g., night, was), children are required to remember the configuration and the mental image of the word. At the same time, most readers use silent speech (inner language) to say the word to themselves. Children with dyslexia have difficulty acquiring word recognition skills and are slow when recalling the spoken representations of the written words (Catts, 1989a). When having to decode a word phonetically, children with dyslexia struggle to assign a phoneme to a letter or letters, blend the speech sounds together, and recognize that the printed letters, when combined in a particular sequence, represent a familiar spoken word.

Phonetic Short-Term Memory

The inability to hold letter strings, word strings, and sentences in short-term memory has been shown to predict reading disability (Mann and Liberman, 1984). Individuals with dyslexia reveal severe deficits in this ability (Mann and Liberman, 1984). When trying to remember a string of printed words, most people will recode the words into silent speech. They remember the consonants and vowels that form the name of each item rather than the visual shape of the letters or the shape of the words.

Individuals with dyslexia do not use silent speech to hold the words in short-term memory (i.e., rehearsal strategy). They seem to have extreme difficulty holding sentences in memory long enough to make sense of them. They have no difficulty remembering nonlinguistic items, such as faces or designs that have no verbal labels (Katz, Shankweiler, and Liberman 1981; Liberman, Mann, Shankweiler, and Werfelman, 1982).

Listening Comprehension

Individuals with dyslexia are found to have deficits in listening comprehension (Byrne, 1981). However, their difficulties are not thought to be due to deficits in syntax or in the understanding of complex sentences. Their problems are thought to involve retention of sufficient words to understand sentences and whole thoughts expressed verbally or in written form (Clark, 1988; Mann, 1991). They have difficulty remembering lengthy sentences (Catts, 1989b).

General Information-Based Reading Comprehension Deficits

Some of the comprehension problems of children with dyslexia have been attributed to a lack of a strong knowledge or information base due to limited reading experience (Stanovich, 1985; Torgesen, 1985). Compounding the problem is a tendency of poor readers to use the text inefficiently. They cannot decode many of the words they encounter, so they rely on the few words in the sentence or paragraph that they can read. They use these words as clues to help themselves comprehend the context and then try to associate these isolated concepts with some related known information (Maria and MacGinitie, 1982). When unable to find familiar words they can use as anchors, they skip large portions of the text and draw inaccurate conclusions without expanding upon information they already know.

Poor verbal memory again interferes when students with dyslexia must cope with written material that contains less redundancy and more complex syntax than is heard in oral communications (Maria and MacGinitie, 1982). While readers with dyslexia must rely on context for meaning, they often cannot comprehend the text because they have a poor information base due to lack of reading experience. They also may have a poor vocabulary because they do not read.

Written Expression

The spelling difficulties of individuals with dyslexia contribute to their severe problems with written expression. They are so caught up in the spelling of words that they lose fluency of thought. They also reveal word-retrieval problems indicated by circumlocutions (e.g., "it meows, it has whiskers, it's furry and cute . . . you know") (Brady and Fowler, 1988; Wagner and Torgesen, 1987). "Poor written expression is one of the distinguishing characteristics of the adolescent with dyslexia" (Clark, 1988, p. 25). Their writing samples are filled with poor punctuation, word omissions, grammatical errors, and poorly organized sentences. Their dictated stories often contain fewer grammatical errors than those written by hand or typed on a word processor (MacArthur and Graham, 1988). Typing or writing requires the integration of motor, perceptual, and sensory systems. The use of inner language and phonological memory is involved, as well.

Etiology

It is generally agreed that dyslexia is due to neurological anomalies. Sophisticated technology (e.g., CT [computed tomography], MRI [magnetic resonance imaging], and BEAM [brain electrical activity mapping]) enables researchers to study the neurological activity of the brain as an individual is reading. These techniques have contributed greatly to our understanding of the reading process, both normal and abnormal.

Anatomical studies have been conducted at Harvard Medical School, Department of Neurology, and the Dyslexia Neuroanatomical Laboratory at Beth Israel Hospital in Boston, Massachusetts, where a "brain bank" was established in 1982 by the Orton Dyslexia Society. Findings by Galaburda (1983, 1985, 1989) suggest that dyslexia is caused by abnormal prenatal development of the areas of the cortex where language, reading, and writing are usually processed (Hynd and Semrud-Clikeman, 1989). Also reported were abnormalities of neurological pathways that carry visual stimuli to the visual cortex of the brain ("Dyslexia's cause," 1987; "Study links," 1991). Other studies revealed a genetic basis for dyslexia (DeFries and Decker, 1982; Lewitter, DeFries, and Elston, 1980).

Long-Range View

Whether dyslexia is caused by brain abnormalities, heredity, or neurological anomalies, the teacher is concerned with the language deficits that reveal themselves in the classroom and the emotional damage to the intelligent student who does not learn to read.

A number of remedial techniques are used for teaching decoding, oral reading skills, and spelling skills to students with dyslexia, including the Orton-Gillingham Method, the Glass Analysis Method, the Slingerland Multisensory Approach, the Fernold Method, the Orton-based multisensory total language arts program, the Writing Road to Reading, and the use of micro-computer technology. With appropriate support systems by qualified reading teachers, learning disabilities specialists, and speech-language pathologists, students with dyslexia do learn to read and spell with relative success. Their skills are usually not as proficient as persons who do not have dyslexia (Catts, 1989b). Speech sound awareness might be improved somewhat by reading, since reading experience has been found to substantially increase this skill (Liberman, Rubin, Duques, and Carlisle, 1985; Read, Zhang, Nie, and Ding, 1986). However, long-range studies reveal that the language processing disorder that most often underlies dyslexia continues to manifest itself in other ways throughout school years and adulthood (Blalock, 1982; Campbell and Butterworth, 1985).

Dyslexia becomes more pervasive as the child grows older, affecting academic, social, and emotional development. It is important for educators to anticipate problems in many areas of functioning as the child grows older. The underlying linguistic processing deficits of individuals with dyslexia must be addressed. There is a tendency to retract the services of the speech-language pathologist for students in the higher grades. A student with dyslexia requires this service especially in the higher grades when the linguistic demands are greatest.

Lindamood, Bell, and Lindamood (1992) reported that an alarming number of adults involved in teaching have phonological processing dysfunction, and some have moderate to severe degrees of dysfunction. These teachers are generally not identified, yet are teaching, testing, or remediating students with reading difficulties. The ramifications of this finding with regard to students with dyslexia and other serious reading disabilities warrants investigation.

ATTENTION DEFICIT/HYPERACTIVITY DISORDER (ADHD)

Attention deficit/hyperactivity disorder is a neurological disorder that is characterized by three types of behaviors: 1. excessive motor activity (hyperactivity); 2. inability to focus and sustain attention to specific stimuli while disregarding irrelevant stimuli (distractibility); and 3. inability to use inner language to reflect on possible responses before acting on a stimulus (impulsivity).

Criteria for Diagnosis

ADHD is also considered a syndrome (i.e., a collection of behaviors or symptoms that are prevalent among a particular population of children and adults). The syndrome is described in the American Psychiatric Association (1987) publication, *Diagnostic Statistical Manual of Mental Disorders, 3rd edition, Revised (DSM-III-R)*. In that publication, criteria were established for identification of children with attention deficit/hyperactivity disorder. Prior to 1987, the syndrome had been called attention deficit disorder (ADD), with and without the presence of hyperactivity. When the disorder was renamed attention deficit/hyperactivity disorder, the child with the disorder who was not hyperactive was included under the separate category of "Undifferentiated Attention Deficit Disorder" (UADD).

Because of criticism regarding the lack of distinction between the two patterns of behavior (i.e., ADHD and UADD), the 1993 draft for DSM-IV-R contains separate categories: "Attention-deficit/Hyperactivity Disorder, Predominantly Inattentive Type," "Attention-deficit/Hyperactivity Disorder, Predominantly Hyperactive-Impulsive Type," and "Attention-deficit/Hyperactivity Disorder, Combined Type." These classifications are indeed important because, as mentioned previously, there is currently no specific category under which a child with this disorder can receive greatly needed special services. Also, unless there is clear distinction between children who are inattentive and distractable without ADHD and children who are inattentive and distractable with ADHD, an appropriate educational program cannot be designed for either group. In this chapter, children with and without hyperactivity will be discussed separately for the sake of clarity.

Table 9.1 presents the final draft criteria for ADHD proposed by the American Psychiatric Association (1993). As detailed in the table, children exhibiting at least 6 of the 9 symptoms listed under A(1) can be classified as having Attention-deficit/Hyperactivity

Disorder, Predominantly Inattentive Type. Children exhibiting at least 6 of the 9 symptoms listed under A(2) can be classified as having Attention-deficit/Hyperactivity Disorder, Predominantly Hyperactive-Impulsive Type. Children exhibiting at least 6 of the 9 symptoms under A(1) and 6 of the 9 symptoms under A(2) can be classified as having Attention-deficit/Hyperactivity Disorder, Combined Type. Children who have attentional deficits or symptoms of hyperactivity-impulsivity but do not meet the criteria for Attention Deficit/Hyperactivity Disorder described in Table 9.1 are classified in the 1993 DSM-IV Draft Criteria as Attention-deficit/Hyperactivity Disorder Not Otherwise Specified. Children who have attentional deficits but not to the degree described in the DSM-IV Draft, should be assessed for possible learning disabilities, particularly if these symptoms are not pervasive and appear during specific activities and in school, but not at home.

Table 9.1

Final DSM-IV Draft Criteria for Attention Deficit/Hyperactivity Disorder

A. Either 1 or 2:

1. Inattention: At least six of the following symptoms of inattention have persisted for at least six months to a degree that is maladaptive and inconsistent with developmental level:

   a. often fails to give close attention to details or makes careless mistakes in schoolwork, work, or other activities.

   b. often has difficulty sustaining attention in tasks or play activities

   c. often does not seem to listen to what is being said to him or her

   d. often does not follow through on instructions and fails to finish schoolwork, chores, or duties in the workplace (not due to oppositional behavior or failure to understand instructions)

   e. often has difficulties organizing tasks and activities

   f. often avoids or strongly dislikes tasks (such as schoolwork or homework) that require sustained mental effort

   g. often loses things necessary for tasks or activities (e.g., school assignments, pencils, books, tools, or toys)

Continued

Table 9.1—*Continued*

        h. is often easily distracted by extraneous stimuli

        i. often forgetful in daily activities

2. Hyperactivity-Impulsivity: At least six of the following symptoms of hyper-activity-impulsivity have persisted for at least six months to a degree that is maladaptive and inconsistent with developmental level:

Hyperactivity:

        a. often fidgets with hands or feet or squirms in seat

        b. leaves seat in classroom or in other situations in which remaining seated is expected

        c. often runs about or climbs excessively in situations where it is inappropriate (in adolescents or adults, may be limited to subjective feelings of restlessness)

        d. often has difficulty playing or engaging in leisure activities quietly

        e. often talks excessively

        f. often acts as if "driven by a motor" and cannot remain still

Impulsivity

        g. often blurts out answers to questions before the questions have been completed

        h. often has difficulty waiting in lines or awaiting turn in games or group situations

        i. often interrupts or intrudes on others

B. Onset no later than seven years of age.

C. Symptoms must be present in two or more situations (e.g., at school, work, and at home).

D. The disturbance causes clinically significant distress or impairment in social, academic, or occupational functioning.

E. Does not occur exclusively during the course of a Pervasive Developmental Disorder, Schizophrenia, or other Psychotic Disorder, and is not better accounted for by a Mood Disorder, Anxiety Disorder, Dissociative Disorder, or a Personality Disorder.

Code based on type:

    314.00 Attention-deficit/Hyperactivity Disorder, Predominantly Inattentive Type: if criterion A(1) is met but not criterion A(2) for the past six months.

    314.01 Attention-deficit/Hyperactivity Disorder, Predominantly Hyperactive-Impulsive Type: if criterion A(2) is met but not criterion A(1) for the past six months

Continued

Table 9.1—*Continued*

314.01 Attention-deficit/Hyperactivity Disorder, Combined Type: if both criterion A(1) and A(2) are met for the past six months

Coding note: for individuals (especially adolescents and adults) who currently have symptoms that no longer meet full criteria, "in partial remission" should be specified.

314.9 Attention-deficit/Hyperactivity Disorder Not Otherwise Specified This category is for disorders with prominent symptoms of attention-deficit or hyperactivity-impulsivity that do not meet criteria for Attention-deficit/Hyperactivity Disorder.

From *DSM-IV Draft Criteria (3/1/93)* by the American Psychiatric Association, 1993, Washington, DC: APA. ©1993 by the American Psychiatric Association. Reprinted by permission.

Even though learning disabilities and attention deficit/hyperactivity disorder are often present in the same child, "attention disorders and learning disabilities are distinct problems" (Conti, 1991, p. 94). They are currently considered two separate disorders (Shaywitz and Shaywitz, 1988). Silver (1990) also suggests that ADHD should be considered as a separate entity, different from learning disabilities. He argues that ADHD does not interfere with the necessary psychological processes needed to learn. ADHD interferes with the individual's "availability" for learning.

Prevalence

It is estimated that attention deficit/hyperactivity disorder affects 10%–20% of the school-age population (Shaywitz and Shaywitz, 1988). The prevalence is three times more common in boys than girls (Conti, 1991). Underidentification of girls with ADHD is becoming a major concern (Shaywitz and Shaywitz, 1988).

Categories of ADHD Language and Behavior Characteristics

Attention Deficit/Hyperactive Disorder Without Hyperactivity (Predominantly Inattentive Type)

Girls are more frequently included among the group of children with attention deficit/hyperactivity disorder who are not hyperactive. Research results indicate that children having ADHD without hyperactivity demonstrate significantly different behavioral, academic, and social patterns from those with characteristics of hyperactivity and impulsivity (Shaywitz and Shaywitz, 1988). Although they reveal attentional problems similar to those of boys with ADHD, girls are less intrusive and exhibit fewer aggressive symptoms.

These youngsters often appear passive and can go for long periods of time without movement. They are often described as "dreamers." However, they do not sustain attention to any topic for more than a few moments. They may not move, but their eyes dart from one object to another. They do not seem to know what is going on and do not remember instructions by the teacher. They rarely smile and do not enjoy interaction with other children; they are often socially withdrawn. They do not cause any trouble for the teacher, are not disruptive in class, and are less likely to be diagnosed or receive special educational services. Children with attention deficits without hyperactivity may represent an underidentified, under-served group of children who are at significant risk for long-term academic, social, and emotional difficulties (Berry, Shaywitz, and Shaywitz, 1985; Sandoval and Lambert, 1984; Shaywitz and Shaywitz, 1988).

Attention Deficit/Hyperactivity Disorder with Hyperactivity (Predominantly Hyperactive-Impulsive Type)

Reports by parents and reports in the literature (Ross and Ross, 1982) describe infants who were hyperactive while still in utero and who are "squirmers and screamers" from birth. One longitudinal study (Campbell, Breaux, Ewing, and Szumowski, 1986) reported that high-risk toddlers often demonstrate a number of problems including inattention, impulsivity, disobedience, and aggression through the preschool years. Richman, Stevenson, and Graham (1982) found that family stress can exacerbate the child's behavior.

Ironically, the child's behavior often exacerbates the family's stress. The stress of the school environment exacerbates all the behaviors listed above. Hyperactive children are indeed a disruptive influence in the classroom (Cohen, Sullivan, Minde, Novak, and Helwig, 1981).

Hyperactive infants do not develop turn-taking skills and close interrelationships with adults. They do not sustain face-to-face interaction with the unique gaze of young infants. Most likely, they do not sustain attention long enough to discriminate or imitate the facial expressions or gestures of their caregivers. They do not learn to relate emotions and feelings to facial expressions in others and in themselves. They are unaware of others' feelings.

The children with attention deficit/hyperactivity disorder with hyperactivity are always moving or climbing or fidgeting, often disrupting activities and damaging anything and anyone in their path. These are sad and unhappy children, who rarely smile, cry easily, and are fearful, irritable, often out of control, and easily frustrated.

Children with ADHD are easily distracted and have difficulty concentrating on schoolwork. Thoughts are disorganized; information that is learned is incomplete. Impulsivity is also a striking characteristic of the youngster with ADHD, who often acts without thinking and frequently interrupts the class. The child often speaks out impulsively and at inappropriate times (Atkins, Pelham, and Licht, 1985; Shaywitz and Shaywitz, 1988). There is need for a great deal of supervision because the child can suddenly dash across the room to retrieve something that is momentarily interesting, oblivious of other children or adults who are engaged in activities. There is little or no control, and it is almost impossible for the child to wait a turn in games or group activities.

The hyperactive child's ability to form and maintain friendships is greatly impaired. Pragmatic abilities are seriously disordered. They are often aggressive and intrusive and annoy their peers. They have difficulty empathizing with people in their personal relationships.

They also cannot understand characters in a story who are unhappy, embarrassed, or frightened. They do not focus or attend to tones of voice, stress of words, or inflections in the utterances spoken by others. They are not aware that they have angered or annoyed their peers, for example, until they are literally knocked down. They are usually disliked and rejected by their peers.

Although the child with ADHD is often observed to talk a great deal, the quality of the spoken language is poor with regard to sentence complexity, appropriateness, relevance of utterances, and richness of vocabulary. Inability to focus attention and sustain attention to a whole communication interferes with the acquisition of new information. The child does not complete a communication or sustain attention long enough to listen to a complete thought expressed by the speaker. There is little or no concern for the listener's needs. The child is intrusive and does not read "privacy markers" (e.g., "back away, you are in my private space," "leave me alone"). This child typically has no friends and is not welcome in any group activity.

Children with ADHD are often observed asking questions, but not for the purpose of clarification. The questions often indicate clearly that the child has no idea of the topic of conversation or instruction. Children with ADHD speak in phrases or broken-off sentences. They often do not complete an utterance because they are so easily distracted by the slightest noise or movement. Children with this disorder have not learned and often never learn the communicative rules established for a particular classroom. They do not seem to know when to speak and when to listen. They frequently call out or raise their hands to ask questions that have no relevance to the discussions going on at the moment. They impulsively respond to the teacher's questions without having listened to or accurately processed the questions. Children with ADHD often fail in school, fail in interpersonal relationships, and fail in their relationships with their family members.

Intervention Planning: Emphasis on Underlying Deficits

Certain inferences can be drawn from the research findings described earlier in this chapter and in previous chapters regarding potential language deficits of children with attention deficit/hyperactivity disorder. Basic concept development requires ability to focus on attributes of objects, people, and events. Lack of selective attention will probably result in the child's attending to irrelevant stimuli, often at the expense of relevant stimuli. Deferred imitation, object constancy, object permanence, and means-ends behaviors all require selective attention, ability to focus, and ability to sustain attention (see Chapter 3). The child stores the irrelevant or incomplete stimuli in memory in a disorganized, "bits and pieces" fashion. There may be little attempt to classify, categorize, or expand on concepts already formed. The information that is stored in memory by a child with ADHD will probably be inadequate and not organized in an efficient manner that allows for easy accessibility.

The child with ADHD is easily distracted so that information acquisition is spotty and incomplete. As a result, the child will probably have an inadequate information base and limited general world knowledge. Vocabulary may remain concrete and inflexible. Narrative ability (oral and written) may also be deficient.

Teachers should anticipate that children with ADHD will have specific problems related to learning to decode, reading comprehension, and problem-solving ability, all of which require the ability to focus, select details and information worthy of processing, sustain attention, and store newly acquired information in an organized manner. Educational placements and management techniques are the same as for students with learning disabilities, or emotional or behavioral problems (Silver, 1990). Evidence indicates that cognitive behavior modification techniques may be effective in improving sustained attention, impulse control, hyperactivity, and self-concept (Fiore, Becker, and Nero, 1993). (See Chapter 8.) Educational intervention, however, must be based on the individual child's specific needs.

Although the disorder may change in its manifestations as the child matures, "it does not go away" (Shaywitz and Shaywitz, 1991). Overall, studies indicate that adolescents and adults continue to have many of the same symptoms they had when they were young children, i.e., inattention, restlessness, fidgetiness, impulsivity, poor self-esteem, and difficulties establishing social relationships (Weiss, Hechtman, Milroy, and Perlman, 1985). The language deficits caused by an attentional disorder remain long after the hyperactivity subsides.

ADHD Services Clarified

In PL 94-142, attention deficit/hyperactivity disorder was not classified as a disorder and did not entitle students to special services. Children had to fail in academic subjects to the extent that the discrepancy between their intellectual potential and their academic performance was significant enough to fulfill the requirements for classification as learning disabled or their behaviors deviant enough to be labeled emotionally or behaviorally disordered. Only then could their underlying linguistic, conceptual, and cognitive deficits be addressed.

On September 16, 1991, a clarification policy memorandum was released by the U.S. Department of Education. The memorandum

- clarified the circumstances under which children with ADHD are eligible for special educational services under Part B of IDEA and the requirements for evaluation of such children's unique educational needs;

- clarified the responsibilities of local education agencies to provide appropriate regular and special educational services to those children with ADHD who are not eligible under Part B, but who fall within the definition of "handicapped person" under Section 504 of the Rehabilitation Act of 1973; and

- distinguished ADHD from other disabilities, such as specific learning disabilities or seriously emotionally disturbed, while reiteration the current legal requirement that children with both ADHD and any other Part B disability receive appropriate educational services to meet the needs of each disability.

Congress and the U.S. Education Department recognize the need to provide information and assistance to teachers, administrators, parents, and other interested persons regarding the identification, evaluation, and instructional needs of children with ADHD. Funds have been appropriated by Congress to implement these programs.

NONVERBAL INFORMATION PROCESSING DISORDER

Children with nonverbal information processing disorder do not interpret the nonverbal, paralinguistic information, such as tone of voice, inflection, intensity of voice, and all the indicators of emotion embedded within the voice. In addition, they have great difficulty determining the significance of facial expression and body posture of others that carry essential communicative information. The deficit is not in perception of faces, but rather in the identification of expression (Borod, Koff, and Caron, 1983). They experience difficulty on tasks requiring the matching of facial expressions or gestures with verbal content (Ozols and Rourke, 1985). They also do not respect personal space between themselves and other people.

In a number of studies by Byron Rourke and his colleagues (Ozols and Rourke, 1985; Rourke, 1982, 1989; Rourke and Strang, 1983; Strang and Rourke, 1983, 1985), the term **nonverbal perceptual-organizational-output disability (NPOOD)** was used to refer to children who have well-developed, rote verbal abilities and adequate word recognition, decoding, and spelling skills. However, they exhibit severe social interactional problems with their peers.

Research by Bender and Golden (1990), Korhonen (1991), and Van der Vlugt (1991) supports the classification of a subtype such as NPOOD. Semrud-Clikeman and Hynd (1990) suggest that "nonverbal disorders may be more handicapping than verbal learning disabilities, as verbal deficits have little effect on nonverbal experience, but nonverbal deficits may make major contributions to the mis-reading of verbalization" (p. 198). Children with nonverbal infor-mation processing disorder are almost always labeled "learning dis-abled," "language disordered," "behaviorally disordered," or a com-bination of these. Research seems to indicate that the problems are most likely present from birth and become more and more appar-ent as the child develops (Semrud-Clikeman and Hynd, 1990; Strang and Rourke, 1983, 1985).

Preschool Years

In the histories of these students, as provided by their parents, they are described as speaking early and using adult-like language at very early ages (Foss, 1991). They all revealed at early ages clear indications of severe visual perceptual deficits. Parents reported that they rarely played with puzzles, blocks, or construction-type toys. They revealed poor perception of space and were clumsy, with poor gross and fine motor control. Their histories also revealed social problems even as toddlers.

Elementary School Years

When these children enter school, they do well in word reading, decoding, and spelling, but they have difficulty learning to write, and their handwriting is barely legible. They lack appropriate facial expression denoting feelings and emotions. Their voices tend to have a monotonic and expressionless quality. They speak a great deal, but the quality of their expressive language is immature. They do not understand humor and are oversensitive to criticism (Foss, 1991).

Because of their visual and spatial perceptual deficits, they probably perceive their world in a distorted fashion. Their basic concepts are inadequate and inaccurate. They do not benefit as well as they should from past experiences and do not have an adequate information base (Rourke, 1982). They have difficulty applying what they have learned from past experiences to novel and different situations.

These students have difficulty describing their experiences in oral and written narratives. They often have difficulty retrieving *specific* words and phrases to describe events and situations in their narratives. Descriptions of characters' actions, motives, and emotions quickly reveal their lack of empathy and understanding of social relationships. If they cannot understand the feelings, relationships, and cause-effect aspects of their own actions, they will not understand these factors in fictional stories.

Severe Pragmatic Deficits

The primary problem of children with nonverbal information processing disorder is their inability to interact with others and establish friendships. They hurt and distress people inadvertently because they cannot read nonverbal messages. They do not know how to initiate a conversation, how to uphold the communicant's role in maintaining a conversation, and how to repair a conversation that has broken down. They do not assess novel situations and adapt quickly to them. They do not have the social skills necessary to conform to the demands of different contexts and different social requirements. Most important, they are not aware of the needs of other people and give the impression that they do not care about those needs.

The fact that they are very verbal and express themselves fairly well orally hides a multitude of problems (Thompson, 1985). They have strong decoding skills and word recognition skills, but when they reach the higher elementary grades, they often begin to fail, particularly in reading comprehension, written expression, and in many specific content areas. Mathematics continues to elude them. Their handwriting remains unintelligible. They are not able to excel in sports because of their awkwardness and spatial perceptual deficits.

Junior High School and High School Years

In junior high and high school, they continue to write illegibly and slowly. They have difficulty with note taking. They continue to perform poorly in all content areas, despite their apparent verbal language ability. They usually begin to fail at this academic level. The greater linguistic demands, memory requirements, and attentional requirements become overwhelming. They are less and less able to adapt to novel situations and the social responsibilities that accompany these situations. At a time when peer acceptance is especially important, they continue to have few, if any, friends because of their inability to "read" the nonverbal clues indicating distress, annoyance, or sadness.

Early Identification

Rourke (1989) stresses that students with the symptoms and behaviors described reveal the syndrome of right hemispheric dysfunction. Visual/spatial perceptual information, mathematical concepts, and nonverbal, paralinguistic information have been shown to be processed in the right hemisphere, whereas verbal information, written and oral, is usually processed in the left hemisphere of the brain by most individuals. In addition, "the ability to recognize and identify emotion in others as well as in ourselves, to control and stimulate motivation, to sustain attention to a task, to control our moods, to understand the emotional impact of events upon ourselves and others, and to interpret emotional experiences and keep them in proper perspective, are all controlled by the right hemisphere of the human brain" (Ratner, 1991, p. 372). In studies by Badian (1986, 1992), children with suspected right hemispheric dysfunction who were referred for brain electrical activity mapping (BEAM) revealed abnormal right hemispheric activity. Interestingly, 50% of the children in Rourke's study who exhibited this particular type of learning disability were females, a distinct difference from the usual 4:1 incidence in favor of males that is apparent in other types of learning disabilities (Rourke, 1982).

Because of their verbal strengths and their at least normal intelligence, they are good candidates for cognitive behavior modification techniques described in Chapter 8. There is no question of their need for psychological counseling and for intervention by teachers with special training in learning disabilities. However, these desperately needed services will have to wait until these children with a nonverbal information processing disorder begin to fail in content areas. Only then can they be classified with a definable learning disability and be eligible for appropriate special education services (Badian, 1986). Despite their oral language "abilities," they would also benefit from the services of the speech-language pathologist with regard to their superficial verbiage and nonverbal language deficits.

Long-range research studies are revealing that individuals with nonverbal information processing disorder are at high risk for severe depression (Rourke, Young, and Leenaars, 1989; Semrud-Clikeman and Hynd, 1990). Waiting for the child to fail in school, in social interactions, in development of self-esteem and estimation of self-worth exacerbate the situation. Early identification and intervention are vital.

SUMMARY

Three neurologically based disorders have been described in this chapter—dyslexia, attention deficit/hyperactivity disorder, and nonverbal information processing disorder. The latter two of the three disorders are not included under any legal classification that entitles the student to the special services they need.

Dyslexia was defined as a specific learning disability in PL 94-142 and IDEA, but was not clearly differentiated from other reading disabilities. In fact, it is a unique language-based, severe reading disorder requiring specialized intervention techniques. These remedial techniques are different from those that are appropriate for other severe reading disabilities.

Children with ADHD are eligible for special education services under Part B of IDEA. ADHD is distinguished from other Part B disabilities, such as specific learning disabilities and emotional disorders. Each disability must receive appropriate educational services. Children with ADHD who do not meet the requirements for services under Part B of IDEA may fall within the definition of "handicapped person" under Section 504 of the Rehabilitation Act of 1973.

Nonverbal information processing disorder is not classified as a specific disorder. Often, the symptoms can be identified early, despite the presence of verbal "ability." The children's social imperception, their poor coordination, their lack of empathy, their insensitivity to the feelings and needs of others, and the lack of emotion in their affect are obvious even as toddlers. These children require very specific intervention strategies. They have been shown to benefit from cognitive behavior modification techniques. They require intensive language intervention despite their superficial verbiage. There is presently no legal classification entitling them to these necessary services. They, too, have to fail to be classified as "learning disabled." Their self-esteem is dangerously low because they are socially unsuccessful. Failure can only add to their severe depression and feelings of worthlessness.

Individuals with any of these three disorders have been shown to be high risk for severe depression. Early identification and appropriate intervention can prevent far-reaching, damaging effects.

SUGGESTED READINGS

Barkley, R. (1990). *Attention-deficit Hyperactivity Disorder: A Handbook for Diagnosis and Treatment.* New York: Guilford.

Valletutti, P., and Dummett, L. (1992). *Cognitive Development: A Functional Approach.* San Diego, CA: Singular Publishing Group.

Thomson, M., and Watkins, E. (1990). *Dyslexia: A Teaching Handbook.* London: Whurr Publishers.

10 THE NATURE OF LANGUAGE DISORDERS AMONG CHILDREN WITH COGNITIVE DISABILITIES

Mental retardation is a disorder affecting cognitive (i.e., intellectual) functioning and **adaptive behavior,** or the ability to adjust to new and novel situations. The more current terminology, *cognitive disabilities* and *developmentally delayed*, is used in this textbook. The quality of overall functioning can differ greatly among individuals, ranging from those who do not respond to any extraneous stimuli and who do not express any language to those who speak and function in regular classrooms and in regular jobs, although their language skills are depressed. The latter group comprises approximately 80–90 percent of the population with cognitive deficits (Grossman, 1983).

In the past, individuals with cognitive disabilities were grouped together under two general categories: They were considered either *educable* with limitations or *trainable* for limited adaptation in the community. Their deficits were not expected to improve appreciably during their lifetime, and educators had low expectations which were reflected in the restricted goals of the special educational programs designed for this population. Many moderately and severely retarded individuals were placed in institutions (Schiefelbusch, 1993). Others were placed in programs segregated from the nondisabled school population.

Extensive research has been conducted in the past twenty years, and some important changes have taken place with regard to expectations and attitudes toward individuals with cognitive disabilities. As a result, language specialists have changed their priorities. Emphasis is being placed upon communicative needs that are relevant to the daily activities of children and adolescents with severe language deficits related to cognitive disabilities. There is also increasing awareness of the variation and range of capabilities.

Programming for individuals with cognitive disabilities has also changed due to provisions of PL 94-142 (IDEA). The least restrictive environment (LRE) provision requires that all children are to be educated with their peers to the "maximum extent possible." The child's academic and social strengths and individual needs should determine how much intervention should be provided within a "regular" classroom setting (McCormick and Schiefelbusch, 1990). Children who do not have disabilities can model age-appropriate social and communicative skills. Students with cognitive disabilities are no longer to be physically segregated from the total school population and their education is everyone's responsibility. (A full discussion of IDEA and LRE can be found in Chapter 15.)

Serious language deficits are indeed apparent among individuals with cognitive disabilities. The language disability is considered to be one of many "symptoms" of retardation (McCormick and Schiefelbusch, 1990). This is a more positive and constructive orientation that reflects the attitude that the symptoms of language deficit can be modified and improved. Intervention programs now emphasize communicative skills that are necessary to function in increasingly less restrictive environments (McCormick and Schiefelbusch, 1990). Artificial limitations on expectations of intellectual and social development are no longer acceptable.

When individuals with cognitive disabilities are given a means of expressing their feelings to others in their environment and learn how to indicate what they want to do, what they do not want to do, and what they need, they gain more control over their actions and do not have to resort to inappropriate behaviors to obtain these objectives. Research has also indicated that learned skills are retained longer and are more easily generalized to other related skills and contexts if they are taught in the course of "transactional" situations, that is, through interactions with other individuals in a natural environment and in the course of natural, not contrived, activities (Owens, 1989; Schiefelbusch, 1993). Highly structured settings do not encourage spontaneity and restrict opportunities for a variety of communicative interactions.

The severity and characteristics of language disorders among individuals with cognitive disabilities vary greatly. Chapter 10 describes the nature of language disorders among children with cognitive disabilities by

1. defining cognitive disabilities and components of the disorder and describing tools for determining the presence of this condition;

2. presenting factors known to cause cognitive disabilities;

3. examining basic cognitive skills of individuals with cognitive disabilities;

4. discussing language development in each component area and factors influencing a range of language abilities; and

5. providing alternative strategies for language intervention.

DEFINITION OF COGNITIVE DISABILITIES

The American Association on Mental Deficiency (AAMD) uses the term *mental retardation* and defines it very specifically as having at least 3 components:

1. significantly subaverage general intellectual functioning, with an IQ of 70 or below;

2. depressed ability to adjust or adapt to novel situations and achieve personal independence with respect to cultural expectations and chronological age; and

3. the existence of the condition during the developmental period (i.e., from birth to 18 years of age) (Grossman, 1983). For example, if an individual is functioning as though severely cognitively disabled after suffering a stroke or having been in an accident that caused trauma to the brain at the age of 25 years, the condition did not exist during the developmental period.

All three requirements must be met before the condition can be classified as "mental retardation" (Grossman, 1983).

Intellectual functioning is evaluated by standardized intelligence tests, such as the *Wechsler Preschool and Primary Scale of Intelligence (WPPSI)* (Wechsler, 1974a), *Wechsler Intelligence Scale for Children-Revised (WISC-R)* (Wechsler, 1974b), the *Wechsler Adult Intelligence Scale-Revised (WAIS-R)* (Wechsler, 1981), the *Leiter International Performance Scale* (Leiter, 1979), and the *Stanford-Binet Intelligence Scale* (Terman and Merrill, 1973). The IQ score alone is not sufficient to make a diagnosis of mental retardation because the performance by children and adults with language delays, regardless of the etiology, on currently used tests of intelligence do not always reflect their true intellectual ability (Miller, 1993). The IQs indicating retardation range from 55 to 70 (mild), 40 to 55 (moderate), 25 to 40 (severe), and below 25 (profound) (Grossman, 1983). There is a tremendous variation and range of intellectual ability within and among each of these categories.

Adaptive functioning is evaluated by the use of tests, such as the *Vineland Social Maturity Scale* (Doll, 1965), the *Vineland Adaptive Behavior Scale* (Sparrow, Balla, and Cicchetti, 1984), the *American Association on Mental Deficiency* (AAMD) *Adaptive Behavior Scale* (Nihira, Foster, Shellhaas, and Leland, 1974), and the *Cain-Levine Social Competency Scale* (Cain, Levine, and Elzey, 1963). In addition to these tests, there are numerous scales that evaluate skills considered to be appropriate for individuals of different ages. Adaptive functioning can be further evaluated by analyzing actual maladaptive behaviors (e.g., destructive, disruptive, or violent behaviors and/or self-injurious behaviors) (Schiefelbusch and Lloyd, 1988).

Informal Observations

Cognitive disability is considered "pervasive," in that it affects the individual's ability to function across all types of activities. This overall depressed functioning is quite different from learning disabilities, which are manifested in several, but not all areas of intellectual and social functioning. Individuals with learning disabilities function at normal and even superior levels of performance on tasks requiring specific abilities that are not depressed by neurological involvement. It should be noted that adaptive and social behaviors rely heavily on language skills. The results of tests administered by speech-language pathologists and their informal observations regarding linguistic knowledge and communicative abilities should be added to observations by parents, teachers, psychologists, and other professionals who observe and work with the student daily. All of this information must be carefully evaluated before a diagnosis of *cognitive disabilities* is made.

Hearing Loss

Although information processing takes place in the cortex of the brain, the information itself is first received through the primary senses (e.g., hearing, vision, touch, smell, and taste). The integrity of the bony and neural structures within the ear and the neurological system responsible for carrying the auditory stimulus in the form of electrical impulses to the brain is crucial for the development of speech and the acquisition of the verbal code used by individuals in a linguistic community. (The impact of hearing loss is discussed in detail in Chapter 12.)

Cognitive disabilities and sensorineural hearing loss have common etiologies (e.g., maternal rubella, Rh-incompatibility, meningitis, drugs and alcohol ingestion by pregnant mother, and child abuse).

The fact that there is a high incidence of sensorineural hearing loss among individuals with cognitive disabilities is no surprise. Audiological testing of children with cognitive disabilities can detect sensorineural hearing loss. Early detection and the use of amplification can ensure that language development will not be further impeded.

Studies of individuals with Down syndrome ranging from 2 months to 60 years indicate a high incidence of both sensorineural loss and hearing loss due to physiological abnormalities of the ear itself (Down, 1980; Carrow-Woolfolk and Lynch, 1982). The condition is rarely identified in early infancy because the speech of most of these children is seriously delayed and their verbal deficits are attributed to their cognitive disabilities. Only a small percentage of the children identified as having hearing loss receive amplification at an early age. Although it is difficult to administer audiological tests to individuals with cognitive disabilities, especially young children, present technology is capable of detecting middle and inner ear pathology in this population.

In addition to sensorineural loss, children with Down syndrome often have structural malformations of the face, head, and middle ear, and an abnormal alignment of the Eustachian tube, which encourages middle ear infection. *Otitis media,* a condition where fluid accumulates in the middle ear due to respiratory infections and allergies, is common among children with Down Syndrome. The resultant fluctuating hearing loss from otitis media should be anticipated in children with Down syndrome because of their common structural abnormalities. This condition, which hinders sensory reception, can be expected to significantly impede language and conceptual development.

ETIOLOGIES

Cognitive disabilities can be caused by many factors. An estimated 80 percent of retarded individuals have unknown etiologies (Scott, 1980).

Genetic Causes

Several hundred genetic disorders are associated with cognitive disabilities (Carrow-Woolfolk and Lynch, 1982). One genetic form of retardation is Down syndrome, which accounts for approximately 10% of all children diagnosed with mental retardation (Carrow-Woolfolk and Lynch, 1982). An extra set of genes on chromosome #21 or a chromosomal abnormality can cause *Down syndrome,* a condition resulting in cognitive disabilities, skeletal malformations, respiratory disorders, heart disorders, and hearing disorders. Degrees of intellectual functioning among individuals with Down syndrome can range from mild to moderate.

Another group of genetic disorders result in biochemical imbalance which in turn can cause damage to the brain. A disorder of this type is *phenylketonuria* (PKU). All newborn infants in neonatal nurseries in the United States are routinely screened for this disorder. The effects of PKU can be controlled by restricted diet, and cognitive disabilities can be prevented if the condition is identified.

Toxic Agents

Excessive exposure to or ingestion of lead or mercury can cause severe retardation and many other disorders in children. Drugs and alcohol are also suspected of causing serious brain damage in the unborn fetus (see Chapter 14 for a detailed discussion).

Viral Infections

The brain of the fetus begins to develop about 3 weeks after fertilization of the ovum. In the first trimester of pregnancy, the cortical development of the fetus is highly vulnerable to disease. Cognitive disabilities and other serious conditions can result if a pregnant woman contracts a disease, such as rubella (German measles), during this period of her pregnancy. Meningitis and encephalitis, viral diseases affecting the brain and its coverings, can also cause cognitive disabilities in children.

Developmental Delay

Sometimes there are no observable medical reasons to account for mild retardation. The *developmental theory* refers to a group of intellectually low-functioning children who are nonverbal or seriously language delayed. Included in this population are youngsters from impoverished learning environments and those who come from families with other intellectually low-functioning members. With appropriate language intervention and educational support, the language development of many of these children is observed to progress in a normal sequence, only at a slower rate (Zigler and Balla, 1982; Zigler and Hodapp, 1986).

COGNITION AND COGNITIVE DISABILITIES

As discussed in Chapter 3, some of the basic cognitive abilities that are important for learning and developing intellectually, socially, and emotionally, include the following:

- perception
- attention
- organization
- memory
- generalization

Perception

Visual and auditory perceptual learning disabilities can occur concomitantly with cognitive disabilities. A number of etiologies causing deficits in cognitive functioning also cause minimal damage to the areas of the cortex that process perceptual information. As a result, the child with retardation may perceive visual and auditory stimuli in a distorted fashion, further inhibiting conceptual development.

Attention

In general, individuals with cognitive disabilities have been found to have the capacity to attend to a task or to an event as well as nondisabled individuals of the same **mental age** (i.e., an expression of the developmental level of an individual that is characteristic of a particular chronological age, usually a younger child). However, persons with cognitive disabilities have difficulty selecting the relevant information that requires attention (Ford and Mirenda, 1984; Noonan and Siegel-Causey, 1990); they may scan an array of stimuli and focus indiscriminately and inconsistently, without considering whether they are relevant to the task at hand. Even when objects or aspects of an event are pointed out, children often have difficulty sustaining attention to these relevant aspects for the amount of time necessary to take appropriate action.

Organization of New Information

For learned information to be available for future need, it has to be stored in long-term memory in an organized fashion. For example, when young children with no disability encounter a ball, they store the concept of *ballness* into memory under categories such as *round things*, *things that roll*, and *things that bounce*. Every time a ball is encountered with a different attribute, such as color, size, surface texture, bouncability, or ownership (*Jimmy's ball, my ball*), the child adds the new information under the appropriate categories for future retrieval and expansion of meaning. Otherwise, every ball the child encounters would be considered a new entity, the child's memory capacity would be filled unnecessarily, and the child would not have easy access to the information as needed.

The child organizes concepts by categorizing them. In nondisabled children, this organization is learned from personal experience in different contexts. In addition, every language has rules that govern the way ideas can be categorized for the purpose of talking about them, and these rules vary across cultures (McCormick and Schiefelbusch, 1990). Children with cognitive disabilities usually are able to categorize concrete objects, such as a ball, but have great difficulty categorizing concepts that they cannot see or hold in their hands, such as love and other emotions, because they are abstract.

Long-Term Memory for Learned Information

Without selective attention to pertinent aspects of the task at hand, the child will have difficulty selecting similar information learned from past experiences (Meador, 1984; McCormick and Schiefelbusch, 1990). This is necessary if the new information is to be added in an organized fashion to knowledge already stored in long-term memory. In this way, knowledge is expanded, made accessible, retrieved, and generalized to new situations.

Individuals with mild and moderate cognitive disabilities can retain learned information in long-term memory if it is organized by the teacher first and explained explicitly (Merrill, 1985; Owens, 1989; Schiefelbusch, 1993). They learn slowly, and need more instruction and more practice to understand the task and learn what it is they have to do. Once they understand, they can learn the required skill and retain the information for later retrieval (McCormick and Schiefelbusch, 1990).

Short-Term Memory

Individuals with cognitive disabilities have been found to have poor short-term memories. They often have difficulty holding new information or a stream of instructions in mind long enough to act on them. Observations during research studies reveal that they do not use strategies to help themselves hold on to small bits of information for a short time. Strategies commonly used to retain information in short-term memory include (Gutowski and Chechile, 1987) the following:

1. *Rehearsal strategies*—repeating the information to oneself in silent language.

2. *Association strategies*—grouping words or thoughts according to relationships.

3. *Clustering strategies*—organizing nine items into 3-3-3 separate groups, which are easier to remember than a list of nine separate, unrelated items.

As is true for all individuals, persons with cognitive disabilities can improve short-term memory if taught to use such strategies (Burger, Blackman, and Tan, 1980; Reid, 1980; Turner and Bray, 1985).

Generalization

Individuals with cognitive disabilities have difficulty generalizing or transferring newly learned information to a new situation (Horner, Sprague, and Wilcox, 1982; Noonan and Siegel-Causey, 1990). According to Burger, Blackman, and Clark (1981), to generalize, the person must

1. understand which aspect of the newly learned information can be applied in the new situation; and

2. understand the similarities between the learned information acquired in a particular context and the new situation.

In other words, they must use selective attention appropriately. Also, both new and old situations have to be meaningful to the individual.

LANGUAGE DEVELOPMENT AND COGNITIVE DISABILITIES

Language impairment is observed among all individuals with cognitive disabilities. Increasing evidence indicates, however, that the language of children with cognitive disabilities is best described as delayed rather than deviant, and is characterized by later onset and slower progress (Kamhi and Johnston, 1982; Lobato, Barrera, and Feldman, 1981; Ratner, 1989; Rosenberg, 1982). However, there is a range of linguistic abilities found among this population.

Morphological Knowledge

Acquisition of morphologic forms and rules progresses in the same sequence as that of children without cognitive disabilities.

However, the pattern of development seems to be severely delayed (Klink, Gerstman, Raphael, Schlanger, and Newsome, 1986; Moran, Money, and Leonard, 1984).

Phonological Knowledge

Acquisition of phonological rules is delayed and progresses at a slower rate than for children without cognitive disabilities. There is also a higher incidence of articulation disorders, particularly among the Down syndrome population (Mahoney, Glover, and Finger, 1981). This is partly due to inadequate phonological awareness and partly due to a higher incidence of anatomical abnormalities of the jaw, teeth, and tongue among children with Down syndrome.

Syntactic Knowledge

In general, children with cognitive disabilities are delayed in their acquisition of more complex syntactic forms as compared to nondisabled children of the same chronological ages. Children with mild retardation do acquire more complex syntactic forms, but are observed to use them less frequently (McLeavey, Toomey, and Dempsey, 1982; Owens and MacDonald, 1982).

Semantic Knowledge

Word meanings are more concrete than those held by nondisabled children of the same chronological age. However, vocabulary of individuals with mild and moderate cognitive disabilities can be enriched in the course of interaction with others in natural and meaningful situations (Schiefelbusch, 1993).

Pragmatic Knowledge

Among the most debilitating problems shared by individuals with cognitive disabilities are those related to pragmatic deficits. To help these individuals develop socially and functionally, teachers and other professionals need to understand the extent of their communicative difficulties.

Mild-to-Moderate Cognitive Disabilities

Individuals with mild cognitive disabilities have been observed to learn to take turns appropriately, request information if needed, maintain the topic, change topics, and respond appropriately to their conversational partners' comments if the topic is within their understanding. The problems they encounter are most often related to the topic itself, more than to linguistic difficulties (Abbeduto and Rosenberg, 1980). They have particular difficulties with topics that involve past experiences and subjects that are not actually present, but are being discussed.

Moderate-to-Severe Cognitive Disabilities

Children usually learn pragmatic skills from infancy, and with each new experience, their knowledge about the individual differences among people and contexts expands. This knowledge is necessary for interpreting the verbal and nonverbal messages conveyed by the participants in a communication. Individuals with cognitive disabilities do not appear to gain these skills through their experiences. They appear to have particular difficulty making sense of what happens around them and what people mean (McTear and Conti-Ramsden, 1992).

One of the problems contributing to this confusion is the tendency for individuals with cognitive disabilities to be less accurate labeling facial expressions denoting attitudes and emotions of people with whom they are communicating (Maurer and Newbrough, 1987). They also have difficulty comprehending orally expressed emotions (Marcell and Jett, 1985). The listener's affect can help the speaker with cognitive disabilities to monitor his or her behavior and modify this behavior so that it is more appropriate and acceptable to the listener (e.g., over-friendliness or over-aggressiveness). This information is also important to formulate an appropriate response or comment (Adams and Markham, 1991; Marcell and Jett, 1985; Owens, 1989).

Individuals with cognitive disabilities also have a tendency to initiate and focus on topics primarily about themselves (Bedrosian, 1993). Topic switching is also found to be difficult. There is a tendency to frequently introduce and reintroduce the same topic (Bedrosian, 1988). In addition, persons with cognitive disabilities frequently have difficulty communicating intended meaning (Kernan and Sabsay, 1989; Sabsay and Kernan, 1993).

Individuals with cognitive disabilities tend to be passive communicants, that is, they do not usually initiate verbal exchanges, and they respond infrequently in conversational interactions unless prodded. In attempting to analyze the cause of this tendency, Cunningham, Reuler, Blackwell, and Deck (1981) observed parent-child interactions with young children who were cognitively disabled. These interactions reveal that the parents of these children tend to be less responsive and give less feedback. They also tend to be "teacher-like" when interacting with their children (Petersen and Sherrod, 1982). Children with cognitive disabilities and developmental delays are often not encouraged to respond and actively participate when interacting with their parents. As they grow older, they continue to be passive communicators (Kamhi and Masterson, 1989).

Severe-to-Profound Cognitive Disabilities

Children with severe language impairment who are severely cognitively disabled demonstrate a considerable range of ability with regard to understanding the functions of communicative interaction. Often cursory observations of these children's behaviors reveal limited pragmatic skills. Joint focus on topics and referents and turn-taking patterns are often fleeting or nonexistent. However, careful analysis of their behaviors by McLean and Snyder-McLean (1988) and by Cirrin and Rowland (1985) revealed valid indications that they may not be deviant behaviors. Instead, they may be severely delayed with regard to pragmatic development and more closely resemble those of very young, nondisabled children. The intentional, nonverbal communicative acts and gestures of the children observed in these research studies indicated understanding of the effect their behaviors had on the actions of other people (e.g., when they offer a cup, tug at an adult, or place another person's hand on an object, they are influencing the actions of that other person) (Cirrin and Rowland, 1985).

While there are obvious quantitative differences between the pragmatic behaviors of normally developing children and language-deficient children with severe cognitive disabilities, the sequential pattern of development is similar. On the basis of their research findings, McLean and Snyder-McLean (1988) suggest that intervention strategies should follow the sequences and patterns of normally developing children rather than arbitrary sequences selected on the basis of conventional perceptions of the abilities of children with severe cognitive disabilities.

FACTORS INFLUENCING LANGUAGE DEVELOPMENT

There is a high degree of diversity among children with severe cognitive disabilities. Some are delayed in the acquisition of speech, but learn to talk in simple phrases or sentences and understand most of what is said to them (McCormick and Schiefelbusch, 1990). Some severely impaired individuals do not speak, and communicate with gestures. Others do not understand speech and make little or no attempt to communicate. Many factors contribute to the tremendous variations among individuals with cognitive disabilities.

Cultural Diversity

Cultural diversity and the primary language of the family of the individual affect semantic, syntactic, morphologic, and phonological development. The quality of the special educational program and the professionals who coordinate the input of both languages is of utmost importance.

Enriching Experiences

The quantity and quality of the experiences these children have in their home environments and in the community have important influential value. A number of adults are observed not to read to children with cognitive disabilities because they feel that the child will not understand the story. Infants with such disabilities often have accompanying multiple handicaps and are not as responsive to attempts by adults to play and cuddle as nondisabled infants. Adults often become tired and frustrated when they receive little or no feedback from their youngsters who are disabled.

Children with cognitive disabilities who are taken on family excursions or into the community for shopping often are not drawn into communications with shopkeepers or friends; they are often inadvertently ignored. The "experiences" of a holiday, a trip to the zoo with the family, or shopping in the community will have little value if they are not accompanied by communicative interaction. In those instances, the chance to enrich the vocabulary, the verbal expressions, and the communicative skills of the child with cognitive disabilities in a natural and functional context is lost.

LANGUAGE INTERVENTION

Cognitive Hypothesis

As previously discussed in Chapter 3, Piaget (1952, 1954, 1962) together with Inhelder (1969, 1971) argued that until children could mentally represent with a symbol an object that was not actually present, they could not comprehend symbolic language. They advocated that children needed to experience relationships between objects, to act on them, and perceive the changes that take place as a result of their actions before a symbolic language could be expressed. According to Piaget, milestones such as symbolic play, deferred imitation, object permanence, and means-ends mental manipulations are essential prerequisites to the use of linguistic symbols. Piaget advocated that until these milestones are passed, children cannot acquire symbolic language skills.

Piaget's cognitive hypothesis has been questioned. Theorists do not agree that language development is contingent upon mastery of specific cognitive abilities. Investigators have found that the cognitive knowledge alleged to be the basis for language does not always precede words or word combinations (Casby, 1992; Rice, 1983). There are many important language concepts that children can learn only through exposure to language and through social interactions (e.g., the meanings of nonverbal behaviors during interactions; the clues that indicate that the topic of a communication has changed; the perception that there is a need to rephrase a comment because the listener does not understand (Cole, Dale, and Mills, 1990; Miller, 1981b).

It is more likely that linguistic and cognitive development may progress in parallel (Gopnik and Meltzoff, 1984) and in some instances in an unrelated fashion (Cromer, 1988; Curtiss, 1981; Miller, 1981b). Currently, there is little support for the practice of teaching specific cognitive skills for the purpose of preparing children for language acquisition (Ratner, 1989).

Child language is now viewed as a social learning process (Bates, Bretherton, and Snyder, 1988; Snyder and Silverstein, 1988). This view recognizes that children indicate communicative intentions long before they are able to verbally express these intentions. The young child's one-word and two-word utterances represent complex concepts and thoughts. Children are observed to represent objects and events with symbolic language considerably earlier than suggested by Piaget.

Change in Emphasis

The current perspective emphasizes the development of pragmatic skills and suggests that humans are predisposed to communicating with other humans. Chapter 3 discussed behaviors from birth that indicate a motivation to communicate and an actual need to interact with others in order to survive, as well as to develop emotionally and cognitively. The young, developing child must learn to express these social intentions in a manner that is culturally appropriate and pragmatically effective (McLean and Snyder-McLean, 1988).

This view of language as a social learning process has influenced the change in orientation regarding intervention. Emphasis is now placed upon developing communicative interaction skills for individuals with cognitive disabilities. Specific linguistic skills related to syntax, morphology, semantics, and phonology are remediated in the communicative context, in a natural, functional setting (Rice, 1986; Schiefelbusch and Lloyd, 1988). The remedial techniques using single isolated components of language have been shown to be unsatisfactory (Kaiser and Warren, 1988). Language training should be taught in situations where there is an actual need for language to be used (Creaghead, 1984; Culatta, 1984; Halle, 1984; Hart, 1981; McLean and Snyder-McLean, 1984a, 1984b; Snyder-McLean, Solomonson, McLean, and Sack, 1984; Wulz, Hall, and Klein, 1983).

Also in the context of a natural, functional setting, children and adolescents with cognitive disabilities should receive formal training in affect recognition. Clinical observations have revealed that whereas children usually acquire the ability to recognize emotions in the affect of other individuals through simple exposure over time to faces expressing emotions, children with cognitive disabilities and developmental disabilities are less able to learn this skill passively (Adams and Markham, 1991; Maurer and Newbrough, 1987; Walden and Field, 1982; Wiggers and van Lieshout, 1985).

Language Intervention for the Bilingual, Bicultural Child with Cognitive Disabilities

Intervention programs differ considerably from school district to school district. Intervention depends upon the severity of the handicap, attitude and involvement of the family, available resources, and available bilingual professionals who communicate in the primary language of the child's family. In many states, educators and other professionals who speak in Vietnamese, Chinese, Japanese, Russian, Portuguese, and other languages and even dialects from within the same country are not available. Most programs provide intervention in English (Erickson and Walker, 1983). This poses considerable problems when counseling and attempting to draw parents into the intervention program. Parental communication with their children is a crucial component of such a program (see Chapter 5 for further discussion).

Augmentative and Alternative Systems for Persons with Moderate and Severe Cognitive Disabilities

When an individual has limited ability to communicate feelings and desires, the resulting frustration may lead to the development of unconventional or socially unacceptable means of communicating such as aggression, tantrums, self-abuse, and destruction of property (Donnellan, Mirenda, Mesaros, and Fassbender, 1984; Prizant and Wetherby, 1985; Wetherby, 1986).

Carr and Durand (1985) found that when inappropriate behaviors were interpreted not as deviant behaviors, but as nonverbal communicative behaviors to obtain attention or something that is wanted, intervention could be more constructive and successful. When an individual with cognitive disabilities does not speak or uses unintelligible speech due to concomitant physical limitations, other means of communication should be made available. The implementation of an augmentative communication system can provide the means with which to interact with others and develop socially. Refer to Chapter 2 for a discussion of various communicative devices.

The degree of socially unacceptable behaviors increases proportionately with the degree of cognitive disability and the degree of speech and language impairment (Burke, 1990; Jacobson, 1982). Providing nonverbal children or adolescents with an alternative or augmentative communication system will not only reduce the frustrations that develop when individuals cannot express their needs or cannot obtain the attention they require, but will enable them to develop socially acceptable and more effective means of communicating with others (La Vigna, 1987; Prizant and Schuler, 1987; Smith, 1985; Wetherby and Prizant, 1989).

In the past, there have been concerns that the child will become dependent on an augmentative language system and will not develop speech or language skills. Conclusions from numerous research studies indicate that an alternative or augmentative communication system will not interfere with the acquisition of natural speech (Daniloff, Noll, Fristoe, and Lloyd, 1982; Silverman, 1980.) In fact, there are reports of improved speech and increased development of linguistic concepts (Shane, 1985).

Sign Language

Several studies have demonstrated the benefits of sign language as an alternative communication system for individuals with moderate-to-severe cognitive disabilities. Karlan and Lloyd (1983) found that "comprehension recall . . . was significantly improved by the use of signed cues during the learning task" (p. 330). Signs that were functionally useful to the individual (i.e., those that resulted in obtaining something that was wanted or needed) were learned faster and maintained longer that nonfunctional signs (Dennis, Reichle, Williams, and Vogelsberg, 1982; Reichle, Williams, and Ryan, 1981; Romski, Sevcik, and

Rumbaugh, 1985). (A full description of sign language is provided in Chapter 12.)

Augmentative Devices

An augmentative device is a device that displays a language code and enables a nonspeaking individual to communicate with others in their environment. These devices have proven to be very helpful to individuals with cognitive disabilities who cannot speak or whose speech is unintelligible because of physiological abnormalities. Such a device can consist of a board using pictures, written words, symbols such as Rebus, or Blissymbolics. It can be a simple teacher-constructed communication board or a complex electronic computer with synthetic speech mechanism or printed output mechanism.

Augmentative devices should be individually programmed or designed, with consideration for the individual's needs in "different contexts." Choosing the specific items to be included in the different devices requires a "team" effort—the members of the team consisting of parents or caregivers, the speech-language pathologist, the special education teacher, the occupational therapist, and all specialists who interact with the individual with cognitive disabilities in the course of everyday activities. Not one, but a number of augmentative devices and alternative communication systems (e.g., sign language) may be needed to enable nonspeaking individuals to communicate with "speaking others" in the variety of environments in which they must function on a daily basis.

SUMMARY

Individuals with cognitive disabilities are indeed a heterogeneous population. Common learning characteristics exist:

- They acquire new information slowly, and much repetition is necessary.

- They often fail to identify and differentiate relevant from irrelevant information.

- They do not demonstrate learned skills without prompting. They often wait for someone to tell them what to do.

- They have difficulty organizing newly learned information for easy access at a future time; therefore, they have deficits in long-term memory.

- They do not generalize learned skills to new situations.

Important changes have taken place with regard to educational techniques and expectations of professionals who work with individuals with cognitive disabilities.

Emphasis is currently placed on the development of communicative and interactive skills. Specific linguistic skills related to syntax, morphology, phonology, and semantics are remediated in a natural and functional context and in the course of spontaneous interaction with others. Long-range goals are to enable individuals with cognitive disabilities to function in increasingly less restrictive environments. Artificial limitations are no longer placed on capabilities of this population.

SUGGESTED READINGS

Bates, E., Bretherton, I., and Snyder, L. (1988). *From First Words to Grammar: Individual Differences and Dissociable Mechanisms.* New York: Cambridge University Press.

Carrow-Woolfolk, E., and Lynch, J. (1982). *An Integrative Approach to Language Disorders in Children.* New York: Grune and Stratton.

Schiefelbusch, R., and Lloyd, L. (Eds.). (1988). *Language Perspectives: Acquisition, Retardation, and Intervention* (2nd ed.). Austin, TX: Pro-Ed.

11 THE NATURE OF LANGUAGE DISORDERS AMONG CHILDREN WITH AUTISM

Individuals with the cluster of characteristics which are associated with autism have existed through the ages. However, it wasn't until 1943 that Leo Kanner (1943, 1985a, 1985b), the child psychiatrist, used the term *autistic* to describe youngsters with this syndrome. During the next 50 years, researchers and scientists explored its causes and appropriate intervention. Modifications in its definition and its specific features have been made. By the 1990s, more questions have been raised than answered.

Autism is known to affect more males than females. The male-female ratio of 4:1 has been cited for classic autism (Frith, 1993; Lotter, 1985; Rumsey, 1985). This disorder has attracted considerable attention among professionals. **Autism** has been viewed as an affective or psychological disturbance and as a physiological or organic disorder. All of the affected youngsters have communication, social, and behavioral difficulties. They frequently don't show love or form social attachments. They demonstrate stereotyped and repetitive behavior, function at a retarded level, show a lack of self-awareness, and exhibit difficulty grasping abstract concepts, speech, and other symbols (Lahey, 1988; Macchello, 1986).

There is a wide range of abilities exhibited by children with autism. Some are judged to be extraordinarily intelligent and others are considered profoundly retarded. Some youngsters can speak and others cannot. Some have concomitant disabilities such as hearing, motor, or visual impairments. Furthermore, the individual child can exhibit discrepant abilities. For example, one child may be in constant motion and become easily absorbed in whirling objects but demonstrate more advanced mathematical skills. For that child, some characteristics of autism appear more pronounced and others seem less affected.

There are numerous theories on the possible causes of autism. Environmental pollution, viral infections, genetic irregularities, vitamin and mineral deficiency, metabolic disturbance, and brain stem abnormalities are mentioned in the literature most frequently. Each child with autism exhibits a unique range of abilities which suggest that causal factors may be numerous and affect each child in clusters.

Chapter 11 examines the perplexing disorder of autism by

1. discussing the characteristics of autism as observed by researchers and as currently defined by diagnosticians;

2. differentiating autism from other emotional disturbances;

3. exploring the theories associated with autism over the last few decades and explaining how the professional understanding of the disorder has altered intervention strategies;

4. emphasizing the linguistic and communicative aspects of autism and issues related to using alternative forms of communication; and

5. presenting current perspectives regarding intervention.

DIAGNOSTIC CRITERIA FOR AUTISM

Leo Kanner (1943), the psychiatrist from Johns Hopkins University, who described and named autism, viewed it as a disorder where the children have an innate inability to interact affectively with people. The word *innate* implied a biological base for the disorder. However, the aberrant behaviors that were present in the children were the focus of professional attention and for several decades the syndrome came to be recognized as an emotional disturbance (Bettelheim, 1967; Lahey, 1988; Rutter, 1985).

Kanner (1943) described a number of characteristics of autism based on the eleven youngsters he examined. He noted poor relationships with people. He concluded that children with autism seem to treat people as other objects in the environment. From infancy, they appear aloof and are very difficult to reach. They avoid eye contact and use the hand of a person to obtain desired objects. If the children learn to speak, language is not generally used to convey meaningful messages to the listener. Some children may recite lists and poems at an early age but these are repetitions of memorized material. The words do not seem to communicate feelings or thoughts. They often use **immediate echolalia,** which occurs when the youngster repeats exactly the last word or a stream of words just heard. **Delayed echolalia** also is exhibited by some of the children. They tend to store words and express them at a later time, sometimes in an appropriate context and sometimes for self-stimulation. Kanner describes the language comprehension of these youngsters as being literal. When told to put down a cup, the child might put it on the floor. Another common idiosyncratic use of language by children with autism is the repetition of personal pronouns as they are heard. When the child says, "Are *you* ready for school?", the child may mean, "*I* am ready for school."

Kanner also observed ritualistic and compulsive behaviors among many of the children with autism. The children who exhibit these behaviors try to maintain sameness. If routines or objects are changed, the child can become overly disoriented and agitated. In play sessions, blocks are often aligned in the same arrangement that was seen initially by the child. Activities such as bath time and meal time must be executed in the identical format at each encounter. A crumb on the floor may draw the child's attention and concern. Appropriate spontaneous activities are limited. Only objects that remain constant in appearance and position are accepted by the youngster.

Kanner (1943) felt that the children he examined appeared to have cognitive potential. They had the look of intelligence in their faces. Kanner described the speaking children as exhibiting astounding vocabularies. Certain nonverbal tasks were completed normally in their examination. The physical appearance of the children was normal, although gross motor abilities were inconsistent for many of the youngsters. On some occasions, a child might execute skillful and rapid movements. At other times, the very same movements were labored or difficult to initiate.

In diagnosing autism today, psychiatrists use the *Diagnostic Statistical Manual of Mental Disorders, 3rd edition, Revised (DSM-III-R)* (American Psychiatric Association, 1987). Autistic disorder is defined as a **Pervasive Developmental Disorder** (PDD) because many basic areas of development are simultaneously disturbed to a severe degree. Autism is recognized as the most severe form of PDD. It is considered to be lifelong although severity can change with age. Cognitive and social skills can improve or regress independently of one another. Even the most promising youngsters show some social awkwardness. Diagnostic criteria for autism in the *DMS-III-R* (1987, pp. 33–39) include these:

1. *An impairment in reciprocal social interaction.* This is described as a lack of responsiveness to, or interest in, people.

2. *An impairment in verbal and nonverbal communication, and in imaginative activity.* This may include no speech, echolalia, pronoun reversals, inability to use abstract terms, abnormal speech melody, inability to understand jokes, and absence of fantasy play.

3. *A restricted repertoire of activities and interests.* The child resists change, has motor stereotypies such as hand flapping, and shows a fascination with movement.

4. *Onset during infancy and almost always before 36 months of age.*

Other diagnostic features listed as associated with the disorder are abnormal development of cognitive skills; abnormal posture and motor behavior (e.g., walking on tiptoe, poor motor coordination); odd responses to sensory input; abnormalities in eating and sleeping; abnormalities of mood; self-injurious behavior (e.g., hand biting and head banging) (American Psychiatric Association, 1987, p. 35).

AUTISM AND EMOTIONAL DISTURBANCE

Children with autism appear to lack appropriate self-control, possess communication abnormalities, and exhibit difficulty relating to people. It is understandable that Kanner (1943) would have been asked to examine the children who later became the basis for his study of autism. These youngsters were thought to have a form of childhood psychosis and some had already been diagnosed as schizophrenic.

In both schizophrenia and autism, children relate to other people in an abnormal way. However, children with schizophrenia appear to develop normally until after they are school-age. The onset of schizophrenia also can occur in late adolescence (Erickson, 1978). Children with schizophrenia have delusions and hallucinations (i.e., they hear and see things that are not there). The disorder tends to be degenerative over time.

Even during the 1960s, confusion in differentiating autism and schizophrenia continued. Behaviors such as echolalia, obsession, social isolation, and insistence on sameness can be seen in each of these disorders. Professionals viewed both conditions as psychogenic disturbances. Autism was treated on a psychiatric basis. Bettelheim (1967) believed that children with autism abandoned their world in despair. He stated that the parents of the children wished that their children didn't exist and didn't provide appropriate attention. The "refrigerator mother" became associated with inadequate parenting of youngsters with autism and was considered a causal factor.

Today the diagnosis of autism continues to be confirmed by the child psychiatrist. However, many aspects of the writings of Kanner and Bettelheim have historical validity only. Autism is no longer associated with psychosis or early parent-child interactions. The blame placed upon so called "refrigerator mothers" is no longer considered acceptable by the professional community. Autism is classed as a separate entity under the umbrella of *pervasive developmental disorder*. This term implies multiple causes including the strong possibility of organic abnormality.

THEORIES ASSOCIATED WITH AUTISM

Speech, language, and communication impairment is a central feature of autism. Failure to acquire language at the expected age is the most frequent reason for medical referral. Communication disabilities pervade social and cognitive functioning. Deficient social interaction and limited play routines are observed in early life. Rapin (1991) states that virtually all preschool children with autism have impaired comprehension of language. Nonverbal communication such as gesture or pointing is generally absent (Holmes and Weitzner, 1990). Rather than pointing, they might take the hand of an adult and put it on a desired object. Play tends to lack imagination or the ability to reenact familiar routines like drinking and eating. Toys are not used for pretend play and tend to be placed in arrangements or lined up. Some children focus on one aspect of a toy like a wheel on a truck and spin it incessantly. Youngsters with autism may resist cuddling. They might appear unaware of people and walk past them or fail to respond to attempts to engage them in conversation. They seem to seek social isolation. The relationships among language, cognition, and behavior have spawned a number of theories on the nature of autism.

Cognition and Autism

A cognitive theory was proposed by Rimland (1964) who suggested that children with autism cannot attach meaning to incoming sensations. This affects memory and concept formation which are necessary for information processing.

Memory capability has been studied by Cesaroni and Garber (1991) who report that persons with autism can exhibit an exceptional ability at times in remembering large amounts of information, understanding what it means, and recalling elaborate detail. On other occasions, they have difficulty processing information. These processing differences from people without autism interfere with communication skills. Putting yourself in another person's situation is difficult if you perceive and experience the world differently. In addition, the way the individual with autism experiences a situation may not correspond with the way other people assume he or she is experiencing the situation.

Experiences without meaning create a fragmented view of the world and the child's "self." In short, people learn who they are by engaging in a dialogue with the world. Children with autism have impaired cognitive abilities which underlie emotions, communication, and social interaction (Rutter, 1983).

Socialization and Autism

The importance of social interaction in child development and the focus on pragmatics in language acquisition gave rise to theories of autism with social factors influencing language and cognitive development (Volkmar, 1987). Initial socialization occurs primarily in the facial dialogue between the infant and caregiver. Youngsters with autism may be highly responsive to minute changes in their environment, but the human face and social interaction tend to be avoided. The child displays unusual social attachments in that strangers can receive the same social responses, such as hugs, as close family members. As children with autism mature, social functioning may improve but it rarely becomes "normal."

For individuals with autism, taking the other person's perspective is difficult, resulting in very limited social success. As the children mature, close family members tend to be the principal sources of social contact. Even those youngsters with autism who experience the most promising outcomes are usually described as friendless or deviant in their social interaction (Williams, 1992). One subject in the Cesaroni and Garber (1991) study reported expending enormous energy and control in his efforts to interact with others. However, he achieved very limited success. He often missed cues and appeared unresponsive to others even though he had devoted considerable time trying to develop social relationships.

One explanation for the social ineptness experienced by children with autism has been proposed in the theory of mind (Frith, 1993; Perner, Frith, Leslie, and Leekam, 1989). This theory implies that youngsters with autism have difficulty taking their own mental states into account as well as the mental states of others. For example, children with autism have difficulty comprehending certain facial and body expressions of feeling, which creates problems concerning empathy and understanding another person's point of view. Baron-Cohen (1988) characterizes social and pragmatic deficits in autism as an inability to participate in "two-way reciprocal social interaction." This is related to pragmatics in that children with autism use language instrumentally but not communicatively. He suggests that the youngsters have an impaired theory of mind because they cannot visualize or represent the beliefs or intentions of other individuals as well as their own. This overlaps with cognitive theories of autism which also focus on the child's inability to form accurate concepts.

Pragmatics and Autism

Pragmatic ability is an integral part of linguistic and communication theories of autism. Prizant and Wetherby (1990) state that the primary function of language competence is to regulate one's own behavior and the behavior of others. A person's communication signals, both verbal and nonverbal, can influence the behavior and beliefs of others, can solve problems, and can achieve specific goals. Therefore, language enables children to function both socially and cognitively. Youngsters with autism have fundamental and pervasive linguistic deficits which affect their communicative abilities.

Prizant and Wetherby (1987) present a framework for understanding the interrelationship between social and communicative behavior in autism. They state that **communicative intent** connects social awareness and the ability to affect the behavior and attitudes of others. It requires preplanned behavior to influence other people. The fact that one must engage in an interaction with another person suggests a social encounter. The signals used to affect the behavior of others are the communication. Infants influence the listener unintentionally. They cry and receive food but they may not understand why their body feels uncomfortable. By nine months, babies gesture and coo to affect the listener. These actions are preverbal but intentional. By 18 months, toddlers communicate intentionally. For the child with autism, conventional means of communicating may not be used. There is little pointing and a lot of aberrant behavior such as self-injury and echolalia. When words are used, sometimes they are not meant to communicate a message but rather serve other purposes such as self-stimulation. These signals are not understood or shared by the social community. It takes an individual who is very familiar with the child to understand that head banging might mean the child is anxious or bored (Donnellan, Mirenda, Mesaros, and Fassbender, 1984).

All aberrant behaviors may not have communicative intent, however. Some inappropriate behaviors may reflect automatic and involuntary expressions of frustration or anxiety. Sometimes even very familiar people cannot understand the communicative intent of the movements displayed by the child with autism (Donovan, 1993).

Echolalia and Autism

The use of echolalia can also be explained as an unconventional means of conveying communicative intent. Prizant and Wetherby (1987) suggest that children with autism may select one aspect of a situation to reenact when attempting to replicate the situation. For example, every time one youngster with autism wants juice, the parent's hand may be grabbed and pulled toward the refrigerator, since the parent had held the child's hand the first time the situation occurred. Vocal as well as gestural replication of events can also be demonstrated by the child. The child may ask, "Do you want juice?" This is the verbal utterance that the child is associating with the event of obtaining juice. It is an inappropriate selection of one aspect of the event that the child heard and associates with getting juice. The intent is confusing because the exact utterance the parent had produced during the situation has been lifted out of the event and doesn't exactly fit in the new circumstances. An unfamiliar listener may conclude that the child is expressing meaningless echolalia. The child may be using the question with communicative intent (i.e., to obtain juice) but its meaning is obscured because the rote reiteration of that particular question does not match the child's real intent. Thus, memorized portions of utterances produced by family members or on television may serve to communicate messages that the child with autism is associating with events. The problem is that the listener cannot determine which situation the child is intending to connect to the words. Echolalic utterances often seem to have little apparent relationship to the situations in which they are produced. This type of utterance is often seen, therefore, as bizarre or meaningless. In fact, it may serve a function for the child with autism that is misunderstood by the listener.

Prizant (1987) discusses other functions of echolalia. When children with autism repeat comments just heard in a conversational setting, researchers believe this form of echolalia serves as a turn-taking mechanism. The children know that a response is expected in a communication exchange and inappropriately state what another person just recited during their own conversational turn.

Gestalt Processing

Some children with autism have powerful memory systems and process language and experiences as whole units rather than segmenting them into meaningful units. The echolalic utterances are but one example of whole unit processing. The amount of information taken in is too much for the child with autism to analyze effectively. The entire sentence is stored and then repeated without being segmented and properly processed. Extreme whole unit processing of language and experience has been referred to as **gestalt processing** (Prizant, 1987).

The attempts to correlate the communicative, social, and cognitive factors of autism have not clearly determined which of these is primary and which is secondary. Professionals have concluded, however, that each factor develops in a different manner in children with autism. Therefore, it becomes difficult for the general population to understand the world of individuals with autism. They perceive and process their environment in unusual ways so that their world knowledge cannot be compared to the conceptual framework of people without the disorder.

Autism and Neurological Factors

In more recent years, researchers have been exploring organic causes for autism. Kanner (1985a, 1985b) had suspected brain dysfunction in the eleven children he examined but when EEGs (electroencephalograms) were administered, all but one youngster, who subsequently developed right-sided convulsions, showed normal function. Yet Kanner (1985a, 1985b) stated that the disorder was "innate" and not the result of postnatal psychogenic factors. Rimland (1964, 1985) evaluated extensive published reports on autism and concluded that in time the causes of autism would be found in biologically based deficits. He stated that children with autism behave differently from birth. He also noted research on children with confirmed acquired brain damage that described their behavior as simulating the characteristics of autism. In studies of identical twins with autism, both twins were affected although other siblings were normal and nonautistic. Most parents of children with autism were found to be loving and appropriate and had other children who were not autistic.

In the last several decades, research has explored pharmacological effects in children with autism (Cohen, Caparulo, and Shaywitz, 1985). In these studies, drugs have induced better social skills or decreased repetitive activity but improvement is not sustained and subsequent deterioration has also been observed. Other researchers have looked to vitamin therapy (Rimland, Callaway, and Dreyfus, 1985) and neurochemical studies which involve drug therapy to change the function of transmitters in the brain (Anderson and Hoshino, 1987). Other causes have been researched such as genetic factors including alteration of enzymes or structural proteins (Paul, 1987). Disturbances in motility or motor behavior have also been investigated (Biklen, 1990; Damasio and Maurer, 1985; Rogers, 1992).

Movement Disturbances

Movement disturbance is defined as the inability to organize, control, and move one's body at will (Hill and Leary, 1993). Damasio and Maurer (1985) studied movement disturbances in children with autism. The motor behaviors included **stereotypies**, which are isolated, purposeless, and repetitive movements (e.g., hand flapping, head banging, and slapping), as well as abnormal postures and gait.

Results of their study indicated that youngsters with autism exhibit characteristics similar to those of adults with certain neurological disturbances such as Parkinson's disease (Sacks, 1990). They suggested that areas of the frontal lobe and basal ganglia of the brain were affected. Motor irregularities were also seen in the faces of children with autism when they smiled or spoke spontaneously, which was described as emotionally determined facial paralysis. The researchers suggested that it is these motor irregularities that affect verbal production in autism.

Motor Dysfunction

Damasio and Maurer (1985) discussed the notion that many youngsters with autism are nonverbal. Other children with autism exhibit echolalic speech production. These repeated utterances often have good stress and melody. Yet the very same youngsters, when using nonechoed language, speak in a poorly structured, flat style with a minimum number of words. Even the most verbal children with autism generate language that is spoken in a wooden, stilted, and concrete manner. Respiration during speech is not normal and pauses that should occur between phrases are inappropriately placed. They conclude that these manifestations suggest motor dysfunction.

Praxis

Biklen (1990), in his landmark article, suggests that autism is neurologically based and is a motor disorder. He states that the problem is **praxis**, a neurological condition that affects the ability of a person to perform a motor routine or to implement effective motor planning. Currin and Fitzwater (1993) further explained praxis as a motor skill which requires ideation, planning, and execution of an unlearned motor act.

Speech is a motor activity. Muscles must move to form words. People with autism have unusual speech because there are problems with the "output mechanism." For some people with autism, phrases or words that have been heard and put into the brain can be recited back. The ability to select words and phrases to speak is a more advanced version of speech output. The child with autism has a more difficult time expressing words and ideas. The ideas are inside the child but what comes out does not always resemble those ideas. In short, motor planning and other neurological motoric deficits interfere with the ability of the children to express their innermost knowledge and ideas.

Kinesias

Motor planning difficulties are founded in cerebral dysfunction and neurological disorders. The muscles of the lip, tongue, and palate, as well as the muscles for breath control and facial expression, are intact and not paralyzed. They are not moving as expected because the brain cannot get its commands through the neural pathways to them.

Maurer and Damasio (1982) associated the repetitive stereotyped hand movements (e.g., hand flapping) and body postures found in autism to be tic-like involuntary actions. They discuss **dyskinesia** which is described as difficulty with the initiation, switching, and stopping of movement. Related disturbances are **akinesia,** which is the absence of movement, and **bradykinesia,** which is a general slowness of movement that resembles a slow motion film (Rogers, 1992). An individual who exhibits these kinesias can be rigid on some occasions and agile at other times. It is an "on-off" phenomenon.

A person can have **emotional dyskinesia** as well, where moods cannot be started, executed, switched, or stopped. For example, children with autism can get angry or agitated but they get stuck on the emotion and find it difficult to switch to another emotional state. Therefore, behaviors that look like obsessive or oppositional routines like biting or rocking in a corner may be related to these kinesias (Hill and Leary, 1993). The research of Damasio and Maurer (1985) associated these movement disorders to specific areas of the brain and they were able to document replication of these behaviors in monkeys. Thus, they concluded that neural dysfunction in specific areas of the brain can affect social behavior, verbalization, and body movements.

Sensory Processing

Atypical Sensory Reactions

Damasio and Maurer (1985) examined attentional issues such as atypical reactions to sensory stimulation (i.e., visual, auditory, tactile, taste, and smell). They observed that peripheral vision is used more than central vision. Visual scanning seems less systematic and the children orient to visual stimuli in unpredictable ways. The sensory system can appear less responsive at one moment and hyperresponsive at others. In fact, many children with autism are misjudged as deaf at times. Damasio and Maurer (1985) conclude that many youngsters with autism have the potential for normal perception and memory and that the disorder occurs in higher-level perceptual and memory storage and retrieval systems.

Courchesne (1989) has studied brains of people with autism using magnetic resonance imaging (MRI) technology. He found abnormalities, as did Bauman (1993), in the cerebellum, which regulates movement and the portion of memory that allows individuals to react appropriately to sensory stimulation like bright lights, loud noises, or hot surfaces. He suggests that children with autism are constantly trying to shield themselves from sensory stimulation which, because of neurological abnormalities, seems excessive. For the child with autism, light can be more intense, sound can be louder, surfaces can feel more prickly, and smells can be more pungent. For example, the fragrance of soap on a person's skin or of cleansers in a bathroom can be repugnant to the child with autism. To others, it may not be noticeable at all.

Synesthesia

Cesaroni and Garber (1991) have linked some of these heightened sensory systems to **synesthesia**, which is an intermingling of the senses. The signal may come from one source but the information is received by more than one sense. The stimulation of one sense can also stimulate another. For example, sounds heard conjure colors.

People from many cultures who experience synesthesia say that high sounds are associated with bright colors and low sounds correspond to dark colors. This phenomenon can cause sensory overload to some individuals. The individuals with autism whom Cesaroni and Garber (1991) studied reported synesthesia. For example, when the lower part of the face of one young man was touched, he experienced sound-like sensation as well as the sense of touch. This individual stated that he finds it difficult to describe his sensory processing experiences because there is no language available to him that codes his thoughts on the topic in a way that would be understood by normal people with a different perceptual processing mode. He reports turning off kitchen appliances so he can taste something. He also has premonitions of intense auditory stimuli. He can tell when a train is coming before anyone around can hear it. He describes this multichannel receptivity as disorienting, unpleasant, and frightening for him at times.

Multiple Etiologies

Extensive study of the brains of young people with autism who have died has uncovered two primary areas of abnormality (Bauman, 1993). Research suggests that the Purkinje cells of the cerebellum (the part of the brain responsible for regulating complex movements) and the limbic system (the system which affects multiple areas in the brain that involve memory, learning, emotion, and behavior) appear to cut short their development prior to the thirtieth week of gestation of the child in utero. Bauman (1993) suspects that autism is a disorder with multiple etiologies (e.g. environmental factors, metabolic dysfunctions, and genetic factors) which selectively affect nerve cell development in the brain at a critical time. This corresponds with reports from Leominster, Massachusetts, and Rochester, New York, of a higher incidence of autism associated with suspected exposure to toxic substances in the environment.

In summary, the variety of theories as to which areas of the brain are functioning abnormally in individuals with autism continues to be investigated (Bauman, 1993; Courchesne, Lincoln, Yeung-Courchesne, Elmasian, and Grillon, 1989; Dawson and Lewy, 1989; Ornitz, 1989). Research indicates that there are sensory processing, motoric, and cognitive variations due to neurological differences.

ISSUES IN COMMUNICATION

Years ago, adults assumed when a child was not communicating, the child had nothing to express. There was a time when children with profound hearing loss were called "deaf and dumb." These notions have been stifled by the achievements of brilliant individuals with deafness like Helen Keller. Children with motoric disabilities such as cerebral palsy have also been mistaken for being retarded because there was no physical means for them to communicate. Analysis of the research suggests that approximately half of the youngsters diagnosed as autistic have nonfunctional or no utterances (Macchello, 1986), and about three-quarters of those children who develop oral language exhibit echolalia (Rutter, 1985). Other linguistic irregularities such as pronoun confusion, poor comprehension of abstract concepts, and unusual stress and melody in utterances characterize nearly all children with autism (Baltaxe and Simmons, 1987). Although some researchers associated these irregularities in communication with motoric disorders, many professionals viewed most youngsters with autism as also being retarded. Language is a social and cognitive tool. Without the means to communicate effectively, the youngster appears socially inept and limited cognitively.

Although brain dysfunction or damage is probably associated with a higher incidence of retardation, some professionals believe that a number of nonverbal youngsters with autism might have higher cognitive and linguistic abilities than they can express (Biklen,

Morton, Gold, Berrigan, and Swaminathan, 1992; Crossley, 1992a; Crossley, 1992b). Crossley, working in Australia between 1986–1990, was searching for a means of communication for her clients who were labeled intellectually impaired and/or autistic. These individuals did not speak and had difficulty learning sign language. Although none were judged to have cerebral palsy, they exhibited poor eye/hand coordination, impulsivity, perseveration, low muscle tone, and difficulty pointing. These problems interfered with the ability to select items from a communication display. Crossley held the person's wrist or hand to help with pointing and discovered that of the 431 individuals she evaluated, 70% beyond the age of five could type a comprehensible sentence without a model. Speech and hand function impairments had prevented her clients from demonstrating the knowledge they had acquired.

Children with autism and little expressive language are generally considered "lower functioning." Those children with autism judged to have intelligence in the normal range have been characterized as producing useful language by the age of five (Macchello, 1986). Thus, professionals also link speaking ability to cognitive abilities. This notion correlates with the observation that even nonverbal communication is limited in those youngsters with autism who have little speech. Spontaneous use of gesture and the ability to perform gestures on demand is difficult for them (Lahey, 1988). Nonverbal youngsters with autism exhibit little evidence of linguistic knowledge. Therefore, Crossley's unexpected discovery of "literacy" among nonverbal youngsters with autism has been viewed with skepticism (Calculator, 1992; Silliman, 1992).

These doubts are countered by Biklen (1990). He has proposed a theory which links the unexpected thinking and literacy skills of youngsters with autism to their motoric difficulties which prevent them from expressing what they know. If Biklen's view is accurate, many children with autism who were also considered cognitively disabled should be reevaluated. The intelligence of some of these youngsters could be hidden by their inability to speak. Biklen's movement disturbance theory (1990) has generated a debate concerning the physical support offered to children with autism and whether the language generated is initiated by the child or the person assisting the child.

Facilitated communication is the term applied to the alternative means of communication in which students are given physical and emotional support by another individual so that they can express their thoughts by pointing to pictures, letters of the alphabet, or keys on an electronic keyboard. What concerns the detractors of this communication system is the content and form of the language expressed by the children. It challenges nearly all the traditional assumptions of the disorder.

The Facilitated Communication Controversy

Facilitated communication (FC) is one of several alternative or augmentative forms of communication. Like sign language, computers, and communication boards, it is a method of communication used when oral language is not functional. In the 1990s, FC initially was offered to those youngsters whose motor planning abilities did not allow them to speak, gesture, or even point without support. Assistance might be given to the hand, wrist, arm, or shoulder. This support is gradually reduced or faded as the youngster develops internal confidence and control.

Some of the children with autism who were introduced to this communication system could not point voluntarily with their fingers. They also demonstrated little ability to follow directions, identify letters, or read. When they were offered an alphabet board and physical support, they gradually spelled out words and, with bolstered confidence, they expressed ideas. When did these youngsters learn to read? Facilitators were even more astonished to discover that youngsters who spoke using echolalia, pronoun reversals, or disjointed words, were discarding these linguistic forms during facilitated communication. Whereas most youngsters demonstrated only rote knowledge before being introduced to FC, they displayed much better receptive language than expected after using FC.

The speech-language pathologists who were among the first to work with FC were extremely skeptical initially. Conceptual and vocabulary understanding is developed from birth through the child's interaction with the environment and with other individuals. Children with autism do not engage in these interactions in the same way their nonautistic peers do. They avoid people and manipulate objects inappropriately. Youngsters with autism might be assisted in pointing to the letters of words. However, would they have the depth of comprehension of the words they type that other children do? Would the material they express be a shallow recapitulation of words heard and seen? Many speech-language pathologists were only willing to experiment with FC because they had limited success using other interventions.

Researchers (Biklen and Schubert, 1991) are attempting to understand autism by examining what students are telling them when using facilitated communication and comparing these ideas to research in neurology and cognition such as the studies outlined earlier in this chapter. However, only speculation explains how or why FC works and extensive research is indicated. The unexpected literacy exhibited through FC by the youngsters with autism has altered the way in which they are treated. Some are now viewed as competent individuals whose ideas do not have to be locked in their minds. Open-ended communication is encouraged. However, the youngsters using this mode of communication are selective in their choice of facilitators and require varying amounts of support during each new communication encounter (e.g., holding the elbow, arm, or wrist).

Observers wonder if the facilitators are unconsciously assisting the children in locating letters. However, proponents of FC state that the children are writing information that is unknown to their facilitators, like names of family members, their social security number, and personal information. One youngster was asked why he ate the paste at school. He typed that it tasted like mustard. The facilitator tasted the paste and discovered that it did taste like mustard. Further support for the notion that the children are pointing independently is that they produce unique phonetic spellings and typographical errors. In addition, some students only require support on the elbow or shoulder which makes cuing or direct assistance from the facilitator difficult. Furthermore, the content reflects the distinct personalities of the children (Biklen and Schubert, 1991). Some youngsters have startled their facilitators by swearing at them or telling them negative information. One young boy typed, "You rude." The surprised facilitator asked why he said that. The boy wrote, "You don't let me play in the sand." In fact, the facilitator had taken the child from the sand table when it was his turn to practice facilitated communication.

Youngsters have expressed very personal thoughts using facilitated communication. Frequently, one of the first unsolicited comments by the child with autism is "I'm not stupid" or "I'm not retarded." Other statements often typed are "I don't want to be alone" or "I want people to like me." One young nonverbal child expressed his feelings about autism by saying, "I no in my mind I can talk. My autism is driving me nuts."

Facilitated communication helps individuals with autism to express their ideas and feelings. However, in most instances it does not change apparent deviant behavior. This outcome is unexpected. Professionals (Donnellan, Mirenda, Mesaros, and Fassbender, 1984; Prizant and Schuler, 1987; Prizant and Wetherby, 1990) have stated that acting-out behaviors, self-injury, and assault are attempts by the children with autism to communicate anger, frustration, and confusion. Researchers who initially tried facilitated communication expected that with a better way to express their feelings, the behavior patterns of the youngsters would improve. However, obsessive behaviors, biting, banging, self-mutilation, and rocking persist. Certain movements are difficult to initiate and other actions become repetitive and not easy to switch or stop.

Dawson and Lewy (1989), in their study of brain function, suggest that children with autism have chronic levels of overstimulation or intense responses to novel stimuli. Furthermore, their responses are unpredictable and beyond their control. One youngster who continued biting his hand typed a message requesting that the facilitator tell him when he puts his hand in his mouth because he has no awareness of this "involuntary" action.

If the premise is correct that the children with autism cannot speak because of brain irregularities affecting organized movement and sensory stimulation, it is possible that these youngsters may not have full control of other complex physical actions. Some of the children have communicated to their facilitators that they are unable to control their behaviors all the time. They ask that people stop punishing them for actions that are out of their control. When asked about the help that should be provided when a particular adolescent loses control, he responded, "Be patient. Don't lose control just because I am."

Facilitated communication has generated heated controversy. Proponents of this means of communication have been unable to substantiate their claims with reliable research. Parents and teachers of some youngsters with autism have developed false hopes about the long-range progress of their children. The wide range of abilities of youngsters with autism reinforces the notion that a variety of communicative, educational, and behavioral strategies are appropriate.

Autism Reconsidered

The decade of the 1990s has attempted to integrate conventional theories of autism with the increased volume of personal impressions that have been expressed with the aid of facilitated communication by individuals who have autism. Some people who appear to have minimal functional verbal expression or social knowledge and who are considered severely retarded are typing personal and logical thoughts when provided with physical support to the hand or arm (Biklen and Schubert, 1991). Researchers (Calculator, 1992; Silliman, 1992) question the credibility of the method and whether the thoughts that are typed are subtle, unwitting communications transferred from the facilitator to the individual with autism through the use of a typewriter or computer. It appears improbable that children with autism can suddenly be transformed into active and independent creators of ideas.

Cognition Reconsidered

One outcome since the introduction of facilitated communication is that the cognitive abilities of some youngsters with autism are apparently better than had been suspected. Children who were being taught colors, matching letters, and the concepts of same/different behaved as though they did not know what was going on. This behavior was interpreted as an indication of low cognitive function and an incapacity to learn sophisticated skills. After being introduced to facilitated communication, some of the children demonstrated reading and writing skill and considerable world knowledge. These children consistently state that they want to be recognized as competent. Classroom curricular activities have been drastically altered. A few youngsters who were attending classes for very low functioning children are now being placed in regular classrooms with their facilitators and perform grade or above-grade level work. People are beginning to interact with these youngsters in a different way. They are no longer treated like naughty young children.

Communication Potential

A second outcome since the introduction of facilitated communication is that people believe that a child who does not talk or, at best, speaks in an incomprehensible way, can have a great deal to express. Some children with autism are "conversing" with facilitators, displaying a sense of humor, using sophisticated vocabulary, and expressing ideas. Some youngsters continue to blurt out echolalic or irrelevant utterances while they are simultaneously typing seemingly competent messages. Flexible language, abstract concepts, and proper pronoun usage are exhibited in some of the typed communications. However, the child's concurrent verbalizations are often a series of nonsense words.

Interest in Others

A third outcome is that some individuals with autism who are using facilitated communication indicate that they are concerned about the people around them. The definitive description of autism (American Psychiatric Association, 1987) states that a characteristic of autism is a lack of interest in people. It appears from the facilitated communications that a number of individuals with autism have difficulty in demonstrating their interest in other people. They communicate that they care about others and wish that their behavior was more acceptable to others.

Need for Validation

In short, through facilitated communication the minds of some children with autism have apparently been unlocked. Youngsters are seen who have ideas to communicate, better intelligence than could be determined without a communicative outlet, and a greater range of social and emotional abilities than had been suspected. Extensive research must be undertaken to determine the actual comprehension of the communications being expressed by the children with autism using facilitated communication. A time lag exists between the application of facilitated communication, the information being expressed by the people with autism, and scientific validation. Some researchers are withholding judgment on the information apparently being expressed by the youngsters with autism. Other professionals are eager to apply the communication approach because valuable time for those youngsters who might be helped could be lost. In the interim, other communicative modes such as oral and signed language should continue to be simultaneously employed.

APPROACHES TO INTERVENTION

Children with autism often appear unusual and lacking in social, intellectual, and linguistic abilities. These behaviors create a challenge for integration into mainstream educational settings. If the assumption is correct that more youngsters with autism have greater social, intellectual, and linguistic capabilities than had previously been acknowledged, those children are entitled to an appropriate education.

Early Intervention

Professionals are reconsidering intervention strategies for very young children with autism. Infants and preschoolers with autism experience their immediate environment or interact with others in a unique and limited manner. Their perceptual and motor processing abilities prevent them from obtaining vital information from their world so that concepts in social and cognitive areas can develop. That is, idiosyncratic sensory motor systems interfere with their ability to tolerate the environment. Biologically based regulatory dysfunctions make connections with people and situations extremely difficult. Intervention approaches which engage children with others are being developed to enhance more purposeful and intentional interaction (Greenspan, 1992; Kalmanson, 1992; Shanok, 1992; Wieder, 1992).

Greenspan (1992) focuses on engaging the very young child in reciprocal relationships with others. The parents and a team of professionals collaborate to implement early and intensive intervention programs. Generally the early childhood specialist, speech-language pathologist, occupational therapist, and parents observe and identify elements in the environment that distract or overstimulate the child. Then, through careful development of interactive routines, the child is taught to relate to people and the environment more effectively.

Wieder (1992) outlines the steps toward intentional and purposeful interaction as well as symbolic thought. To attain mutual attention, the adult joins the young child in an activity that the youngster finds pleasurable. The child always leads the reciprocal encounter. The adult helps the child at the activity, accompanying it with verbalizations. For example, the child may line up cars. The adult attempts to assist in this project. The aim is to transform what looks like random behavior into intentional, interactive activities.

The early intervention process gradually advances toward experiences which include higher-level symbolic and representational participation. Symbolic play is based on the child's real-life experiences. Therefore, regular opportunities to interact with children who are developing normally are critical (Shanok, 1992). Relationships with other youngsters as well as adults builds shared experiences to reenact during structured intervention. Children must enter the real world to learn about it. These activities are the foundation for linguistic, emotional, and cognitive development.

Shanok (1992) emphasizes the importance of gradual variation in activities to promote generalization of responses to new situations and to discourage rote nonverbal behaviors. A few children who have received early and intensive intervention, which encourages interaction and symbolic formation as determined by a collaborative team of professionals, have developed to a level which permits successful enrollment in regular kindergarten with professional support services (Greenspan, 1992).

Identifying Specific Learning Needs

The wide range of abilities of children with autism creates many learning needs and different styles of intervention for each child during different development periods. Mesibov (1991) has identified specific educational practices which are important for youngsters with communication difficulties, particularly autism. They include the following:

- **_Developing organizational skills._** An organized individual should understand what needs to be done and develop a plan of implementation. Work routines are facilitated with checklists, visual schedules, visual instructions, and assisted practice in analyzing what has been completed, what needs to be done, and how to proceed.

- **_Reducing distractibility._** Sensory distractions differ considerably among children. Extraneous noises, changes in lighting, and movement can disturb the child's focus on the task at hand. Environmental modifications such as a change in a child's work area can reduce distractions.

- **_Developing sequencing strategies._** A youngster should see relationships between tasks and details to complete them in order. Systematic work routines and visual instructions can develop the appropriate work sequence.

- **_Promoting generalization strategies._** Youngsters should understand the application of learned knowledge to other situations. Parent-community-school collaboration can facilitate generalization (Schopler and Mesibov, 1985).

Sensory Processing Training

Children with autism orient to sensory stimuli in unpredictable ways. At times, they seem oblivious to the noises around them. On other occasions, they respond to sights, touch, sounds, or smells with hypersensitivity. Minimal stimulation like a tap on the shoulder can cause a child to scream, run, or bite. Intervention efforts to regulate and integrate the senses are often incorporated with occupational therapy programs (Ayres, 1985; Fisher, Murray, and Bundy, 1991).

In recent years, **auditory integration training** (AIT) has received media attention as a method of retraining the ear to receive and process sound more efficiently (Stehli, 1992). The work of Berard (1993) in France is being expanded in the United States by Edelson, Rimland, and others. Auditory integration training has produced improvement in those individuals with autism whose audiograms indicate that this reeducation of the hearing mechanism is appropriate.

The first step in AIT is the administration of an audiological exam to determine the individual's ability to hear specific sounds at different pitches and intensities. Based on the audiological results, AIT may be recommended. Those children who demonstrate an intolerance to intense sounds, who run away from certain noises, or who protect their ears with their hands seem to respond well to AIT. An electronic sound device such as the audiokinetron developed by Berard (1993) is used for the training. The youngster with autism listens to music through earphones connected to the audiokinetron. The sounds of specially selected music are filtered so that a certain pitch and loudness range is presented. The listening sessions are scheduled for a two-week period and occur twice daily. The intent of the training is to sensitize and "reeducate" the auditory pathways so that sound can be processed more appropriately. Although auditory processing irregularities are not found in all children with autism, those with confirmed difficulties show improved language and behavior. One recipient of auditory training reported that doors closing, telephone voices, dishes being stacked, and dogs barking were no longer painful. He could reduce the use of earplugs (McKean, 1993). For children with autism, reducing their hypersensitivity to sensory stimuli allows them to attend to activities for extended periods of time without distraction.

Behavior Management

Children with autism exhibit challenging behaviors. Donovan (1993) cites *structure* and *warmth* as important components to appropriate behavior. Structure includes arranging the learning environment to provide organization and predictability for children. The room is arranged spatially to invite involvement and communication. The temporal structure includes schedules to anticipate patterns and transitions between activities. The social climate of the classroom provides opportunities for appropriate interactive skills. Warmth is characterized as teacher-child interactions based on respect. Children's ideas, feelings, and behaviors are acknowledged, and the positive attributes of each person are valued.

Behavior management includes problem-solving strategies (Donovan, 1993). This approach assumes that behaviors are responses that a child learns to cope with experiences. It also assumes that behaviors are communicative and tell us something about the child's ability to manage the demands of the environment. By observing behaviors in their context and analyzing the function of the behavior, the teacher can reinforce or teach positive responses. Donovan (1993) suggests using instructional objectives that are developmentally appropriate and interesting to the child. She also states that when the language of instruction is comprehensible to the youngster, it stimulates better behavior.

Inclusion

Evidence suggests that many youngsters with autism have thoughts to communicate and capability to learn despite their intrusive behaviors (Biklen and Schubert, 1991). Educators are reevaluating appropriate school settings, including regular classrooms, and communication opportunities for the nonverbal child. The presumption is if many more children with autism can communicate (through facilitated communication and other alternative methods), then a social network needs to be established for them. Children who can communicate need people to talk to. The educational setting provides a controlled environment with communicative opportunities for all children. By including youngsters with autism into broader educational environments, they too can utilize their communication skills. The inclusion movement (Biklen, 1989; Biklen and Schubert, 1991) promotes integration of children with autism into natural, mainstream settings because it recognizes that these youngsters want to be with other people and such environments might promote shared learning.

Inclusion, in its broader sense, also refers to involving the students with autism in decisions regarding changes in their own behavior. For example, many educational programs for children with autism rely on reinforcement techniques to modify behavior (Lord, 1985). Techniques used to modify aggressive behavior and oppositional outbursts include time-out routines such as isolating the child for a few minutes so that the child calms down. By removing the child from the environment, the youngster is prevented from expressing a message (either in an acceptable manner or with aberrant behaviors). Conversely, some FC users have typed that time out is helpful because they can reorganize themselves to reduce inappropriate behavior. Thus, time out is most effective when it also includes opportunities for communication between the child with autism and others.

Children with autism are indicating that they get discouraged with emphasis on their negative behavior. If they could get their bodies to perform in a more acceptable way, they would not misbehave. Professionals now realize that they must eliminate blame for negative behavior from the children with autism. By including them in decisions regarding behavior change, aberrant behavior may be reduced more expediently. Children with autism can share in selecting priority behaviors to change; this stimulates their motivation and promotes success.

Inclusion in decision making also enhances self-esteem. The opinion of the child with autism has validity. Sometimes people talk about youngsters with autism in front of them. It is natural to assume that a child who can't speak and appears to be rocking in an isolated world is not listening. However, professionals (Leary, 1992) encourage inclusion of the child with autism in interactions wherever possible. She believes that chatting and reading with the child without expecting a verbal response helps the child to develop relationships. Leary (1992) and others advocate that teachers should never assume that children with autism aren't listening when their behaviors suggest isolation or indifference.

Youngsters with autism who speak may not initiate conversations. That does not mean that they aren't interested in communicating. It is suggested that individuals assume the child with autism would like to engage in social interaction. By assisting the youngster in a difficult communicative encounter, the experience possibly could serve as a model for future, independent success. All children should be treated with respect.

Literacy

The issue of unexpected literacy exhibited by those youngsters provided with facilitated communication has educational implications. Professionals (Goodman, 1986; Wallach and Miller, 1988) state that literacy begins at birth. Exposure to labels, books, television, and signs is an important prerequisite to reading. Much is known about why children have reading difficulties. However, researchers do not agree on the process of learning to read.

Some young children with autism have been diagnosed over the years with **hyperlexia.** This is the advanced ability to recognize words and sound them out without a corresponding ability to comprehend what is read (Silberberg and Silberberg, 1967). Youngsters with autism sometimes develop this skill without direct instruction.

The students with autism who have been introduced to facilitated communication have also baffled their teachers. Many had been presumed incapable of academic learning. Yet their typing reveals unexpected literacy. Parents have tried to reconstruct ways that their children may have learned to read. Incidental learning seems to explain literacy skills. Some parents recall children leafing through books without indicating comprehension. Others became intrigued with game shows on television. Still others watched siblings out of the corners of their eyes while the family members spoke, did homework, and played. Educators, therefore, should not dismiss the benefits of incidental learning of academic, linguistic, and social skills.

SUMMARY

Children with autism display behaviors that are poorly understood. Since the middle of the 20th century, scientists have proposed that the disorder has psychological and physiological origins. The aspects of intellectual, linguistic, and social behaviors of the child vary considerably. Diagnostic criteria include impairment of social interaction, impairment of verbal and nonverbal communication, restricted repertoire of activities and interests, and other motor, sensory, and cognitive irregularities. Self-injurious behaviors are also frequent.

Nearly half of the youngsters with autism are nonverbal or have no useful verbal language. This condition has been associated with motoric dysfunction that affects the entire body. Researchers suggest that the difficulties are caused by specific neurological disturbances which are being examined using advanced radiological devices. A heightened sensory system and an intermingling of the senses have been linked to the disorder as well.

Poor verbal abilities led professionals to seek alternate forms of communication. One such method, facilitated communication, has generated intense controversy over the nature of autism. Since its introduction, children who appeared to have limited linguistic, social, and intellectual ability have expressed profound ideas regarding the nature of autism. The unexpected literacy demonstrated by these youngsters is being challenged by professionals who have no scientific explanation for the extraordinary results produced by some youngsters with autism. Facilitated communication reinforces the notion that the observable behaviors of the children with autism may not represent what is locked within their bodies and minds.

The facilitated communication controversy has implications in the educational setting. If many children with autism have intellectual and verbal strengths, then social opportunities in the educational environment are critical. Principles of inclusion in decision making, social situations, and academic opportunities are essential. Continued research and observation of this perplexing disorder are needed. Scientific facts are often determined by belief systems. What is known and not known about autism suggests that new theories are necessary to explain new observations.

SUGGESTED READINGS

Barron, J., and Barron S. (1992). *There's a Boy in Here*. New York: Simon and Schuster.

Cesaroni, L., and Garber, M. (1991). Exploring the Experience of Autism Through Firsthand Accounts. *Journal of Autism and Developmental Disorders, 21*(3), 303–313.

Williams, D. (1992). *Nobody, Nowhere*. New York: Times Books.

12 THE NATURE OF LANGUAGE DISORDERS AMONG CHILDREN WITH HEARING IMPAIRMENT

Comprehension of language and the development of speech to express a child's thoughts and needs usually are acquired by listening. Deaf infants generally do not acquire speech unless they are taught. Some of them never learn speech, regardless of the intensity of instruction. However, they can acquire rich and complex linguistic concepts if their parents communicate with them in a language they can see, a signed language.

The vast majority of children with hearing impairment have hearing parents who can only communicate with them orally. They use a spoken language that their children cannot adequately hear. Unless a hearing impairment is diagnosed early in infancy and children receive appropriate habilitation, it can be predicted that their concept development, their spoken language comprehension, and their speech production will be deleteriously affected. Contributing to these deficits are deficient hearing acuity and deficient linguistic stimulation during the first two years of life. When these children enter school, they can be predicted to have severely delayed linguistic development.

The ramifications of hearing loss extend into every aspect of the child's life. Chapter 12 explores these ramifications by

1. defining hearing impairment and the global impact of hearing loss;

2. describing the factors affecting language acquisition in terms of rate and quality;

3. presenting alternative modes of communication used to teach language when spoken language is not naturally acquired;

4. contrasting language development of children who are hearing impaired in families with deaf parents versus hearing parents;

5. examining the impact of concomitant auditory and visual perceptual disabilities and multilingual and multicultural issues; and

6. proposing ideal educational environments and suggesting teaching strategies for students in classroom settings who use various communication modes.

GLOBAL IMPACT OF LOSS OF HEARING

Hearing impairment is a generic term that includes all types and degrees of hearing loss, with mild hearing loss being the lowest degree and severe-to-profound hearing loss, or deaf, being the greatest degree of hearing impairment. When the impairment is caused by damage to the nerves located in the cochlea, or inner ear, or in the nerve pathways to the brain, it is called a **sensorineural hearing impairment**. A **conductive hearing impairment** refers to any dysfunction of the outer or middle ear in the presence of a normal inner ear.

The term **deaf,** when beginning with a lower case *d,* refers to the audiological condition of an individual "whose hearing impairment is so great, even with amplification, that vision becomes the main link to the world and main channel of communication" (Quigley and Paul, 1990, p. 1). **Deaf,** when referring to the community of individuals who share a culture and a language (American Sign Language), is capitalized. The members of this group reside in the United States and Canada (Padden and Humphries, 1988).

Hearing impairment should not be defined only in terms of how loud a sound must be before a person is aware of it. Understanding the global impact of a loss of hearing is more important. Hearing impairment is not a problem that only concerns the ears of the child. The disorder impacts every aspect of the child's development and well-being. Children with hearing impairment are a heterogeneous population. Some students cannot speak and use sign language to communicate; some speak and do not know or use sign language.

This textbook has continuously stressed the importance of intersensory integration. Long before the infant can walk, objects, people, and environments become meaningful because of the dynamic interplay among the visual, auditory, tactile, olfactory, and gustatory stimuli that are unique to specific situations. Concepts develop and are enriched by means of the sensory stimulation experienced by the child. When the infant is partially or entirely deprived of information received through a major sense, particularly during the first two years of life, the effects of the deprivation will be considerable.

Congenital Deafness

Children who are born with a severe-to-profound hearing loss are **congenitally** deaf, meaning the condition is present at birth. These children's early experiences and perceptions will not include most auditory stimuli. People and objects outside the child's range of vision will not exist. When the infant's mother moves out of sight, she has disappeared even though she is still in the same room. When the child is alone, there are no audible sounds in the environment to give pleasure and reassurance (Sanders, 1982).

Among the many sounds in the environment that are not heard by the congenitally deaf infant are the sounds of speech and vocal play that cause normally hearing infants to respond with delight. To a young infant, the inflections, stress, tones of voice, and individual characteristics of mother's voice are even more important than the words that are expressed. Chapter 3 notes that newborn infants orient to a gentle voice and differentiate between mother's voice and that of other women. When a child is born with profound hearing loss, some of this valuable information is lost.

In most cases, young congenitally deaf children have no concept of sound. When they first hear sounds after being fitted with hearing aids, they are irritated, if not alarmed by them. When they first hear speech, they often disregard it as noise and consider it a source of irritation (Sanders, 1982).

When deaf parents sign to their deaf infants from birth in American Sign Language parentese, all the paralinguistic cues signalling moods, emotions, and feelings are expressed by that form of communication. However, unless the parent's face and hands are within the infant's direct view, the communication as well as the parent are lost.

Impact on Schools and Families

Initially, in compliance with PL 94-142, only children with mild-to-moderate hearing losses or those with well-developed expressive and receptive oral communication skills were considered for inclusion in regular classes. Because they could speak, it was assumed for the most part that they understood the teacher's instructions, the classroom discussions, and the language of the textbooks and materials assigned.

Currently, hearing impaired students in the United States are being integrated at least part-time in regular classrooms. In addition, increasingly larger numbers of profoundly deaf children, accompanied by their sign language interpreters, are spending at least part of their school day in regular classes with hearing students (Moores, 1987; Moores and Kluwin, 1986). The interpreter translates the teacher's words into a communicative mode that the child understands and translates the child's signs into verbal representations that the teacher understands. The interpreter usually is not a teacher. The child must interpret the concepts being taught. The teacher must learn to anticipate the problems the child with hearing impairment is bound to encounter. Unfortunately, investigators have found a lack of administrative and professional support and also inadequate preparation for deaf students' classroom teachers (Bench, 1992; Chorost, 1988; Hull and Dilka, 1984; Luckner, 1991; Martin, Bernstein, Daly, and Cody, 1988). In most instances, these teachers have had no experience with deafness nor even minimal special training to teach children with profound hearing loss.

Parents are an integral part of the support team for hearing impaired children who are attending regular classes. Families of hearing impaired children are immigrating to the United States from every nation in the world. These children with serious language deficits in their primary languages are confronted with two additional languages simultaneously, English and sign language. They must also acclimate to American culture and Deaf culture, and still retain the culture of the family system. The classroom teacher has to have an understanding of the cultural attitudes the parents have toward hearing impairment and toward handicapping conditions in general. The parents will require counseling as to the requirements of the school and the special needs of the child.

FACTORS AFFECTING LANGUAGE ACQUISITION OF THE HEARING IMPAIRED CHILD

Several factors affect the rate and quality of language acquisition of the hearing impaired child:

1. degree of hearing loss;

2. pattern of residual hearing;

3. age at onset of hearing impairment;

4. age at which hearing impairment is diagnosed;

5. etiology of hearing impairment; and

6. family environment and quality of linguistic stimulation.

Degree of Hearing Loss

The degree of hearing loss is highly predictive of whether or not the individual will use sign language or speech to communicate. It is an important factor to consider when planning an educational program for the child.

Severe-to-Profound

The person who has a **severe-to-profound hearing impairment**, or is deaf, detects sound only when it is presented at 70–90 decibels (dB) or more in intensity (i.e., loudness). To understand how loud this decibel level is, zero decibels represents the softest sound that can be heard by most young adults with normal hearing. Whispered speech is usually 20–35 decibels (dB), and the average conversational decibel level in American culture is approximately 60–70 dB (Meadow, 1980). Sounds that are 120 dB are extremely loud and can be painful to people with normal hearing; rock music that is amplified is often played at this decibel level.

Among the population of individuals with severe-to-profound hearing loss, there are those who can benefit from high-powered amplification units (i.e., hearing aids) to the extent that, when aided, they can hear some components of speech and some inflections and tones of the voice, as well as environmental sounds.

Children who are born with severe-to-profound hearing impairment or become deaf soon after birth have great difficulty acquiring speech. Spoken language is not acquired naturally by these children, if it is acquired at all. The greater the degree of hearing loss, the more difficult it is to acquire intelligible speech and the more likely it is that the child will communicate by means of a manual language.

In a study of more than 48,000 hearing impaired students reported in the 1992–1993 Annual Survey for Hearing Impaired Children and Youth, 79 percent of the students in the severely impaired hearing range (70–90 dB) communicated by sign language. Ninety percent of the students whose hearing levels were 90 dB or higher were reported to sign (Center for Assessment and Demographic Studies, 1993).

Moderate-to-Severe Hearing Loss

Not every child with a hearing impairment is deaf. When there is a **moderate-to-severe hearing impairment,** 55–70 dB is required for sounds to be barely detected. Verbal conversation may be heard but cannot be understood without amplification.

Mild-to-Moderate Hearing Loss

Some individuals have **mild-to-moderate sensorineural hearing losses** indicating that nerve damage is less severe. They can detect sounds including speech sounds that are at least 40–55 dB in intensity unaided. They can usually benefit from amplification and can be taught speech, depending upon the pattern of their **residual hearing,** the hearing that is available after sensorineural damage has occurred.

Mild Hearing Loss

Children with a **mild hearing loss** require intensities of 25–40 dB for most sounds to be barely detected and higher decibel levels to understand and discriminate speech. The speech they hear may be distorted. The child may have a great deal of difficulty understanding spoken language in a noisy room. The child with a mild hearing loss usually acquires speech naturally through the auditory channel, but often has noticeable articulation problems and voice quality differences. The hearing levels of children with mild impairment can usually be improved with the aid of amplification and other methods depending upon the specific medical reasons for the hearing loss.

Mild hearing loss can be caused by nerve damage in the inner ear and also by medical conditions other than nerve damage. It is a mistake to consider the effects of these hearing impairments as "mild," however. Long-range ramifications with regard to language development are evident when the conditions are not diagnosed early.

Acute **otitis media with effusion** (OME) is diagnosed when fluid is detected in the middle ear space, sometimes following respiratory illness or symptoms of severe allergies. Many children have severe and recurrent episodes of acute otitis media, and fluid persists in the middle ear for weeks to months after each episode even with antibiotic treatment (Klein, 1986). Most children have impaired hearing while fluid is present (Klein, 1986). Up to 75 percent of episodes of OME are silent with no symptoms and no pain (Marchant, Shurin, Turczyk, Wasikowski, Tutihasi, and Kinney, 1984; Schwartz, Stool, Rodriguez, and Grundfast, 1981). It also has been reported that 3 of every 10 children have repeated episodes of otitis media with effusion. Of every 20 children with otitis media, 1–2 develop chronic middle ear disease, often with hearing loss (Feagans, Blood, and Tubman, 1988).

Otitis media is most frequent during the first three years of life, the period when language is developing. This development is highly dependent upon the acoustic information that the hearing baby is receiving (Menyuk, 1986; Paradise, 1980). After age three, the incidence of otitis media declines. It is relatively uncommon in children seven years of age and older.

In a large scale study following children with chronic middle ear disease, Teele, Klein, and Rosner (1984) consistently demonstrated poor language development. Their findings and those of other investigators point to depressed linguistic and auditory processing abilities (Brandes and Ehinger, 1981; Jerger, Jerger, Alford, and Abrams, 1983; Sak and Ruben, 1981). These symptoms are manifested in impairments of auditory attention, sequential memory, auditory discrimination, and auditory closure skills. Another very insidious outcome of fluctuating hearing loss is that, because of inconsistency of input, the child may learn not to attend to spoken language (Feagans, Blood, and Tubman, 1988). Academic progress is seriously impaired for many children with otitis media and the effects of the fluctuating hearing loss with its concomitant language and attention deficits remain long after the recurrent episodes have subsided and disappeared.

Children with hearing impairment who wear hearing aids and who rely on residual hearing also can have otitis media. When their middle ears are filled with fluid, they cannot benefit from amplification and will probably not be able to hear at all for intermittent periods. Deaf children can also have otitis media with effusion and this fact is often overlooked.

Residual Hearing

Most individuals with moderate-to-profound hearing loss have some residual hearing. The reliance upon residual hearing depends upon which nerves are damaged. These nerves are highly specialized to process specific frequencies of speech and environmental sounds. "Frequencies" of sounds are perceived as changes in pitch. The damage rarely occurs equally across all intensities and all frequencies of speech. Consonants carry the information of speech in the English language and are heard as high-pitched, relatively weak sounds. Unfortunately, ability to hear these high-frequency sounds is most often greatly diminished by nerve damage in individuals with hearing impairment.

Whatever sensitivity is still available from residual hearing can and should be utilized. Many speech sounds and environmental sounds can be amplified to within hearing range by hearing aids, although hearing aids cannot make hearing normal as eye glasses can make vision normal. Even when wearing hearing aids, individuals with moderate-to-severe hearing impairment hear voices and speech of others only partially and with distortion.

Age at Onset

Another factor that affects the rate and quality of language acquisition is **age at onset** or the age at which the condition causing the hearing impairment occurred. By two years of age, normally hearing children are sophisticated language users. They understand a great many individual word meanings even when the words are embedded in complex sentence structure. They understand the nonverbal cues perceived in tone, inflection, emphasis, and loudness of voice that provide additional information to aid comprehension.

If a child is born with a hearing impairment, the effect is a reduction in the amount of auditory information available during a critical period for language development. If the degree of impairment is severe-to-profound, the child may be referred to as a **prelingually deaf child,** or deafened before language acquisition. The infant cannot hear speech or most environmental sounds. Serious language delay will result unless the child's parents communicate immediately to the infant in a visual, manual language (i.e., sign language). In that case, the child will receive linguistic concepts just as rich as those heard by normally hearing children.

If the child is born with normal hearing and, after the age of two years, is in an accident or is afflicted with a viral disease causing serious damage to the nerves of the inner ear, language will have developed prior to the damage. The child will probably be able to speak to some degree, but further development will be seriously delayed unless amplification, special education, and habilitation are provided as soon as possible after onset of the hearing loss. If the degree of hearing impairment is severe-to-profound, the child may be referred to as a **postlingually deaf child**, or deafened after language acquisition.

Age of Diagnosis

Deaf infants look the same as infants who are born with normal hearing. They are just as beautiful, charming, and animated, especially when a familiar adult or a shiny object is within their visual field. They will gaze into the adult's eyes, and are fascinated by the adult's face, just the same as an infant with normal hearing. Within a few weeks after birth, they will reach for an attractive bright object that they see, the same as a normally hearing infant.

However, they will not turn to or follow sound when they cannot see the source of the sound. They will respond to their mother's smile, but not to her voice. They will not respond to noise in the environment, not even a loud noise that would cause a normally hearing young infant to scream.

Although parents may suspect that their child cannot hear, they often prolong seeking professional confirmation of their suspicions. Children with considerable residual hearing in the low frequencies (i.e., low-pitched sounds) may respond to many or most environmental sounds. Ironically, the infants with more extensive residual hearing may escape notice because they are aware of their environment (Sanders, 1982). However, infants with severe-to-profound hearing loss will usually ignore environmental sounds.

If audiological testing is done as soon as suspicions are aroused, and a hearing impairment is diagnosed in early infancy, appropriate steps can be taken to ensure that speech and language will develop as normally and naturally as possible. Long delays in acquiring official confirmation of the diagnosis are the norm, but they are not always because of parental procrastination. Pediatricians with little or no experience with deaf children often attribute these fears to "over-anxious parents."

If the hearing impairment is diagnosed after the age of two years, the child will have spent those two years in a silent world with little or no auditory stimulation and very limited acquisition of auditory information. Electric amplifying hearing aids became available in the early 1900s. The rationale behind providing hearing aids to very young children is that speech should be made accessible as early in the first year as possible (Bench, 1992).

Etiology

The importance of knowing the etiology or cause of a prelinguistic hearing loss has to do with preparation and prevention. According to the 1992–1993 Annual Survey for Hearing Impaired Children and Youth conducted by the Center for Assessment and Demographic Studies at Gallaudet University, 14 percent of the 48,000 hearing impaired students reported were known to have hearing impairments due to hereditary, or genetic causes. Genetic awareness could improve early identification of some forms of hearing impairment. Appropriate education can be planned for the children and counseling can serve to educate, inform, and provide emotional support to their families.

Infectious diseases are capable of causing prelingual hearing loss and are preventable. Maternal rubella (German measles), meningitis, herpes, cytomegalovirus (CMV), infantile congenital syphilis, infectious mononucleosis, small pox, mumps, and some influenza viruses are all known causes of prelingual hearing impairment. All can be medically treated and others, such as mumps, rubella, and smallpox, can be eliminated with immunization by available vaccines (Bergstrom, 1988; Glasscock, McKennan, and Levine, 1988).

Prenatal medical care can also identify and possibly prevent congenital hearing impairment. The discovery of Rh-immune globulin has resulted in a marked reduction of Rh-incompatibility of the newborn, a condition which often leads to sensorineural hearing loss.

Any situation during the birth process that can deprive the fetus or newborn of oxygen can result in damage to the inner ear and middle ear structures (Fischler, 1988). Premature infants have a greater likelihood of suffering complications than full-term infants. In addition, infants with fetal alcohol syndrome are reported as high risk for sensorineural hearing loss (see Chapter 14). Child abuse is another cause of hearing impairment that must not be overlooked (Fischler, 1988).

A federally appointed panel of experts assembled by the National Institutes of Health has recommended that all infants be screened for signs of hearing impairment before they are discharged from newborn nurseries or within the first three months of life (Leary, 1993). Presently, newborns who are known to have been exposed to viral diseases in utero, to be genetically at risk, or to be born prematurely with a low birth weight are often, but not always, routinely screened either in the intensive care neonatal nurseries or privately by pediatricians. The average age for identifying deaf or severely hearing impaired children in the United States is when they are almost three years old and lesser degrees of hearing loss go undetected even longer (Leary, 1993).

Early detection of hearing impairment is important for medical treatment and subsequent educational intervention (Fischler, 1988). In a position statement by the Joint Committee on Infant Hearing, the American Speech-Language-Hearing Association established criteria for identifying infants at high risk for hearing impairment (ASHA, 1982).

Preventive medicine, special educational planning, amplification, and early language saturation for the young infant with hearing impairment are advantages gained from the acquisition of etiological information. In the 1992–1993 Annual Survey (Center for Assessment and Demographic Studies, 1993), the etiology of 53 percent of the reported 48,000 students with hearing impairment was unknown. One can only wait and see, or guess at the types of problems these children will encounter.

Family System and Linguistic Stimulation

Approximately 5–10 percent of the total population of children with hearing impairment have parents who are hearing impaired. The majority of children with hearing impairment have families consisting of two hearing parents, hearing siblings, hearing grandparents, and hearing aunts and uncles. Their families socialize with hearing friends. Probably all the families that live on their streets or in their apartment houses are hearing. Most likely the parents have never met or known a deaf person.

In the past, when the term *hearing family* was used, it implied that the one hearing impaired member of the family was deviant. Currently, the term used to describe the family of a hearing impaired child is *family system*, which includes hearing and deaf members. The term implies that deafness does not belong to the child alone, but to the whole family (Henderson and Hendershott, 1991).

Deaf Children of Hearing Parents

Statistical evidence indicates that the deaf child in the family system described above is, in fact, isolated in many ways. Communicative difficulties are the most overwhelming of the many problems confronting individuals who are deaf. Unless the etiology was known to be genetic or the child was considered as "high risk" for hearing impairment, the family was probably completely unprepared for such a problem. Most likely, the infant was not screened for hearing impairment within the first three months of life. Most likely, by the time the suspicions of the parents were aroused and the diagnosis made and finally confirmed, the major portion of the crucial first two years of life was spent without auditory stimulation, including speech and language.

Very important choices must be made soon after the diagnosis. These choices include the selection of appropriate amplification for the child and appropriate language stimulation and aural habilitation programs. Immediate decisions also must be made as to which mode of communication is to be used consistently with the child both at home and at all education facilities with which the child is involved. The choices should be made for the entire family, not just for the deaf child. For example, if simultaneous communication is the mode selected, then the "whole" family should commit themselves to learning and using that particular combination of sign language and spoken language with the child.

Interaction between the deaf child, hearing parents, and hearing siblings is difficult at best, and nonexistent or gestural most often. The emotional reactions and concerns regarding their deaf child "affect hearing parents' judgments and, worst of all, are often communicated to the child" (Schein, 1989, p. 107). Parents turn to professionals for counseling and are often confronted with conflicting opinions, particularly with regard to the use of sign language, oral language only, simultaneous communication, and the type of educational program most appropriate for their child.

The everyday demands and pressures caused by the special needs of the deaf child are often unintentionally relayed to the child by facial expressions, body language, irritability, and stress. Medical and audiological attention, as well as hearing aids, hearing aid batteries, and repairs contribute to the pressures and financial burdens of the family.

Often hearing siblings are not willing to learn and do not have the patience to use signed communication. When using oral communication, children's speech is often not clearly enunciated and very rapid. They often talk while running and assume that their hearing impaired sibling understands what they say.

Family interactions at the dinner table and at other times when all family members gather together often do not include the deaf child, who is not so much ignored, as left out of these conversations. The child cannot participate because spoken language is not understood. Also, the need for constant concentration to comprehend what is going on is exhausting. There is danger that children who are hearing impaired in family systems where all other members are hearing might perceive that they are different or inferior to other members of the family.

Unexplained phenomena are frightening to children. Raymond Stevens (1987), principal of a school for deaf children, describes the underlying fears that can occur when there is lack of communication:

> When a grandfather dies, the hearing child may learn about death through a story that mother reads. Parents select the book that reflects their attitudes toward death, and the hearing child learns that attitude through the real experience of grandfather's death and through the symbolic experience of the story. When the deaf child's grandfather dies, little is said and less is understood. (p. 184)

When parents can explain to the child in a language that can be understood what has happened and what can be expected to happen, fear, at least, can be eliminated from the many emotions that are experienced.

When a deaf child of hearing parents is taken shopping, the conversations between the shopkeepers and the hearing parent are conducted orally. If the parent meets a friend or acquaintance, the conversation is conducted orally. The deaf child cannot understand the major portion of the interactions, is left out entirely, and often inadvertently ignored.

By the time hearing children enter kindergarten, they have developed sophisticated expressive and receptive language and an impressive information base, particularly if they come from homes where they are read to and are included in family interactions and activities. They have acquired language incidentally through natural communication within the family and around the community. The situation is quite different for a deaf child from a family system in which all but the child are hearing. When this deaf child enters school at an equivalent age, there is usually inadequate concept development, severely delayed linguistic development, and an inadequate information base, mostly because of language deprivation.

Deaf Children of Deaf Parents

The small group of deaf children having deaf parents tend to attain higher levels of social skills, basic world knowledge, conceptual development, and academic proficiency than deaf children from families in which all but the deaf child can hear (Meadow, 1980). The difference appears related to the linguistic environment of most deaf families (not all deaf adults communicate in sign language), and also to the acceptance of deafness as a natural phenomenon with which the parents have a great deal of experience. Deafness is not considered a crisis or a tragedy. Deaf parents are keenly aware of their deaf child's communicative needs, probably because they are able to recall the isolation felt when they were children. (Recall that 90–95 percent of deaf children are members of family systems including two hearing parents).

The deaf parents who communicate immediately with their deaf infant in American Sign Language (the language of the Deaf community) initiate a rich, visually accessible communicative environment. Research by Erting, Prezioso, and Hynes (1990) and Rea, Bonvillian, and Richards (1988) reveals that deaf parents use "parentese" when signing to their deaf infants. The signs are modified in that they are slower, clearer, and grammatically simpler with much repetition. There is a great deal of smiling, touching, and stroking. Deaf signing parents are able to obtain and maintain their infants' attention. They appear instinctively to sit with their hands and faces within view (Kantor, 1982).

Deaf babies of deaf signing parents, observed by Petitto and Marentette (1991) at McGill University in Montreal, babbled with their hands in the same rhythmic, repetitive fashion as hearing infants who babble with their voices. The deaf babies who presumably watch the sign language of their parents start their manual babbles before they are 10 months old, the same age hearing children begin stringing sounds together (Petitto and Marentette, 1991). These babbles consist of about 13 different hand motions used over and over again. Nearly all of them have been identified as actual elements of American Sign Language.

As the deaf child of deaf parents develops, there are constant opportunities for discussions with competent sign language users on a variety of topics. American Sign Language is the natural language used by most signing deaf families in the course of spontaneous interactions during everyday activities. Young deaf children of deaf parents have indicated that they find hearing people "strange" because they communicate by moving their mouths (Padden and Humphries, 1988).

Self-image is found to be significantly more positive for deaf children of deaf parents than for deaf children whose parents have normal hearing. Their parents frequently interact with other deaf individuals, and this has a positive effect, especially when deaf children are drawn into the signed conversation. Self-image is found to be significantly more positive for those children whose parents are particularly active in the Deaf community (Meadow, 1980).

Many deaf children attend a residential school from an early age. Usually these state-funded schools are specifically for deaf children from preschool through high school. The schools often serve communities throughout a state, and the distance from the children's homes necessitates their staying at the school throughout the week and going home for weekends and holidays. In the dormitories, children learn American Sign Language, appropriate social interaction within the Deaf community, and Deaf culture (Padden and Humphries, 1988). These social interactions are the means by which deaf children and adolescents become members of the Deaf community. The deaf parents of children attending the residential schools probably attended one themselves. When the child comes home on the weekend, the ASL communications continue naturally. Deaf culture is reinforced in the family environment. On the other hand, when the deaf child returns home to hearing parents, there is little if any understanding of the Deaf community, Deaf culture, and the language of the Deaf community, American Sign Language.

LANGUAGE MODE

Spoken language is not acquired naturally by most prelingual, moderate-to-profound hearing impaired children. Unless they are deaf children of deaf parents who communicate in ASL, they usually do not learn either ASL or forms of manual English until they attend school. This is quite a different situation than is found with hearing children who begin to acquire their language from the day of birth. Deaf infants of deaf signing parents, on the other hand, acquire sign language at the same age as hearing infants acquire oral language or earlier, presumably because the motor control of arms, hands, and fingers develops earlier than the control of speech musculature (Bonvillian, Orlansky, and Novak, 1983). There are also similarities between the developmental stages of oral and signed language (e.g., overgeneralizations of morphological rules in ASL that are similar to *gived* and *eated* in young, hearing children acquiring Standard English).

Children with hearing impairment, particularly those with moderate-to-profound hearing loss, cannot acquire language through the process of listening as hearing children normally acquire language. Therefore, they must be taught a mode of communication in an environment where they have ample opportunity to interact with other children and adults using that mode of communication. Hearing parents who must make decisions regarding the mode of communication they want used in the educational setting for their child need appropriate counseling. Such counseling should include the pros and cons of *all* of the linguistic options available, without bias.

Oral Method

The mode of communication referred to as the **oral method** includes the teaching of spoken English and speech reading. Inherent in this method, also, are the following aspects (Calvert, 1986):

1. emphasis on early diagnosis of hearing impairment prior to two years of age;

2. early fitting of hearing aids;

3. emphasis on the use of spoken English without accompanying gestural language;

4. involvement of parents, teachers, and others in the deaf child's environment;

5. use of technical equipment for teaching and for amplifying spoken language;

6. efforts to develop residual hearing; and

7. individualized approaches considering the deaf child's personality, motivation, and abilities.

Aural habilitation is a term sometimes used to describe a program that incorporates various components just listed. The advocates of oralism contend that "selected profoundly deaf children with a high IQ, when consistently and persistently provided with excellent teachers, can develop satisfactory language and reading" (Connor, 1986, p. 123). However, most the children with hearing impairment who have been successful at learning to speak intelligibly and learning to understand spoken communication are those who have a significant degree of residual hearing and a lesser degree of hearing loss (Osberger, 1990; Paterson, 1986; Smith and Richards, 1990).

Speech Reading

Whenever a significant hearing loss results in reduction of understanding of the speech of others, the listener must look for supplementary cues. These cues are often found in the environmental context in which the communication occurs, the visually observable points of articulation, and the oral configurations of the speaker. In addition, nonverbal stimuli, such as body position, gestures, and facial expressions convey a great deal of information. Use of these supplementary cues is known as **speech reading.**

Oral configurations and **points of articulation** refer to movement and positions of the jaw, lips, tongue, soft palate, and teeth when producing various speech sounds. Some sounds are highly visible on the mouth, such as *b, p, m, sh, f, v, w*. Other sounds look the same on the mouth (e.g., *p, b, m; s* and *z; f* and *v; t* and *d*). Some sounds are produced in the back of the mouth and have poor visibility (e.g., *g* and *y*). The sound of *h* has no visible characteristic. Often, there are too many similarities to be able to rely solely on "lip reading" for message understanding. Individuals learn to anticipate the speaker's comments related to the topic. This ability depends upon their experiences, knowledge of the language being spoken, knowledge of the topic, the physical environment in which the message is communicated, and the people in the environment (Sanders, 1982). Listeners (signers) also need to observe facial expressions and body positions to glean information about attitudes, emotions, and feelings of the speaker. Additional information is found in natural gestures, which do not mean the same as sign language (e.g., nodding the head and shrugging the shoulders). Gestures are used to emphasize meaning.

All individuals who speak also speech read, even when they can hear. Everyone having a conversation with a friend in a school cafeteria, a crowded restaurant, a subway, or a gym, will speech read. If they can only hear the subject, verb, and object and no other parts of the sentence, they can usually fill in the missing words and general meaning based upon the limited kinds of words that are grammatically possible. For example, in the sentence, *I hope you can come . . .*, only a limited number of phrases fit (e.g., *to the party, on vacation, with us*).

Deaf individuals who know English vocabulary and English sentence structure can learn to speech read. Deaf individuals who communicate in ASL do not speech read because the sentence structure is very different. They cannot "fill in" missing words. After they have learned English syntax, they may be able to speech read to some degree, but they have never heard the spoken words adequately and do not relate words to the sounds associated with them. Prelingually deaf individuals "have no auditory image, no idea of what speech sounds like" (Sacks, 1989, p. 26). They have not spoken the words themselves and have not experienced the tactile sensations related to the articulation.

Methods for teaching speech reading were developed for hard-of-hearing adults who already had acquired a mastery of spoken language. The speech-reading task is far different for deaf children who have no oral language to draw from. The following is a good rule when predicting a child's ability to speech read: When a person has acquired an oral language, has knowledge of the syntax of the language, has had personal experience with motor planning and motor/tactile sensations associated with speaking, and has heard, even in the past, the sounds of the words that are spoken, then the person can "fill in" missing portions of the sentence to speech read. Children with mild-to-moderate hearing loss can also benefit from speech-reading training.

Cued Speech

Cued speech was devised by Orin Cornett in 1966 to help deaf youngsters discriminate speech sounds that have the same appearance on the face when spoken (e.g., *mat, bat,* and *pat*). **Cued speech** consists of hand signals that the speakers use while speaking. The technique also is employed in the process of teaching speech to young children with hearing impairment (Quenin and Blood, 1989). It uses four hand positions to distinguish eleven English vowels, and eight hand shapes to differentiate 25 consonant sounds, as well as hand movements for some diphthongs (Cornett, 1967; Schein, 1984). The "signs" or hand shapes are placed in different locations on or near the face. The technique is meant to clarify words and statements that look alike on the mouth and which may be misread due to difficulty in distinguishing mouth configurations. There has been little systematic study of its effectiveness in the years following its introduction (Quigley and Kretschmer, 1982). Available information is not sufficient to indicate whether cued speech improves speech-reading skills. Also, the roles played by other factors, such as vocabulary, cognitive ability, and linguistic ability of the deaf student have not been clarified.

Manual Coded English

Manual Coded English has taken the base signs of American Sign Language and superimposed them on English vocabulary and English sentence structure. It is an artificial language as opposed to American Sign Language, which is a natural language that evolved through use by deaf individuals in Deaf communities in the United States over the past two hundred years. This distinction is very important because ASL is not by any means an artificially constructed language.

The purpose of Manual Coded English is to make the spoken language visible to children with hearing impairment. One of several forms of Manual Coded English is Signing Exact English (SEE 2) (Gustason, 1983; Gustason, Pfetzing, and Zawolkow, 1980). Signs in SEE 2 are designated to depict the same syntactical structure, the same grammar, and the same punctuation as spoken and written English. Many of the signs, particularly those for punctuation, are made up because there are no representative signs in ASL. There is evidence that in the course of communicating, many parents and teachers fail to include a number of the important features of English in their SEE 2 signed sentences, thus limiting or distorting the child's exposure to English (Swisher, 1985). This situation occurs because signing every single plural designation (*s* and *es*), every period, and every single auxiliary verb is tedious and takes too much time.

Manual Coded English is the most common form of manual communication used in the United States because it is easier for English-speaking, hearing parents and hearing teachers to learn than ASL (Hoffmeister, 1982). To learn ASL, one must learn a different grammar. To learn Manual Coded English, one only has to learn the manual equivalents of English words.

Studies do not support the view that the development of sign language will either delay, discourage, or impede the development of oral language. When hearing parents of deaf children use some simultaneous combination of signed and spoken English, vocabulary growth, grammatical complexity, and syntactic structure all progress in the same sequence as for hearing children, only slower (Acredolo and Goodwyn, 1985; Holmes and Holmes, 1980).

Pidgin Sign English

Pidgins develop spontaneously when users of two separate languages improvise to communicate. Deaf signers who are informally conversing with hearing friends who do not know ASL may use signs and fingerspelling in Standard English word order, but will leave off the inflections, such as verb endings *ing* and *ed* (Bench, 1992).

For prelingually deaf children with hearing family systems, the first language appears to be a mixture of English and sign, referred to as **Pidgin Sign English**. Its use and similarity to English is dependent upon factors such as home and school environment, degree of hearing loss, and contact with the Deaf community (Epstein, 1985). Pidgin Sign English is often observed in many classrooms in interactions between deaf children and hearing teachers, but in a form that is more complex than the kinds of Pidgins used at informal occasions (Lucas and Valli, 1989). Each time teachers of deaf children leave off the punctuation marks in their signed Manual Coded English communications, they have reverted to a Pidgin Sign English. This practice is not conducive to language acquisition by a deaf child because it is not a consistently used, syntactically rule-governed, or morphologically rule-governed mode of communication, and certainly cannot be considered a true "language."

Total Communication

In the mid-to-late 1960s, a combination of oral and signing approaches was introduced into classrooms in schools and educational programs for deaf children. This philosophy of communication came to be known as total communication (Schlesinger, 1986), and the method itself is often referred to as **simultaneous communication** (Newell, Stinson, Castle, Mallery-Ruganis, and Holcomb, 1990). **Total communication** is used to describe "the philosophy or system which permits any and all methods of communication to be used with deaf children" (Quigley and Paul, 1990, p. 25).

The main goals of total communication are as follows:

1. to accelerate overall language acquisition (Schlesinger, 1986);

2. to hasten the acquisition of English by helping children who are deaf to improve grammar and learn English morphemes (Bornstein, Saulnier, and Hamilton, 1980; Gustason, Pfetzing, and Zawolkow, 1980);

3. to promote spontaneous production of language (Knell and Klonoff, 1983); and

4. to promote speech production (Silberman-Miller, 1981).

Academic achievement, psychological growth, and ability to live in the adult world with both hearing and deaf individuals are also goals for the use of total communication (Champie, 1984; Giangreco and Giangreco, 1980).

Research over the long history of simultaneous communication has revealed disappointing results. The addition of speech to manual communication does not increase the deaf students' ability to learn the information, but depresses it slightly. Children appear to lose information by having to shift attention between speech and the manual signals or they experience perceptual overload. There is evidence that deaf children cannot process speech, speech reading, and signs at the same time. The signs often do not synchronize with the movement of the mouth.

Deaf children using simultaneous communication have been observed to communicate predominantly in manual language and to disregard speech (Bench, 1992). Geers, Moog, and Schick (1984) found that profoundly deaf children educated by simultaneous communication experienced problems in speech production. These children did not acquire English syntax more rapidly or accurately than deaf children educated in the oral/aural method.

Teachers in kindergarten to fourth grade educational programs were observed to produce the exact signed English representation of spoken language when using simultaneous communication. However, as the linguistic demands became greater for more complex language in the higher grades, the manual communication accompanying the speech deteriorated into a pidgin representation (Mayer and Lowenbraun, 1990). Thompson and Swisher (1985) argue that simultaneous communication is suitable for providing immediate and consistent language for very young deaf children who do not need lengthy or complex linguistic inputs. The trend is to continue with the total communication approach in educational programs until further research is concluded (Bench, 1992).

American Sign Language (ASL)

Like all true languages, **American Sign Language** consists of a symbolic code that has been assigned meaning arbitrarily by the language users of the community. It is rule-governed and has a different grammatical and syntactical structure from spoken and written English.

One cannot separate ASL from Deaf culture. Members of the Deaf community identify themselves through the use of ASL, since one of the requirements for membership is fluency in the use of this language. Prior to 1960, ASL was considered a means of manually encoding English (Schein, 1989) or a "prosthesis" that deaf people use because they cannot speak or hear (Humphries, 1993).

In 1960, William Stokoe, a linguist and professor of English at Gallaudet College, analyzed the grammatical and syntactical components of ASL (Stokoe, 1960). A dictionary was developed from this research (Stokoe, Casterline, and Croneberg, 1965), and from that time on, ASL has been considered a true language in its own right (Schein, 1989). ASL is a natural and very complex language that evolved through use by deaf people in the Deaf linguistic community.

Virtually all concepts can be expressed in ASL. Not only abstract thoughts, facts, and opinions are communicated, but also the culture of the Deaf community is taught and transmitted from one generation to another.

Signs are constructed by arranging the fingers and configuration of the hands in particular ways to designate specific meanings and concepts. Each sign requires a particular movement of the hands and arms. Also, the position of the hands on or near a particular area of the body is an integral part of the sign. There are also signs for the neutral space in front of the body.

Ursula Bellugi and her colleagues at the Laboratory for Language and Cognitive Studies at Salk Institute have studied extensively the morphological processes in ASL. Their research has added significant knowledge about its complex structure. By altering and modulating movement of the hands and arms, and by structuring space according to unique morphological rules, the signer has infinite ways of extending and enriching vocabulary (Bellugi, 1987; Klima and Bellugi, 1979). Facial expressions, essential components of individual signs, contribute meaning related to the intensity of feelings, emotions, and attitudes. Movements of the eyes, eyebrows, face and head often function as adverbs, adjectives, and pronouns, and are actual parts of the sign (Baker, 1985).

Eye contact is an important element in ASL. In a conversation between normally hearing individuals, listeners and speakers periodically glance away. When a deaf listener glances away from a signing speaker, the communication is immediately interrupted, and the speaker may interpret this behavior as "rude." Hearing people continue to hear the spoken message even when they are no longer looking at the speaker. Deaf people cannot continue to communicate unless the listener looks at the deaf speaker. In American hearing culture, children are taught that staring is inappropriate. However, in ASL conversations, Deaf culture clearly specifies rules regarding the appropriate use of the eyes (Schein, 1989).

Speech cannot accompany ASL as it can for Manually Coded English. One cannot speak and simultaneously sign a different language. The hands are considered "sacred" by deaf people. They are used for communication to convey meaning and thoughts. Many individuals who are deaf are strongly opposed to the use of what they call "nonsense" use of hands, such as cued speech (Padden, 1980). When considering cued speech as an educational technique for deaf children of deaf parents, the teacher should make every attempt to ascertain the parents' attitudes in this regard.

ASL is the only mode of communication which cannot be considered a practical option with regard to the choice of an educational program. In the early 1990s, only five educational programs in the United States used ASL as the mode of communication in teaching (D. Bergstrom, personal communication, August 1993). In these programs, reading and language are taught in English; all other subjects are taught in ASL. This is known as the Bi-Bi Approach (i.e., bilingual/bicultural).

LANGUAGE DEVELOPMENT

If parents of deaf children have normal hearing acuity, they typically communicate using spoken English or a pidgin form of signed

English. Most often, they are found to use labels for objects accompanied by mime. Parents are often found to be hesitant about using signs that may be inaccurate. Nevertheless, even if they learn just a few signed utterances, they can help their children acquire expressive vocabulary. Bates, O'Connell, and Shore (1987) reported that several young children in their studies acquired expressive sign vocabulary approaching the 50-word mark by 18 months of age. They found that even inaccurate hand shapes or actions did not necessarily interfere with the ability of mother and child to share meanings. Accurate productions, intact grammatical forms, and fluency (whether in Manual Coded English or American Sign Language) become more important when modeling language for babies who have progressed beyond initial stages of one- and two-word sign utterances (Spencer, 1993).

In studies of deaf children of deaf parents who are exposed to sign language, "all the major milestones of communicative development (use of first sign, size of vocabulary at 12 months, use of first two- and then three-sign combinations) are several months advanced for first language signers over first language speakers" (Snow, 1981, p. 203). In addition to often showing an earlier onset of expressive communication, sign-learning children have often been found to be accelerated in their rate of vocabulary acquisition when compared to children who are learning only speech (Orlansky and Bonvillian, 1988). Syntactic and pragmatic development and the sequence of acquisition are similar to those reported for hearing children despite the differences in modality and syntax.

The acceleration in the attainment of certain linguistic milestones appears to apply only to the earliest steps of language production. When the acquisition of later, more complex linguistic constructions is studied, sign-learning children are found to closely approximate the ages and patterns of language acquisition of normally hearing speakers (Newport and Meier, 1985).

Role of Residual Hearing in Utero

Residual hearing usually consists of the lower frequencies of sound, including those of speech. The lower frequencies of speech carry prosodic information (i.e., inflection, tone of voice) and vowels. Studies of intrauterine sound transmission and fetal hearing suggest that prelingual learning about spoken language begins with the mother's voice and her prosodic cues while the fetus is still in utero (De Casper and Spence, 1986; Locke, 1993; Spence and De Casper, 1987). When the pregnant mother speaks, the components of her voice and speech are carried through her bones, tissues, and fluids to the ears and brain of the fetus. It is thought that normally hearing fetuses in utero respond more frequently to the lower frequencies of their mother's voice, which bear the prosodic information (Locke, 1993). It has been suggested that there is some relationship between intrauterine fetal awareness of prosody in the mother's voice and the evident enjoyment by normally hearing newborn infants of motherese, which contains so much variation in pitch and durational cues (Fernald, 1985, 1991; Fernald and Kuhl, 1987). Fetuses who have acquired auditory sensorineural damage in utero may possibly have some low frequency residual hearing and may be able to hear some of these sounds.

Newborn infants, only a few hours old, indicate clearly that they can discriminate their mother's voice from that of other women; they have been listening to that voice for a number of months. Moon and Fifer (1990) found in their research that normally hearing newborn infants responded positively to their own mother's voice and were aware of her voice as opposed to silence. If hearing impaired newborns' residual hearing allows them to respond to the lower frequencies of their mother's melodic motherese, if only to the extent that they can differentiate the speaking voice from silence, that would be important information for later communication use. Further research is warranted in this area.

Mother-Child Interaction

Mothers are usually observed to moderate their responses so they do not interrupt when infants are responding. Gregory and Mogford (1981) have observed that interactions between hearing impaired children and their mothers exhibit more "vocal clashes" because the children cannot hear when the mother's voice either lowers at the end of a comment or stops when waiting for the child to respond. They emphasize that the breakdown of smooth turn-taking skills may be very serious in their long-term effects.

"Joint reference" stimulates early communications between mother and child. The mother of a hearing child easily alters her language and topic of communication to fit the child's changing interests and perceptions of objects in the environment. For a deaf baby, however, joint reference and maternal comments about the referent cannot occur at the same time. When looking at a joint referent, or object of interest to both mother and child, the child must avert gaze from the mother. Communication then ceases, because little or no auditory input is available when the child with a hearing loss is looking away from the speaker's face or the signer's face and hands. Interaction between mother and deaf infant regarding joint referents is often disjointed because, unlike the hearing infant, the deaf infant cannot hear the mother's comment and explore the referential object of interest at the same time (Bamford and Saunders, 1991).

When a hearing mother interacts orally with a deaf baby, comprehension soon begins to falter primarily because the deaf baby does not speak and does not sustain attention to the speaking face. When this happens, communication becomes more difficult and one-sided. Hearing mothers who communicate orally are often observed to interrupt the deaf child's ongoing activities to direct attention and teach the child language skills. This type of controlled communication does not allow natural turn-taking interaction between mother and child (Bamford and Saunders, 1991; Meadow, 1980; Meadow, Greenberg, Erting, and Carmichael, 1981). In addition, these mothers tend not to ask questions for the purpose of specifically seeking information, but to instruct, without expecting an answer (Kretschmer and Kretschmer, 1988, 1989). High levels of maternal control are also associated with delayed social development in deaf children (Meadow, Greenberg, Erting, and Carmichael, 1981; Musselman and Churchill, 1991; White and White, 1984). Investigations of long-term effects of overcontrol by parents indicate that the children are likely to become passive, low in motivation, and poor at self-regulation in learning and problem solving (Wood, 1986). High levels of maternal control have been associated with slower language development (Snow, 1983; Wells, 1981; Wood, 1981).

Deaf parents are not as overprotective as many hearing parents of hearing children. If they are a family that spends time together, interacts easily with each other in ASL, and envelopes their deaf child in a rich linguistic environment, they will not have a tendency to be overcontrolling of their child's natural desire to communicate. Certainly some deaf parents are overcontrolling and overly concerned about their deaf child. Deaf preschoolers of deaf parents have been observed to have more mature and complex interactions with their parents than do those deaf children who have hearing parents (Meadow, Greenberg, Erting, and Carmichael, 1981).

EDUCATIONAL ENVIRONMENTS FOR CHILDREN WITH HEARING IMPAIRMENT

One important question that must be considered is: "Should English be established before beginning formal reading instruction or can it be learned through the reading and writing process?" Maxwell (1986) suggests that deaf children cannot read because they lack competency in the language they are trying to read. Quigley and King (1982) reported that deaf children often are faced with learning a language (English) and learning to read at the same time, since few of them have adequate mastery of English in any form by the time reading instruction begins. They enter school with poor metalinguistic awareness. Metalinguistic knowledge can be learned through reading and telling stories. Deaf children generally lack a background of conversational exchange with their hearing parents and thus they do not understand conversation. They have access to environmental print, but are unlikely to have anyone interpret it for them.

Most deaf children reach beginning reading with very limited background knowledge on a variety of common subjects. Among the reasons for their poor "world knowledge" are the following (Quigley and King, 1982):

1. Hearing adults usually do not read to young deaf children because they feel that they would not understand what they are reading, especially since the children do not ask questions or comment on the characters in the story.

2. Deaf children are usually not included in oral family discussions on a variety of topics.

3. If deaf children are taken places and allowed to participate in an event, no one accompanies the activity with ongoing commentary about what it means, what is happening, and what can be expected to happen.

Teacher Input

Studies of classroom communication patterns in classes for children who are deaf have typically shown that communication is teacher-dominated and teacher-controlled (Crandall and Albertini, 1980; Kluwin, 1983; Wood, Griffiths, Howarth, and Howarth, 1982). In school, overcontrol emerges in the form of frequent questions by the teacher, usually demanding short, factual answers (Wood, Wood, Griffiths, and Howarth, 1986). Children (both hearing and hearing impaired) in classrooms where teachers are overcontrolling, often ask few questions, seldom elaborate on their answers to questions, and generally say and contribute little. Teachers in this type of classroom are also found to speak in short, literal, and concrete utterances. Children with such teachers are seldom exposed to communications that involve speculation, argument, negotiation, or experimentation (i.e., a stimulating pragmatic environment).

Teaching Techniques

Language is acquired through interaction in contexts that are meaningful to the child. On the contrary, teachers of children with hearing impairment tend to focus on syntax and vocabulary, often out of context and not accompanying any relevant activity. This is reflected in sentence-by-sentence instructional models adopted in classrooms and programs for hearing impaired children (Baran and van Houten, 1988; Wood, Wood, Griffiths, and Howarth, 1986). National surveys on teaching methods for language and reading clearly show that the vast majority of teachers of hearing impaired children in programs throughout the United States rely on syntax/semantics-based teaching procedures and not the functional use of language (King, 1984; La Sasso, 1987).

Individual sentence-by-sentence learning is not the way children acquire syntax or vocabulary (Kretschmer and Kretschmer, 1989). They have to use these forms and expressions for particular purposes (e.g., to influence the individual with whom they are interacting). If their utterances are successful, they will repeat them in other contexts and expand their meaning. If the language has not fulfilled the purpose for which it was expressed, children will use different words and sentence structures to phrase their thoughts in ways that are more effective. Language is acquired and developed through interaction, not through drill.

In the case of hearing impaired children, language delay is due primarily to deprivation of pragmatic experiences. For many deaf children from deaf families, there is the problem of having to learn in a language in school that is quite different from their primary language (ASL), particularly in grammatical structure. In addition, children must learn the pragmatic rules governing social communication and classroom behavior and interaction (Button and Lee, 1987; Wardhaugh, 1985). These rules may be different from those established by the language community and the cultural community of the child.

English is a structured turn-taking system where two people cannot speak at the same time. Such behavior is not acceptable in the English language community, and also not in the Deaf community, where turn-taking is required in a signed communication. Interruptions are tolerated only for good reason. Turn-taking is governed not only linguistically, but by nonverbal expression as well (i.e., through body posture, pauses, gestures, head nods, and eye gaze) (Button and Lee, 1987; Kretschmer and Kretschmer, 1989). There is also an expectation that participants in a conversation that has broken down will try to determine the reason for the breakdown and repair it. They will rephrase their utterances and make them clearer for the listener. Deaf children must become competent in these skills or their deficits will impact on social development.

Hearing children from birth are exposed to communication with their caregivers and they learn through a variety of interactions how to conform to the pragmatic rules of their society. Most deaf children do not have the quantity and quality of linguistic experiences to learn these pragmatic rules unless they have parents who communicated with them in Manual Coded English or ASL immediately after birth. Thus, the educational classroom must provide this type of language-learning experience. Syntactic and semantic components of language can be learned simultaneously by using skills in context (Kretschmer and Kretschmer, 1989). Children with hearing impairment must also learn metapragmatic awareness. They must not only produce language, they must develop the ability to judge whether their efforts have been effective or not.

This ability is acquired through purposeful interaction with others in a variety of contexts.

Amplification Commonly Used in Learning Environments

In the past, special types of acoustic systems used for students who have hearing impairments were associated only with special lessons in auditory training and speech-language therapy. Deaf students were rarely in regular education classes and, therefore, there was not a need for mobile amplification systems other than the child's personal hearing aids. Educational amplification systems were developed because the quality of sound necessary to permit learning of academic content in a normally noisy educational environment far exceeded the specifications of personal hearing aids, which do not block out ambient noise (Sanders, 1982).

With the trend toward inclusion of hearing impaired students into regular education classes, these amplification systems became especially important to enhance the sound quality of the teacher's voice and peers' voices while blocking out ambient noises that interfere with intelligibility of the spoken message. Such systems were designed to accommodate the different amplification needs of groups of children within the class. Teachers and other professionals will probably be asked to use these devices. The two most commonly used educational amplification systems available are the induction-loop system and the frequency-modulated system.

Induction-Loop Amplification System

The induction-loop amplification system, designed for small classrooms, uses a wire or cable long enough to circle the room. The wire is attached to the speaker of an amplifier, which is hooked up to a microphone. The teacher speaks into the microphone and, by means of a special receiver or induction coil connected to the student's personal hearing aids, the speaker is clearly heard without background noise. In most newer models, the microphone used by the teacher is wireless. The students use their own hearing aids. There can be complete mobility by the student and the teacher within the room.

Frequency-Modulated (FM) System

The frequency-modulated system (FM) system is most frequently used when students must be mobile, in classes where the distance between teacher and student can be considerable, where students work in different groups situated relatively close to each other, and/or where noise and reverberation can interfere with speaker intelligibility. The FM system is a miniature FM radio station which broadcasts the teacher's voice to each student wearing an FM hearing aid (often referred to as an auditory trainer). Teachers wear the transmitter microphone around their necks or clipped to their shirts or lapels. The microphone contains a built-in antenna that broadcasts the spoken message to receiver packs, which are connected to hearing aids. These receiver packs are worn on the belt or on the chest. There are no wires around the room or between the teacher's microphone and the student's auditory trainer. The teacher and students have complete mobility. The microphone is never further than six inches from the teacher's mouth. No matter where the teacher walks in the room or how far from the student, the distance between mouth and microphone remains the same.

The strength of the signal received by the student remains the same. The receiver can be switched to FM only, to external microphone only in order to hear discussions in the class, or to a combination of both. Multiple channels in a single classroom are also possible. A teacher's aide, a speech-language pathologist, and a classroom teacher can be conducting small group sessions in different parts of the room without distraction. The sounds in the background are not heard. Each of the teachers wears a microphone set at an FM channel that is different from that worn by the others. The students' receiver units are tuned to the same channel as the teacher who is working with them.

The FM system is very effective in a whole language environment where students are working in groups and at many different tasks within the classroom. By simply switching channels, the child can join different groups or go to different classrooms. The specific channels must correspond to the channel used by the teacher's microphone. The units can also be used by teacher and student on field trips. Power is provided by rechargeable batteries. The teacher might be required to wear a microphone and might be called upon to recharge the unit each night. This is an easy and quick procedure.

VISUAL DISORDERS AMONG INDIVIDUALS WITH HEARING IMPAIRMENT

Extensive investigations have determined that the incidence of vision problems is greater in the deaf population than it is in the general population (Prickett and Prickett, 1992). The incidence of significant vision problems is 0.08 percent in the general school-age population, but 6 percent for deaf students of school age (Wolff and Harkins, 1986). Johnson and Whitehead (1989) found that 51 percent of 1,055 students at the National Technical Institute for the Deaf had correctable or noncorrectable vision problems and/or pathologies. Since more and more deaf students are included into regular classrooms, teachers should be aware of the possible visual acuity problems of these children. The commonly held view that children who lose their sense of hearing will have a strong sense of vision is a myth. A survey conducted by Prickett and Prickett (1992) revealed that teachers of deaf students, including students with known vision problems, are not adequately trained and do not have information necessary to meet their special needs.

Visual Perceptual Learning Disabilities Among Students with Hearing Impairment

Ratner (1988a, 1988b, 1993) has reported that 17 percent of the approximately 3000 deaf children in her research have visual and spatial perceptual disabilities that seriously affect their ability to learn and communicate in sign language. (A description of visual perceptual learning disabilities can be found in Chapter 8.) Learning disabilities, specifically visual perceptual learning disabilities, in normally hearing children have serious ramifications affecting many academic and social areas. When deaf children have visual perceptual deficits, the effects can be devastating (Ratner, 1985, 1988a, 1988b, 1988c, 1988d, 1990). The most serious ramification of this visual perceptual disorder is the effect it has on deaf children's ability to communicate and understand a message that is manually signed.

Children with visual perceptual deficits may have incomplete and faulty knowledge of their own bodies, resulting in an inaccurate awareness of body parts, their boundaries, and their left and right sides. Children with a poor body image cannot point to various parts of the body (Gaddes, 1985; Johnson and Myklebust, 1967). Such children may have serious problems differentiating each of the fingers from the whole hand and perceiving how a signer's fingers are positioned when the signer is facing them. Consequently, these children have difficulty learning to use sign language and reading the messages conveyed by sign. They may not discriminate the fine changes in size, shape, or movement of the facial features of a person who is signing, features that are essential to meaning in American Sign Language.

The ability to perceive changing and moving hand shapes and also body boundaries are essential skills for comprehending all types of sign language. However, spatial relationships are actually built into the syntax of American Sign Language. Each ASL signer uses space as a setting of a stage or a platform. When ASL speakers discuss people or things that are not actually present, they assign a place on that imaginary platform for each of the people being discussed. The signer then carries on an entire conversation by referring to these subjects. Their specific positions on that invisible platform must be visualized by the viewer. Moreover, their assigned positions in space and their spatial relationships must be accurately perceived or the sense of the conversation will be misunderstood. Among the many ramifications of such a communication problem are serious social and emotional disorders among deaf adolescents and adults (Ratner, 1990, 1991). Ratner (1988a, 1988d) found that 45 percent of the deaf students in her studies who were identified as having these forms of visual perceptual disabilities did not learn or comprehend sign language.

Speech-reading ability is strongly affected by a visual perceptual disability. Children who have difficulty distinguishing between shapes such as a circle and an oval, or a square and a rectangle (which are stationary), will certainly have difficulty distinguishing moving and changing oral configurations when speech reading. In addition, they do not effectively use facial expression or body language as cues to enhance the information received through speech alone and through simultaneous communication. To speech read, one must have a good grasp of linguistic concepts to "fill in" when articulation is imprecise. The deaf child's linguistic concepts of the oral English language are not sufficient without the help of nonverbal clues to accomplish this task. Visual perceptual deficits can undermine this skill as well.

Cued speech is also impacted by a visual perceptual disability. The child may not be able to determine the specific hand shape denoting a particular sound of consonant or vowel, and the small differences in position on the face or near the face that differentiate the cues. Failure to communicate, emotional difficulties, and serious social problems can result from these visual perceptual learning disabilities (Ratner, 1991).

Effect of Visual Perceptual Disabilities
On Intelligence Quotients of Children with Hearing Impairment

There has been increasing concern about appropriate services for hearing impaired children with learning disabilities. One indicator of a learning disability is a discrepancy between the child's level of intellectual function and academic achievement. Intelligence classifications for children with hearing impairment are usually based entirely upon performance scales of intelligence tests, such as the *Wechsler Intelligence Scale for Children-Revised (WISC-R)* (Wechsler, 1974b), the *Leiter International Performance Scale* (Leiter, 1979), and *Standard Progressive Matrices* (Raven, 1956). Verbal scales are usually not considered appropriate for deaf children because of their severe language deficits.

The tasks on all of the performance subtests of the above mentioned intelligence tests require considerable spatial and other visual perceptual skills, such as the ability to discriminate shapes, forms, and designs, and to match patterns. These are impossible tasks for an individual with shape discrimination deficits.

If deaf children with visual perceptual disabilities are tested only with the "performance" scales to determine their intellectual ability, their specific deficits are likely to reduce their score on the IQ test, resulting in a measure of less than average intelligence. In addition, their visual perceptual disorder may contribute to poor academic performance (Ratner, 1985). Consequently, there will appear to be a very small discrepancy, if any, between the children's apparent level of intellectual functioning (IQ score) and academic achievement. Therefore, many of their learning problems will be attributed not to specific learning disabilities, but to deafness alone or even to cognitive disabilities. Inaccurate conclusions are too often drawn from the tests, conclusions that preclude appropriate professional services for each handicapping condition. This inaccuracy can result in inappropriate class placement or labeling that can ultimately cause irreparable damage to the child. Using performance scales only on intelligence tests for deaf individuals renders the scores invalid unless visual perceptual learning disabilities have been ruled out.

It may no longer be necessary to rely solely upon nonverbal tasks to measure the intelligence of deaf individuals. Miller (1985) has developed translations of the *WISC-R* Verbal Subtests into Manual Coded English, Pidgin Sign English, and American Sign Language. When these tests are administered to deaf children in the students' preferred modes of communication, useful information may be provided regarding their intellectual functioning. Assessment would then be based upon their knowledge of content rather than on their knowledge of English. Using assessment techniques that are sensitive to the specific needs of deaf individuals will reveal a more complete picture of their potential than traditional techniques (Epstein, 1985).

AUDITORY PERCEPTUAL DISABILITIES AMONG CHILDREN WITH HEARING IMPAIRMENT

Hearing impaired children who wear hearing aids and benefit from amplification can be seriously affected by auditory perceptual learning disabilities. Little research has been done to determine the incidence of auditory perceptual disabilities among students who are hearing impaired. However, since the incidence of learning disabilities among the hearing impaired population is so high, this specific type of problem must be anticipated. Auditory perceptual problems are often overlooked in audiological testing because many of these children can detect sound with the help of amplification. Yet they have difficulty in a classroom and in a school environment. Like hearing children with auditory perceptual difficulties, hearing impaired children may have difficulty discriminating speech sounds that are brought within their range of hearing by means of amplification. Unfortunately, amplification itself distorts the incoming speech sounds as well (Sanders, 1982). Children may have difficulty differentiating the speech of the teacher or another student from background noises. They may have difficulty localizing sounds, whether speech or environmental sounds. They also may have difficulty processing the tones of voice and inflection in the amplified voices of others.

Especially important and often overlooked is the fact that they may be able to process auditory stimuli (speech) and may be able to process visual stimuli (signs), but not simultaneously. Learning disabilities affecting intersensory integration will make it extremely difficult, if not impossible, for a deaf child to communicate using simultaneous communication.

ATTENTION DEFICIT/HYPERACTIVITY DISORDER AMONG DEAF CHILDREN

Preliminary studies at the Illinois School for the Deaf indicate that the prevalence of ADHD among the students who are deaf and hard of hearing appear to be similar to that of the general population (Kelly, Kelly, Jones, Moulton, Verhulst, and Bell, 1993). However, students with acquired causes for their hearing impairment (e.g., bacterial meningitis, congenital rubella, cytomegalovirus infection, and extreme prematurity) were rated as high risk for ADHD (Kelly, Forney, Park-Fisher, and Jones, 1993a, 1993b).

Deaf children rely mainly on sustained visual attention in order to interact socially and derive benefit from classroom instruction. Young, deaf children, particularly, tend to move about impulsively in order to "check out" what is happening because they do not have the ability to gain much information auditorially. In addition, the serious communication problems and possible perceptual problems that underlie language deficits of children with hearing impairment may interfere with their ability to follow directions. There is danger that the degree of activity that is not necessarily unusual for children who are deaf might be misdiagnosed as ADHD. In contrast, the behaviors that should be considered significant with regard to possible ADHD may be overlooked or considered as part of the overall difficulties experienced by children with hearing impairment (Kelly, Forney, Parker-Fisher, and Jones, 1993a).

Children who are deaf and hard of hearing are particularly vulnerable to the serious social, academic and emotional affects of ADHD. Early and accurate diagnosis and early intervention are crucial. Educators certified to test, teach, and counsel children with hearing impairment are essential components of this process.

MULTILINGUALISM AND MULTICULTURAL INFLUENCES

There is a wide range of competence among deaf signers using American Sign Language. Most deaf individuals learn ASL as a second language; it is not the language used at home (Quigley and Paul, 1990). ASL is the primary language of most deaf children of deaf parents and also of hearing children of deaf parents.

Exposure to spoken English and Manually Coded English is not considered bilingualism, but simply two forms of the English language (Quigley and Paul, 1990). American Sign Language (ASL) and Manually Coded English are two different languages, and the child who is required to communicate in both languages is bilingual. Children who communicate using American Sign Language and are members of hearing families are at least bicultural and most often are multicultural. All members of the Deaf community learn the behaviors and the values expected of deaf individuals who are an integral part of that cultural community (Humphries, 1993; Padden, 1980; Padden and Humphries, 1988). Most deaf people in the United States, however, become members of the Deaf community when they are teenagers or adults. The vast majority of them come from hearing families (95 percent), who come from as many cultural backgrounds as there are countries and ethnic communities in the world. Culture that is usually transmitted through oral communication is not accessible to these children. As they become older, they will have to learn to balance home culture, the dominant culture of their country, and the culture of the Deaf community.

The sign languages of other nations are not the same as ASL. Although ASL was brought to this country from France by Thomas Gallaudet, American and French sign languages are very different today. While English is spoken in the United States and in England, English Sign Language is very different from ASL. Some nations do not have a national sign language and most of the deaf children of immigrants from those nations to the United States and Canada arrive with no language.

The enrollment of Asian/Pacific Islands hearing impaired children under the age of six in the United States school systems climbed 206 percent during the 1980s (Schildroth, Rawlings, and Allen, 1989). Immigrants from Asia have come from the following areas: China, Taiwan, Hong Kong, Japan, Korea, Philippines, Vietnam, Cambodia, Laos, Malaysia, Singapore, Indonesia, Thailand, India, Pakistan, Bangladesh; those from the Pacific Islands have come from Hawaii, Guam, American Samoa, Tonga, Fiji, and other Micronesian Islands (Cheng, 1993). The main Asian/Pacific Islands languages spoken in the United States are Mandarin, Cantonese, Taiwanese, Tagalog, Illocano, Lao, Lhmer, Hmong, Hindi, Chamorro, and Samoan (Cheng, 1993). Tonal languages, such as Mandarin, Lao, and Vietnamese rely on the differences in inflection and tones of spoken language for meaning. The same word can have several different meanings depending upon the inflection placed upon it by the speaker. Deaf children from families who speak languages such as these do not come to school having had any exposure to sign language. The deaf child from nations where the languages are tonal will probably be mute. Even mildly hearing impaired children from these countries who have auditory perceptual disabilities probably will not be able to communicate because they do not discriminate different tones, even low frequency tones.

Deaf children of deaf families who immigrate to the United States from other countries must not only learn English in the form of written language, they must learn a manual language as well. Most deaf children from Central American and South American countries have had an oral education, if they have been in school at all (Gerner de Garcia, 1993). Most deaf children from Latin America are not detected until well past four years of age and many remain undetected well into their childhood years (Jackson-Maldonado, 1993). The general knowledge of these children is often also impoverished. Although there are total communication programs in Venezuela, Costa Rica, Panama, Columbia, and Ecuador (Gerner de Garcia, 1993), the sign languages used are very different from American Sign Language.

The Hispanic population in the United States is very diverse. Language is an important cultural characteristic of Hispanic life. To help Spanish-speaking parents understand the need for special educational help for their child with hearing impairment and also the need for the family to learn the language their child is learning, bilingual professional support will be required. Bilingual professionals need to consider the dominant language used at home and still encourage the new language being learned by the hearing impaired child.

Hearing impaired children in the United States who represent Caribbean cultures, African cultures, and African American cultures are also multicultural and multilingual. They are exposed to Black English, Standard English, American Sign Language, Manual Coded English, the culture of the Black community, the culture of the white community, and the culture of the Deaf community. African American and Hispanic children represent nearly a third of the hearing impaired children and youth in the United States (Cohen, 1993). In many of the educational programs for deaf students, especially in urban settings, the majority of children are from diverse racial, linguistic, and ethnic backgrounds.

The Native American deaf child is a member of a distinct cultural community. Despite the use of the general term, American Indian or Native American, there is a great deal of cultural diversity among the population. There are 278 reservations and 209 Alaskan villages in the United States and no two tribes share identical cultural characteristics (Hammond and Meiners, 1993). These cultures are extremely important and must be respected.

There is a need for further study regarding the language acquisition of deaf children from Native American Indian language speaking families. These studies must be conducted by investigators who are very familiar with the culture and language of the specific tribe with which the deaf child is associated. Severe-to-profound hearing impaired Native American children are for the most part in special programs off the reservation (Hammond and Meiners, 1993).

INTERVENTION IN REGULAR CLASSROOMS

When students with hearing impairment attend regular classrooms, the teacher should make some general predictions. These predictions enable the teacher to organize and modify the curriculum for better understanding, and to create a successful learning environment.

Hearing Impaired Students Who Communicate Orally

Hearing impaired youngsters who communicate orally most likely have a mild-to-moderate hearing loss. Hopefully, they will be wearing hearing aids, the batteries for their hearing aids will be in working order, and the aids will be turned on. Some children selectively turn their aids off. Teachers should consider this possibility when the child is not paying attention.

These children usually speak and, therefore, a multitude of problems are camouflaged. There are probably underlying syntactic, semantic, and pragmatic language deficits, with accompanying attentional deficits. These children often receive the services of speech-language pathologists because of their articulation distortions and language delays. Often their serious difficulties comprehending the message that is being conveyed is overlooked by the classroom teacher. Because they speak, these students are expected to comprehend spoken and written language. They may not be able to do so without help.

The teacher can predict that hearing impaired students who rely on oral communication will have difficulty understanding oral instructions and directions in a classroom with cinderblock walls, tile floors, nonacoustic ceilings, and noisy heating systems. Such an environment has a great deal of reverberation (i.e., echo).

In an average classroom at a distance greater than four feet, or in a group activity, the student will have some difficulty following normal conversation. In a noisy situation when others are talking, the child's ability to discriminate by hearing alone will diminish even with hearing aids. When the child is 15 feet from the speaker, only a little over half of what is said will be heard clearly even with hearing aids. At this distance in noise, even a child with a mild hearing impairment will barely understand speech. If the speaker is standing in front of a window with the light on the back of the head, or if the ceiling lights are casting a shadow on the speaker's face, speech reading becomes very difficult. The language level of the child with a hearing impairment can predictably be considerably below age expectations. Complex sentences, new vocabulary, and unfamiliar concepts, even under good listening/watching conditions, may cause the child to be confused and frustrated.

Expressive writing will be difficult for this student, and the teacher can anticipate syntactical and morphological deficits. These students often exhibit difficulties comprehending textbook vocabulary and complex sentence structure, especially since the language of textbooks is often above grade level. Group conversations are also difficult because the children must face the speaker to comprehend spoken messages. Even with hearing aids, the child will probably have difficulty hearing high-pitched speech sounds, such as *s, z, f, v, sh, ch, t,* and *th.* The student with hearing impairment will probably have difficulty understanding taped recordings, including the voices on videotape and TV. Speech reading from a TV monitor is difficult. The student probably will have difficulty understanding all new material presented orally and will need help from resource personnel.

The following suggestions may ease the difficulties encountered by hearing impaired students who rely on oral communication:

1. Write orally presented directions on a chalkboard or overhead transparency.

2. When writing on a chalkboard or overhead transparency, stop talking.

3. Ask a volunteer peer to share notes regarding new instructions and new topics.

4. Repeat important messages to ensure that the student has heard and is paying attention.

5. Face students when communicating to help provide visual clues for message decoding.

6. Seat the student directly in the front of the classroom rather than to one side, and never next to cooling and heating systems or open windows (because of the competing noise).

7. Stand close to the student, but not too close when the student is seated (neck muscles fatigue when having to look up for long periods of time).

8. Be aware of ambient noises in the classroom, such as discussions in other parts of the room, which may interfere with the hearing of instructions. In the gym, reverberations distort speech sounds. When physical education is held outside, a child who is hearing impaired will have difficulty hearing.

9. When the lights are turned off and slides or movies are projected onto the screen, stand next to or close to the screen while speaking to prevent the student from having to turn to

several parts of the room to keep track of two messages spoken simultaneously.

10. Keep hands from covering your mouth while speaking.

11. Refrain from walking while speaking to aid speech reading.

12. Speak naturally without using exaggerated or extra slow speech (which tends to distort the mouth and make speech reading more difficult).

Hearing Impaired Students Who Communicate in Sign Language

Hearing students are expected to understand the language the teacher is using, unless a child has recently come from a foreign country and speaks a foreign language. Professionals who work with deaf students cannot expect all of them to understand, to the same degree, the concepts, the intent of communication, or even the signs conveying that intent. A group of 10 deaf students will have 10 levels of language ability.

Deaf students, especially in the early grades, are very easily distracted. At the slightest movement at the other end of the room or in the hallway, they turn to look for the cause. They cannot hear, so they must depend upon their vision to "check out" what is happening in their world. They realize a certain amount of power in the ability to stop listening at will by simply turning their eyes away, even closing them, or turning off their hearing aids if they wear them.

Deaf students who rely on signed communication and come to the regular classroom with an interpreter have some specific problems that the teacher can alleviate. These students must look at the interpreter to understand what is being said in the class. If they are involved in a group activity, they must glance back and forth from the teacher to the interpreter, to the materials on the table, to the teacher, back to the interpreter, to the student in the group who is speaking, back to the interpreter, and so forth. Most of the time, they will just focus on the interpreter and hope for the best. Deaf students sometimes go for long periods of time without blinking for fear of missing something. If the class period is toward the end of the school day, the deaf student is often tired and has difficulty focusing and attending. The fatigue factor is frequently present with deaf students.

Deaf signing students who attend regular elementary, junior high, and high school classes need support services from either an itinerant teacher of the deaf or teacher of the deaf from their residential school or self-contained class. Reinforcing vocabulary related to curriculum and complex concepts related to topics under study has to be a cooperative effort. Test questions have to be signed by an interpreter for the student and responses also interpreted for the teacher. The deaf student may require more time to prepare reports. However, modifications do not mean lowering the standards and expectations for students with hearing impairment.

SUMMARY

The problems confronting the child with hearing impairment are complex. Hearing impaired students are a heterogeneous population. Some speak, some communicate by using one or more of a number of manually coded languages. Their parents may be deaf or hearing. The age at which their hearing impairment is identified and the steps taken to initiate the necessary support services are most important. If amplification and/or a visual communication mode are made available in infancy, the child with hearing impairment probably will develop conceptually, cognitively, linguistically, socially, and emotionally. Unfortunately, this is not the case in most instances. Most children who are hearing impaired enter school with an inadequate information base, experiential deficits, and little or no language of any kind.

Many students with hearing impairment are currently attending regular classes in compliance with IDEA. It is important that teachers understand the complex problems these students bring with them. Teachers must modify the physical arrangements in the classroom, their personal actions, and their educational techniques to prevent or at least minimize some of these problems. Use of educational techniques and materials that are functional and meaningful is critical for improving language and cognition.

SUGGESTED READINGS

Padden, C., and Humphries, T. (1988). *Deaf in America: Voices from a Culture.* Cambridge, MA: Harvard University Press.

Schein, J. (1989). *At Home Among Strangers.* Washington, DC: Gallaudet University Press.

Sacks, O. (1989). *Seeing Voices: A Journey into the World of the Deaf.* Berkeley, CA: University of California Press.

13

THE NATURE OF LANGUAGE DISORDERS AMONG CHILDREN WITH VISUAL IMPAIRMENT

Educational professionals and service providers who teach and counsel children with visual impairments and their families are becoming increasingly aware of the importance of the quality of language acquisition during the first three years of life. Only in the past twenty years or less have educators and investigators considered the impact a vision loss has on the linguistic, conceptual, and cognitive development of an infant. When children with visual impairments hear and speak, they are often assumed to be developing normally in these respects. However, a number of serious linguistic deficits among children who were born without usable vision have been detected and studied.

Inclusion of children with different degrees of visual impairment within regular education continues to be a main thrust in meeting the total needs of the child. Classroom teachers can best serve the needs of these students if they understand the ramifications of sensory deprivation with regard to cognition, communication, and academic skills.

In this regard, Chapter 13 does the following:

1. defines terms related to visual handicaps;

2. examines the effect of vision on the child's cognitive and social development.

3. discusses the importance of tactile, kinesthetic, and proprioceptive awareness as it relates to the child's language development;

4. explores the impact of concomitant visual impairment and learning disabilities on the child's development; and

5. Presents service delivery models and teacher responsibilities for educating children with visual impairment.

TERMINOLOGY

The term *visually handicapped* is used to denote a group of children who have structural or functional impairments of the eye, regardless of the extent of the impairment. The term was adopted by Congress in 1981 as official terminology used by the Office of Education to refer to the total group of children who require special educational services because of visual problems (Barraga, 1983).

Visual impairment denotes all pathological conditions of the eye(s) or visual system that affect eye structure or functioning and result in less than normal vision (Barraga, 1983). A person's ability to visually discriminate objects and symbols at a clinically measured distance for near and distant objects is referred to as **visual acuity** (Barraga, 1983). **Blind** refers to those who have only light perception or to those who have no vision (Barraga, 1983). The World Health Organization defines **low vision** as a condition in which a child is still severely visually impaired even with correction, but who has significant functional vision (Faye, 1976). The National Accreditation Council (1981) attributes this reduced visual acuity to a disorder in the visual system.

EARLY COGNITIVE DEVELOPMENT

The early cognitive development of children who are missing the stimulation of a vital sense (i.e., vision) is affected substantially. The degree of impact of this deprivation depends upon these factors:

1. the age at which blindness or severe visual impairment occurs;

2. the degree of the impairment;

3. other handicapping conditions; and

4. the linguistic and communicative environment in which the child develops.

As with all children, the first three years of life are the most crucial with regard to concept and language development.

Reach-On-Sight

Sighted newborns attend selectively to objects that touch the skin, that are bright or shiny, and that move. Although grasping is an innate ability and motion development enables the infant to reach out within weeks of birth, the motivation required to do so is usually a shiny, moving, visually attractive stimulus. All moving objects attract sighted infants and hold their attention. The author spent weeks attempting to identify the apparently invisible object that attracted her infant son, who reached out frequently and tried to grasp it. She finally understood the puzzling behavior when she noticed he was reaching for the sunbeams that filled the sunlit nursery. Blind children are not motivated to move toward an attractive looking object. When there is no motivation to grasp an object out of reach, crawling is inhibited (Adelson, 1983).

Reach-On-Sound

Sound cues are not as effective as visual cues for motivating a child to reach and attempt to grasp. "Reach-on-sound" may not occur until 10–11 months of age (Fraiberg, 1977). The blind child is observed to be very "passive" compared to the sighted infant, whose gaze is drawn to colorful toys, pictures, and shapes. Blind, premobile infants are not aware of the variety of elements in their environment unless someone puts objects into their hands for exploration. The blind child may not realize that an object or another person exists at all if it is silent. Even when sound is emanating from the object, the blind child has to be taught through language and experience that there is a relationship between that object and the sound that it makes; otherwise, only noise is perceived. The sighted child makes the connection between sight and sound immediately and simultaneously, giving meaning to each experience.

Body and Object Awareness

Having sight provides infants with information about their body and the relationship between their body and the objects in their environment. Blind children who have not yet become mobile have poor understanding of where their body ends and another object begins. They generally have poor body concepts, and thus it takes them longer to know the capabilities of their bodies.

Sighted infants spend a great deal of time observing their fingers and their hands. Initially, it is apparent that they perceive these objects as unattached and separate from themselves. Through reaching, grasping, and controlling objects by manipulation, they develop a sense of their own body boundaries and body parts.

Proprioception is an inner sensory system that provides awareness of the body and each of its parts, and of the position of the body in space. Kolb and Whishaw (1985) used the term, **perception of body space** to describe awareness of the body in relation to other objects in space and spatial orientation (e.g., the body has a left side, right side, and the feet are rooted in the ground). Proprioceptive integrity enables children with visual impairment to achieve object permanence, to understand spatial relationships between objects in the environment, including themselves, to have a clear and accurate body image, and to develop cognitively.

Sensory Integration

The importance of integrating the incoming information from "all" the senses cannot be underestimated. The process of internalizing the world requires organizing all incoming information about objects and events in an efficient manner so that it can be stored in the brain for retrieval when needed for problem solving, thinking, reminiscing, communicating, and learning new applications. This process, cognition, is dependent upon the quality of the detailed information that is stored in memory. The sighted child simultaneously sees, hears, and feels. Sensory integration has to be meaningfully taught and nurtured in blind children (Rogow, 1988). Sensations tend to remain fragmentary. Blind children with normal hearing can hear birds singing, telephones ringing, rain beating on a window pane, and automobiles starting, but the sounds are isolated bits of noise without meaning and tend to be ignored.

Children who are blind have a more difficult task than sighted children when trying to make sense out of relationships between objects. These relationships appear to be comprehended more readily when objects are perceived simultaneously, as they are by sighted persons, than when they are perceived in succession, as they must be when manually explored by blind persons. In the latter case, one must rely on memory (Stephens and Grube, 1982). The caregiver must supply a running verbal commentary and label the objects and their accompanying sounds. However, unless blind infants also experience the world through movement of their bodies and contact with objects, the words they hear have no referents (Barraga, 1983; Hall, 1981). Language helps to clarify and confirm sensory impressions. But the bricks and mortar that are necessary for building impressions are the bits of concrete information received through the integrated functioning of intact senses.

Imagery

When sighted children become mobile and begin to crawl, they learn to integrate the visual, auditory, tactile, and kinesthetic sensations and develop concepts of the various objects in their environment. Through physical experiences with objects, they perceive the color, sound, size, shape, hardness or softness, consistency, surface texture, graspability, resilience, function, position in space, and spatial relationship with regard to other objects. Repeated experiences with these objects are required to form internal images. These images can then be retrieved when the objects are no longer in view.

The blind child builds an internal "image" of an object, based upon kinesthetic, tactile, and auditory experiences. The awareness of muscle tone, joint movement, and even slight pressure by the muscles and tendons of the fingers and arms when exploring an object is referred to as **kinesthetic awareness**. **Tactile sensation** is information received through the skin, such as that caused by wind on the face, heat or cold on the skin, or rain falling on the face or body.

Haptic perception, the combination of tactile and kinesthetic awareness, requires direct contact with an object, and time to physically explore its three-dimensional surface contours and other attributes by squeezing, pressing, pushing, and mouthing it. Children explore an object haptically by putting their fingers and hands around all sides of a block or other object (Rogow, 1987).

The haptic information obtained by grasping an object contributes to the blind child's understanding of its shape, texture, consistency, resiliency, and position in space (Gerhardt, 1982). However, until infants become mobile and actually have opportunities to manipulate objects, they cannot derive full benefit from the haptic information available. The lack of these experiences also hinders the blind child's development of auditory, tactile, and olfactory senses. Repeated scientific investigations indicate that blind individuals cannot develop their intact senses to a "superior" degree; however, blind children can be taught to use their intact senses more efficiently (Dunlea, 1989).

Concept Formation

Attributes of objects alone do not contribute sufficient information for concept development. The haptic information that a beach ball is round, smooth, resilient to pressure, and bounces is restricted to beach balls, not to *balls* as a category or to *round things* or to *objects that bounce.* The full complement of attributes that are associated with *balls* requires further exploration with basketballs, baseballs, and handballs, whose size, hardness, graspability, bouncability, resiliency, and surface texture are quite different from those of beach balls.

Concepts of tables and chairs are not available to blind children until such time that they can crawl to them, pull themselves up, and experience the height, width, general size, and the differences between the haptic feedback from wood, metal, and upholstered seats. Mobility and orientation are keys to concept development for the blind child. Mobility and orientation also help to establish a sense of "body space" concepts (e.g., *front/back, right/left*) and positional concepts (e.g., *above, between, next to*) (Tapp, Wilhelm, and Loveless, 1991).

Hands: A Blind Child's "Eyes"

The coordination of fingers and palms of *both* hands is necessary for fine manipulations (Elliott and Connolly, 1984; Williams, 1983, 1984). From birth, the neurologically normal infant can reflexively grasp objects that come in contact with them. The voluntary grasp soon replaces the reflexive grasp, and by age 40 weeks, infants actively use their hands to reach, grasp, and hold a variety of objects (Williams, 1983) (see Chapter 3). When children do not actively use their hands to explore and manipulate, they do not develop concepts about things in their environment. Rogow (1987) investigated object manipulation and manual dexterity among 148 blind, visually impaired, and visually impaired/multiplihandicapped children and found a significant relationship between object manipulation and language ability.

Object Permanence

Children with visual impairments do achieve object permanence, but later than children with sight, perhaps because the development of object permanence relies substantially on experience, especially visual experience (Bigelow, 1990; Rogers and Puchalski, 1984). Some vision, even minimal vision, stimulates the development of object permanence to near normal limits; that is, limited ability to see shapes helps to motivate search strategies, locate objects, and develop the understanding that objects can exist even when they cannot be seen or felt (Bigelow, 1990).

Symbolic Play

When children can represent an event, a person, or an object internally, they have reached a stage of symbolic thought. They substitute images of the real thing in their mind's eye and no longer have to rely on the actual object or the "here and now." Piaget (1954, 1962) proposed that memories, images, concepts, and words are all forms of representative or symbolic thought.

When children can remember events or objects through images, they can engage in symbolic play (Zukow, 1984). They can pretend that they are feeding a baby (using a doll) or having tea with a friend (using a teddy bear). They can recall "tea conversation" or "baby nurturing" by retrieving images of actual experiences or observations. Blind children do not "play" with objects; they explore objects haptically and auditorially (Fraiberg, 1977). Their only way of representing an event when they are young children is through the language patterns associated with it (Dunlea, 1989). Symbolic play, the acts of giving, showing, pointing, and reaching on request, which form the basis for early games and turn-taking patterns, is virtually absent in blind children (Rowland, 1984).

SOCIAL DEVELOPMENT

Sighted infants, from the day of birth, direct the type and extent of interaction with their caregivers by use of their gaze, imitation of facial expressions, the intense attention to the adult's face, and, within a few weeks after birth, their intentional smile. As discussed in Chapter 3, the infants' explorations of the adult's affect is an important step in establishing a relationship of attachment with a particular caregiver.

Motivation to Communicate

Sighted newborn infants can identify their mother's face and differentiate that face from that of another woman. Her voice is recognizable while still in the womb and again within hours of birth. In addition, they can identify their mother's particular smell. It is the combination of stimuli from all senses that result in the recognition of the entity, "my Mom." The entire image, as well as its sensory components are stored in memory. Blind infants can identify their mothers by voice, smell, and touch. However, motivation to communicate must be deliberately stimulated by a great deal of prompting. Parentese, with its exaggerated intonation, raised pitch, almost musical tones, and slow rate will help to stimulate the blind infant's response to the voice of the adult.

Interactions with Blind Infants

Infants who are blind establish attachments, but through a very different route than that used by sighted infants. They do not direct the course of interaction, but remain passive recipients of verbal and tactile communication and stimulation. For a relatively long period, their interactions with adults are one-sided. Infants who are blind do not initiate any vocal dialogues (Fraiberg, 1974). They cannot maintain eye contact, observe the adult's facial expressions, or learn to recognize and respond to the pleasure displayed by the adult's smile and general affect. Very young blind infants rarely smile deliberately. There is also a lack of vocal exchange so often observed between young sighted infants and their caregivers. Infants who are blind often remain silent when their mothers try to talk with them and encourage sound production.

In their studies, Landau and Gleitman (1985) observed this silence among children who were visually impaired. They surmised that when the mother vocalizes, the blind infant gives the sounds she is making undivided attention. The babies stop vocalizing because it is difficult to process competing auditory information. Yet blind infants are reported to vocalize a great deal when left alone (Landau and Gleitman, 1985).

When an infant does not respond to nurturance and play by smiling or sustaining intense eye contact, the mother often misinterprets the child's behavior as indicating a lack of enjoyment from touching, cuddling, and vocalizing (Fraiberg, 1974). The tendency to stop displaying affection and body contact is a frequent result when, in fact, more touching, stroking, and cuddling are necessary to help the baby feel and hear the interaction rather than see it.

Referential Communication

Infants become adept at drawing the attention of an adult to themselves. Attracting attention to self is developmentally one of the earliest steps in learning to refer (Mulford, 1983).When premobile sighted infants want an object, they will use distinct nonverbal communication to indicate the desire to have that object (e.g., gaze, gestures such as pointing and reaching, and crying). The adult follows the child's gaze or gesture and responds by giving the infant the object. This results in a definite communication between adult and child on a topic of joint interest. Gestures that are visually guided, such as pointing, reaching, and giving are important aspects of prelinguistic interactions. These behaviors may not be included in the repertoire of the blind or visually impaired child. As a result, the opportunities for interaction over shared referents are severely constrained (McGurk, 1983).

Relating Utterances to Events

Blind children are capable of attracting attention to themselves, but they are not capable of attracting attention to others. Once the attention of the parent is obtained by the infant's crying and by the older toddler's speech, it is up to the parent to determine what the child wants. The parent must direct the interaction and help make the determination.

If blind children are exposed to an environment where they hear communication between family members that does not include themselves or are placed in front of a radio or television set to listen to speech with no personal interaction, echolalia (i.e., repeating the sounds and language heard exactly, with no communicative intent) can result (Barraga, 1983). Blind children's utterances may appear to be irrelevant and unrelated to ongoing events. Sometimes blind children engage in "private speech play" apparently unrelated to what is happening around them; such behavior is sometimes interpreted as asocial or autistic-like (Barraga, 1983). Children with visual impairments should be encouraged to participate in discussions and interactions between family members.

Emotions and Affect

Young sighted children learn within the first few months to observe a person's body posture and facial expressions and to determine the affect being expressed (e.g., sadness, fear, anger, anxiety, fatigue, excitement, pleasure). Blind children do not have access to these nonverbal clues that are shared by a society. Blind children also are deprived of opportunities to relate their own feelings to the facial expressions on their caregivers' faces (see Chapter 3). As a result, they have difficulty identifying their own emotions and those of others. The adult's tone of voice is not as strong a clue to underlying affect as facial expression. Blind children are also deprived of the adult's facial expressions that indicate whether there is reason to be frightened in an unfamiliar environment or situation.

LANGUAGE DEVELOPMENT

Dunlea (1989) observed in the course of her longitudinal investigations that blind children apparently progress through the same stages of language as sighted children, but seem to acquire lexical forms without having developed the underlying conceptual framework. They progress from one- to two-word utterances, but these do not encode the range of meanings expressed by sighted children at the same stages of linguistic development (Dunlea, 1989).

Blind, normally hearing children, like sighted children, begin to express one-word utterances around the time of their first birthday. The content of the early vocabularies of both blind and sighted children appear to be similar in terms of the kinds of words used (e.g., object words, action words, names of specific family members and pets) (Dunlea, 1989; Landau and Gleitman, 1985; Mulford, 1986). However, the quality of the language expressed by blind children in terms of complexity, creativity, and abstract usage, is considerably deficient. Blind children also use language mainly for the purpose of obtaining information, rather than for interacting with other individuals (Erin, 1990).

Dunlea (1984, 1989) concluded from her studies that the absence of visual information leads to significant cognitive and linguistic deficits. The limited information available to the blind child inhibits the development of a realistic conception of the world, and this in turn leads to deficits in the development of language. In addition, congenital absence of vision results in experiential deprivation. Blind children reveal a paucity of world knowledge (Dunlea, 1989).

Early Pragmatic Development

Adult-Child Interaction

Adult-child interaction is essential for pragmatic language acquisition (Van der Geest, 1983). Such interaction is particularly important between caregiver and blind child. Any vocal exchange between caregiver and child includes the silent pauses between vocalizations. Constant vocalizations with no pauses violate the pattern of normal conversational turn-taking. The contrast between adult vocalization and silence can be taught by tactile cues (Tapp, Wilhelm, and Loveless, 1991). Rowland (1983, 1984) observed in her studies that many mothers interacting with their blind infants provided almost constant vocal stimulation. Rowland explained this tendency as a natural consequence of their desire to prod their infants to respond. The result, however, was the reverse. When the mother vocalized, the blind infant's undivided attention, reflected by silence, was the response.

In their investigations, Landau and Gleitman (1985) observed that mothers' speech to their blind children contains a high proportion of directives and statements and a low proportion of yes-no questions requiring a response. Landau and Gleitman attributed this tendency to use a disproportionate amount of directive language to the unique needs of their blind infants. Children who are blind often do not know what is going on in their immediate environment. Their mothers cannot ask them questions about ongoing events, objects or people in that environment and, therefore, they frequently tell the child what to do and how to do it. Also, the adults tend to be repetitive in their requests, presumably because the blind children have difficulty interpreting the adults' messages in the absence of visual information. In addition, the adult often has difficulty assessing the focus of the blind child's attention because the blind child does not use visually guided gestures, such as gaze and pointing, and, when they are used, they are not necessarily relevant to the context of ongoing events. Therefore, the adult takes the lead in directing the blind child's attention. In their studies, Landau and Gleitman (1985) found that blind children revealed delays in their understanding of syntactic structures denoting questions.

The Meaning of Auditory and Nonverbal Clues

Normally seeing and hearing children acquire knowledge about the meaning that is conveyed by tone of voice, rate of speech, volume, emphasis, and pitch of a spoken message. These are the auditory clues contained in spoken language that carry important message value. Most often, they convey emotions and feelings. When a person is sad, the rate of speech is usually slower and the volume is less intense than when the person is feeling contented. Anger often results in a louder and higher-pitched voice. Fear is also frequently indicated by a high-pitched voice and more rapid speech. These emotions can often be detected in the voice of a familiar person when speaking on a telephone.

Sighted children learn very early in their lives the meaning of auditory clues which, when combined with facial expression, body language, and contextual clues, give clear unmistakable messages. Blind youngsters learn to rely on auditory clues also. However, it is a mistake to assume that they acquire even greater sensitivity to the clues' underlying messages as compared with sighted individuals. In fact, blind children must be taught to listen and identify the auditory clues contained in spoken language.

Blind children cannot use the visual cues expressed by affect that are so helpful in determining when an individual with whom they are speaking is confused, annoyed, pleased, interested, bored, or even present. These are subtle but vital bits of information that are not available to them. Auditory vocal tones confirm the emotions observed on the human face. Misinterpretations or incorrect assumptions can result when the visual source of communicative information is missing.

Semantic Development

The first words of blind children are similar to those of sighted children in that they usually consist of labels for objects they can physically manipulate (Mulford, 1986; Urwin, 1983). Almost all of blind children's early word combinations relate to themselves; there appears to be a striking lack of decentration in their single- and multi-word utterances (Dunlea, 1989). Names for specific people, such as Mommy, Daddy, Grandma, and Grandpa, and their pet cat, dog, or hamster are part of the blind child's first lexicon as they are for the sighted child (Bigelow, 1986; Dunlea, 1989; Landau and Gleitman, 1985; Mulford, 1986).

When sighted children extract many attributes of an object and apply the label to other objects that share any one of these attributes, they are said to be "overextending." The extent of generalizations by blind children is very limited when compared to sighted children and applies only to one or two additional referents. The dominant attributes used by blind children in their overextensions consist mainly of tactile information (e.g., texture and three-dimensional contours).

Blind children's early lexicons include action words, but they use them exclusively to refer to their own movements (Dunlea, 1989). Sighted children use action words to describe the actions of other people, animals, and objects as well as their own (Urwin, 1978). Their ability to comment on others' actions is prompted by their seeing them do various things. Blind children do not see what other people are doing and, therefore, do not comment on the actions of others, especially when they are not involved in the activities themselves. However, blind children can use "relational words" in reference to their own actions. Relational terms include *all gone, again, mine, all done,* and *more,* to name a few. Dunlea (1989) points out that some of these terms are often tied to specific situations such as eating.

Landau and Gleitman (1985) observed that Kelli, a blind child participating in their investigations, responded to the directions, *Look up, Look down, Look behind you,* by reaching either up, down, or behind her body with her hands and "exploring" the area. She *looked* with her hands instead of her eyes. When directed to touch the wall or the floor, she literally touched the areas with her fingers, indicating that she distinguished between the words accurately, only differently from sighted children.

Young children without vision are usually limited to understanding and talking about those elements of an event that directly involve themselves. They do not talk about the roles of other people unless they request things or discuss shared past events, again with the emphasis on their own roles (Dunlea, 1989).

Syntactic Development

One developmental delay which appears to be universal in blind children is the acquisition of *I* as a stable pronoun and the ability to use *you* to refer to the other party in the interaction. Blind children tend to encode things from the adult's perspective. Almost all self-references used by young blind children occur as *you* unless they use their proper names, e.g., *You want some juice* instead of *I want some juice* (Fraiberg and Adelson, 1975).

In Mulford's (1983) studies, blind children had difficulty with pronouns *he* and *she*. They relied on voices to distinguish five-year-old boys from five-year-old girls. All young children have high-pitched voices, and it is often difficult to distinguish them. The blind children were confused by the inconsistent information perceived and, therefore, had difficulty applying the appropriate pronoun with consistency. The voices of elderly women or men might also cause some difficulty for the blind child. Women's voices often become lower in pitch with increasing age and men's voices often become higher. Sometimes it is difficult to determine the gender of an elderly individual on the basis of voice alone.

Phonological Development

The absence of visual stimuli seems to be responsible for the large number of articulatory errors among young children who are blind. (Elstner, 1983). There seems to be lack of precision in the articulation of particular visible phonemes (e.g., /m/, /b/, /p/, /f/, /v/, /θ/).

VISUAL IMPAIRMENT WITH CONCOMITANT DISABILITIES

Some of the etiologies contributing to visual and neurological impairments are the same for learning disabilities (see Chapter 8). Neurologically impaired children are at high-risk for learning disabilities (Karchmer, 1985; Wolff and Harkins, 1986).

Concomitant Visual Perceptual Deficit

Youngsters with low vision and those having some functional vision can benefit from magnification and prescriptive lenses as well as from a number of other technological devices now available. All of these will contribute to improved functional visual acuity. However, if there are visual perceptual deficits as well as visual acuity deficits, magnification will be of little help. Vision functioning will remain inaccurate or inadequate unless this specific disability is identified and specialized remedial services are provided.

Visual perceptual deficits are caused by damage to the specialized neural cells in the cortex of the brain where visual stimuli are interpreted and stored in memory for future retrieval and use. There are also many opportunities for minimal damage along the complex neural pathways that carry electrical impulses from the retinas of the eyes to these specialized cortical areas. Numerous problems can cause interference and distortions of retinal images being processed. When this occurs, perceptions of the visual scene are inaccurate and resulting images that are stored in long-term memory are inaccurate as well.

If a visually impaired child with low vision has a visual perceptual deficit as well, the problems may interfere with the effective use of residual vision. Linguistic, conceptual, pragmatic, and cognitive development most likely will be curtailed. (See Chapter 3 for information regarding the impact of visual perception on language development.) Visual perceptual deficits can easily be overlooked when a visual acuity impairment is present, and all the child's problems are attributed to visual impairment. The probability of a visual perceptual deficit existing with the visual impairment should be predicted and monitored, particularly if there is a history of prematurity, birth trauma, physical trauma, maternal viral infections during pregnancy, or maternal drug or alcohol abuse during pregnancy.

Concomitant Hearing Impairment and Auditory Processing Deficits

When visually impaired children are also hearing impaired, they may need specialized educational programs. Sign language in the hand as well as other tactile means of communication may be required with visual impairment and concomitant auditory acuity impairment.

Children with visual impairments are at high risk for auditory acuity deficits because both the eye and the ear are developed in the fetus at the same time, during the first trimester of pregnancy. The inner ear with all its delicate nerve endings and their connections to the neural pathways that carry electrical impulses to the brain are as vulnerable to damage as the retinas and their neural pathways. Auditory stimuli are processed in specialized cortical areas of the brain: verbal language in the left hemisphere, and nonverbal communication information and auditory environmental information in the right hemisphere for most individuals. If there is damage to the auditory cortex in either or both hemispheres, auditory processing deficits might result, interfering with understanding of auditory stimuli. Visually impaired children with normal hearing acuity, but with deficient auditory processing, will have great difficulty making sense of the auditory environment and spoken language.

The child with visual impairment depends on auditory perception to differentiate environmental sounds, musical sounds, nonverbal tones, and speech sounds; to localize sound; to isolate a specific sound from background noises; and to associate sound with sound sources. These cues are invaluable to a child who is missing a major sense, such as vision. They enable infants to learn the sounds of the language of their society and to learn about the nuances of spoken language, including the tones and inflections that convey emotion in spoken utterances. Auditory perception is required to store sounds of an event in memory and also to retrieve specific sounds, sound combinations, and sound sequences from memory. Educators of blind and visually impaired youngsters must anticipate the possibility of auditory perceptual deficits. They also cannot assume that the child understands spoken instructions, although the instructions are clearly heard.

Concomitant Proprioceptive Awareness Deficits

When an individual has minimal damage in the parietal lobes of the brain, problems in body image and spatial orientation may result (Gaddes, 1985). The visually impaired youngster relies heavily on awareness of his own body and its position in space, and also on the visual perception of depth of space and amount of space between objects. Visually impaired individuals are at risk for proprioceptive and spatial perceptual learning disabilities.

Some of the problems children might encounter unless compensatory strategies are taught are listed below (Gaddes, 1985):

1. the inability to localize objects in space;

2. the inability to localize their own bodies and their position in relation to other objects in space;

3. the inability to judge the distance of objects from themselves;

4. impaired memory for the location of objects and places, such as the spatial position of furniture in a room;

5. the inability to trace a path or follow a route from one place to another; and

6. disorders of body schema, such as defective identification of the right and left body parts, impaired imagery, and awareness of individual fingers and their relation to each other.

The child might have difficulty coordinating the use of separate fingers in a variety of tasks, manipulating objects, and learning to use a keyboard. Locating objects in the environment requires understanding of the position of things in relation to oneself. A proprioceptive deficit will prevent visually impaired children from localizing objects in relation to their own positions. Such a deficit can hinder progress in mobility and independence. Such a deficit might also impair the child's conceptual development.

PROGRAMS AND SERVICES FOR CHILDREN WITH VISUAL IMPAIRMENT

More than half of school-age children with visual impairment have additional medically diagnosed impairments (Kirchner and Peterson, 1980). As a result of IDEA, the Individuals with Disabilities Education Act, a greater percentage of students with visual impairments are being served in public schools. Children with total blindness as well as children who are blind with severe multiple handicaps may require more specialized services either within the public schools or a special school. The highest percentage of school-age children with visual impairments (75–80%) have some functional vision and attend regular classes (Barraga, 1983). Service delivery in public schools includes

1. full- or part-time self-contained classes;

2. resource room remedial help;

3. services of an itinerant teacher of visually impaired students who provides specialized instruction, adapts school materials, and develops a close working relationship with the student's regular classroom teacher; and

4. full- or part-time residential placement and programming (Barraga, 1983).

Services for children with visual impairments are determined by the needs of the child and documented on the child's Individualized Education Program (IEP).

RESPONSIBILITIES OF CLASSROOM TEACHERS

When a student with visual impairment is in a regular education classroom, it is the teacher's responsibility to create an atmosphere that ensures the student will be accepted by peers. Team effort by all professionals and parents is most important to stimulate and encourage the child to learn and grow in a natural, functional environment. It is also essential for the child's self-esteem that the teacher "maintain high expectations while adapting to the student's special needs" (Tapp, Wilhelm, and Loveless, 1991, p. 16). Close and frequent interaction between the student's regular classroom teacher and the teacher who is specially trained and certified to teach students with visual handicaps will ensure that all the concepts and specific vocabulary in the curriculum are reinforced for better understanding.

Teachers should anticipate linguistic problems in the following areas:

1. Visually impaired students with normal hearing usually speak normally and give no outward indication of any particular linguistic difficulty. However, teachers should not assume that students understand the vocabulary of textbooks and of verbal lectures and instruction.

2. Conceptual development is delayed at best, and may be seriously deficient because of an inadequate information base. The students may have basic experiential deficits that usually result in large gaps in conceptual development.

3. Semantic development may also be deficient. Students' understanding of word meanings and their knowledge of the deeper overall meaning of complex, abstract concepts are often deficient.

4. The student may have difficulty with specific syntactic structures, such as question forms, prepositions, adjectives and pronouns (described earlier in this chapter). Complex sentence structure is often difficult for visually impaired students to process.

5. Students often have serious deficits in nonverbal language and pragmatic understanding. These deficits may cause serious social problems for individuals with impaired vision. If they have difficulty in personal interactions, the teacher can anticipate difficulty understanding interactions between characters in a story they are reading or hearing, the characters' motivations, their relationships to each other, and the cause-effect relationships among events, situations, and people in the story.

6. Although students with visual impairment depend on listening skills, the degree of ability to listen to oral instructions, sustain attention to the message over time, and retrieve physical, auditory, and tactile images of related experiences for association and transfer may not be adequate to process the message.

7. Memory can be a problem when so much depends upon auditory and attentional capacity.

8. Descriptive writing may be somewhat inaccurate or deficient for the student who cannot rely on visual acuity. Verbal imagery should be encouraged, and memory of stimuli from auditory, tactile, olfactory, and gustatory sources should be called upon to enrich their images of experiences for use in descriptive writing.

Metacognitive training is an excellent tool to encourage students with visually impairment to become "active" learners. They have the verbal skills and inner language to self-monitor their use of strategies that enhance learning.

SUMMARY

When a child with visual impairment enters a school learning situation lacking the early developmental skills, the retarding effects are likely to be long-lasting. All professionals working with students who are visually impaired should be aware of the "hidden difficulties" these children may experience. These problems are masked by the ability of most visually impaired children to speak and express thoughts orally. It is a gross error to assume that blindness, or deficits in vision are the only problems these children are experiencing. Severe language and cognitive deficits, as well as learning disabilities, should be anticipated. These children do not acquire quality language and do not develop cognitive skills naturally without intervention.

SUGGESTED READINGS

Barraga, N. (1983). *Visual Handicaps and Learning*. Austin, TX: Pro-Ed.

Dunlea, A. (1989). *Vision and the Emergence of Meaning: Blind and Sighted Children's Early Language*. New York: Cambridge University Press.

Landau, B., and Gleitman, L. (1985). *Language and Experience: Evidence from the Blind Child*. Cambridge, MA: Harvard University Press.

14 THE NATURE OF LANGUAGE DISORDERS AMONG CHILDREN WITH FETAL EXPOSURE TO CHEMICAL SUBSTANCES

By the end of the 1980s, estimates were that between 11 to 25% of women delivering children in the United States had ingested one or more illegal chemical substances during pregnancy (MacDonald, 1992). Women who use and abuse drugs while pregnant frequently ingest chemical substances such as alcohol, tobacco, cocaine, marijuana, heroin (and other opiates), amphetamines, and prescription drugs, often in multiple combinations. Prenatal legal and illegal drug use crosses all ethnic, racial, and socioeconomic classes. All of the chemical substances cited have been linked to physical and behavioral irregularities in children exposed in utero to them.

Hallahan (1992) states that there is an increased incidence of learning problems related to social/cultural changes occurring in all strata of American society. He cites learning problems that are associated with the increasing risk of disruption of growth of the child's central nervous system in utero from the following:

1. maternal use of drugs and alcohol;

2. the lack of adequate prenatal care;

3. widespread pollution; and

4. increasing numbers of children raised in poverty.

In the United States, the poverty rate for children is 20% (Durning, 1992). One out of every five children lives in an environment of substandard housing, inadequate health care, poor nutrition, and high social stress. Thus, the increased ingestion of drugs and

369

chemicals by pregnant women of all socioeconomic groups in combination with spreading poverty with its multiple problems has affected the physical, social, and academic development of large numbers of children.

When defining substance use and abuse, Sparks (1993) discusses variable social attitudes and circumstances. **Abuse** is viewed as drug use which deviates from accepted medical and social practices in a given community. When any chemical is used improperly so that it harms the user or other individuals, it is considered **substance abuse**.

Research regarding prenatal substance abuse by a paternal chemical abuser is inconclusive. However, research (Kronstadt, 1991; Zuckerman, 1991) has confirmed major infant problems associated with maternal chemical abuse. Controversy continues regarding the incidence and severity of fetal effects. Facts are difficult to obtain and sort for specific substances because many mothers are multiple drug users. The impact of chemicals on the developing fetus depends on

- the stage during the pregnancy a given chemical is ingested;

- the length of time it is used; and

- the amount of the chemical that is consumed.

Yet this information is not always known or provided to the researcher. In addition, the issues of nutrition and prenatal medical care can also affect the fetus.

Children are members of a family system. Professionals continue to investigate the effectiveness of early family and child intervention. Zuckerman and Frank (1992) contend that developmental dysfunction can be partially compensated by appropriate and consistent early intervention.

In exploring the effects of fetal exposure to chemical substances on language development, Chapter 14 seeks to

1. define drug, chemical, and substance abuse;

2. examine the organic consequences of prenatal exposure to chemicals in tandem with the influence of the environment on the child exposed to drugs;

3. discuss linguistic, academic, social, and physical development as affected by prenatal exposure to these substances:
   a) alcohol,
   b) crack/cocaine,
   c) tobacco, and
   d) other drugs;

4. propose intervention considerations for mothers and infants; and

5. present issues of concern to educators, medical professionals, and society as a whole in providing adequate intervention for these high-risk children.

WOMEN AND DRUGS

Women do not typically "start" to use drugs after they become pregnant. They ingest chemical substances over time and often they are unaware of their early pregnancy (Sparks, 1993). Some women binge on drugs and others consume them in consistently high levels. Usually, chemicals are ingested simultaneously (e.g., alcohol, tobacco, and tranquilizers; cocaine and marijuana). This is sometimes referred to as *polydrug use*. Those women who are an active part of the drug culture generally do not participate in regular medical examinations (Kronstadt, 1991). When drugs are an integral part of a woman's life, they can override good nutrition and healthy social behavior. Infections and undernourishment are common. Prostitution to obtain drug money in addition to using unsterile needles for drug use puts women at risk for AIDS and other diseases. Approximately 75% of children infected with HIV are born to mothers who were infected by intravenous drug use or sexual activity (Crites, Fischer, McNeish-Stengel, and Seigel, 1992).

If a woman craves a drug, it becomes extremely difficult to discontinue taking it, even if she desires to do so during pregnancy. She often develops a sense of guilt which can cause depression and a greater dependency on drugs. In addition, an unstable emotional state often causes her to delve into the drug culture initially. Childhood physical, verbal, and sexual abuse may have affected her self-esteem and the ability to function effectively. These factors affect the mother's ability to secure appropriate help during pregnancy, should it be available, and utilize adequate parenting skills once the baby is born (Sparks, 1993).

EFFECTS OF PRENATAL DRUG EXPOSURE

Each drug seems to affect the developing fetus in different ways. Because of the high incidence of polydrug ingestion, it is difficult to isolate specific variables for a single drug. The long-term effects of the drugs are still not understood. Yet certain generalizations have been noted concerning drug-exposed infants.

Drugs, especially alcohol, have been classified as **teratogens.** These are substances that can cause malformations, growth deficiency, or even death in children with prenatal exposure. The body and brain of the fetus can form and grow in defective ways from the effects of a teratogen (Olson, Burgess, and Streissguth, 1992).

Cocaine, alcohol, and tobacco affect the fetus by reducing the transfer of nutrients and oxygen from the mother through the placenta. These and other drugs such as opiates and marijuana also cross the barriers, or filters, of the placenta and can affect the central nervous system (CNS) of the fetus directly (Zuckerman, 1991). Children exposed in utero to chemical substances are more likely to have a low birth weight and be born prematurely. A number of infants have a small head circumference. Sometimes this is related to an underdeveloped brain and developmental delays (English and Henry, 1990; Fried and O'Connell, 1987). Babies have greater risk for death at birth and during early infancy. Also, specific facial abnormalities are associated with alcohol consumption. This impaired or abnormal structure is termed a **dysmorphism.** Cardiac and motor impairments have been reported as well (Zuckerman and Bresnahan, 1991). Impairments of the sensory systems are linked to prenatal chemical exposure (Clark, 1989; Cone-Wesson and Wu, 1992; Dixon, Bresnahan, and Zuckerman, 1990). These numerous organic irregularities affect language, learning, attention, and behavior in the young child. Cone-Wesson and Wu (1992) also found that the central auditory system, which has been associated with some learning disabilities, appears to be affected by maternal cocaine use. Zuckerman and Bresnahan (1991) cite studies suggesting that prenatal drug exposure results in impairments to sensorimotor functioning and attentional factors. These barriers to effective interaction between the child and the environment can interfere with normal development.

Despite some organic abnormalities of the central nervous system, brain cells are thought to rejuvenate in a favorable postnatal environment. Researchers (Zuckerman and Bresnahan, 1991) suggest that the brain cells make new connections to compensate for damaged areas. Thus, the CNS of the newborn has the capacity to recover some functions that were diminished due to exposure in utero to chemical substances. This plasticity (i.e., recovery) is facilitated with competent caregiving. The reverse of this theory is that a poor postnatal environment will reduce CNS function further causing more severe disability.

PARENT-INFANT INTERACTION AND DEVELOPMENT

As discussed in Chapter 3, the interaction between infants and their caregivers helps to build infant self-concept, world knowledge, and communication. "Bonding" occurs as an infant develops a sense of trust with consistent caregivers. These secure attachments facilitate confident exploration of the infant's environment. If the baby's central nervous system is impaired, focus and joint attention with the adult become difficult. The infant is fragile and disorganized, which decreases the ability to maintain an alert responsive state needed to interact with the environment and caregiver. The parent can misinterpret the infant's behavior as disinterest. Without professional assistance, caregivers may become frustrated and might ignore the child or provide improper stimulation.

Most babies who were exposed in utero to chemical substances have reduced or altered **cuing ability** (i.e., the ability to indicate likes and dislikes by cues such as eye gaze, smiles, and positioning). Some infants cannot properly execute the changes in posture, facial expression, and eye contact that comprise preverbal communication. The caregiver uses these movements as guides in interactions. Without them, the precursors of language are not developed. (See Chapter 3 for a discussion of preverbal communication.)

Limited movement or disorganized movements prevent the child from exploring and learning about the environment. Critical information which is used as the foundation for building more complicated ideas is lost. Substance-exposed babies with exaggerated reflexes and unpredictable sleeping patterns interfere with parental bonding because they are so hard to handle.

Because communication and general development in infants depends on environmental factors, the total family must be considered. All members of families that have individuals who are drug users require guidance and support so that proper bonding and interaction with the baby can occur. The caregivers need to learn to intercede as follows (Prizant and Meyer, 1993; Sparks, 1989):

1. how to interpret and modify the child's behavior;

2. how to react to infant attempts at communication; and

3. how to help the infant interact with the environment.

THE EFFECTS OF ALCOHOL ON CHILD DEVELOPMENT

In the 1960s, medical textbooks claimed that alcohol had no harmful effects on the growing fetus. Some doctors believed that the higher incidence of mental retardation and epilepsy in children born to alcoholic parents was due to the "bad stock" of alcoholics. A drink before retiring to calm the fetus was sometimes prescribed for pregnant mothers (Abel, 1990; Sparks, 1993). A study published in France by Lemoine, Harousseau, Bortenyu, and Menuet (1968) discussed distinctive features of 127 children born to alcoholic parents. The features included the following:

1. unusual facial formation

2. prematurity

3. low birth weight

4. postnatal growth retardation

5. malformations, especially in the heart, limbs, and palate

6. delayed intellectual development

7. delayed language development

The study was reported in the United States later that year by the March of Dimes but went unnoticed. Yet those were the features, later known as *fetal alcohol syndrome* (FAS), that Lemoine et al. (1968) had described and which were discussed in an article published by Jones and Smith (1973). Not until 1981 were pregnant mothers advised by the Surgeon General of the United States that to prevent birth defects, they should not consume alcohol.

The abnormal features found in FAS can also appear as independent birth defects or be associated with other congenital syndromes not associated with maternal drinking. Therefore, without a confirmation of maternal alcohol consumption, these features can be associated with other factors. However, confirmed heavy and frequent maternal drinking during pregnancy can be responsible for the pattern of abnormalities known as FAS (Abel, 1990).

Some infants exposed in utero to alcohol exhibit some, but not all, of the characteristics associated with FAS. They are known as babies with *fetal alcohol effects* (FAE). The serious educational implications are evident in this group of children as well. Estimates are that FAE occurs with two or three times the frequency of FAS (Sparks, 1993). Both constitute a leading cause of mental retardation in the United States (Olson, Burgess, and Streissguth, 1992). FAS and FAE are most prevalent in Native American communities but alcohol exposure in utero occurs in all segments of the population (Little and Wendt, 1991). It is suspected that the incidence in middle and upper class groups is underreported (Sparks, 1993).

How Alcohol Affects the Fetus

The developmental effects of alcohol, like other teratogens, depends on the amount, timing, and conditions of exposure. Alcohol ingested during pregnancy puts the fetus at risk for physical abnormalities and behavioral deviations. When development of the central nervous system is taking place, alcohol from the mother can cross the placental barrier without difficulty and affect the fetus (Gold and Sherry, 1984). The liver of the fetus is immature and the child in utero cannot metabolize the alcohol as well as an adult. Furthermore, as the fetus excretes alcohol into the amniotic fluid, it is ingested repeatedly. The blood alcohol levels remain high for longer periods of time so the fetus keeps reabsorbing the alcohol, which can affect brain and physical development (Sparks, 1993).

There are critical periods for development of varying sections of the brain during the gestation period. That is, certain portions of the brain grow more quickly in the initial stages of pregnancy. Alcohol can cause brain malformations early in pregnancy which produce behavior disturbance and intellectual impairment thereafter (Sparks, 1993). In follow-up studies of youngsters with FAS (Spohr and Steinhausen, 1987), researchers found that the effects of resultant CNS dysfunction contributed significantly to poor educational performance. Persistent short attention span, distractibility, and hyperactivity have lasting ramifications on the child's learning process (Gold and Sherry, 1984; Van Dyke and Fox, 1990).

Physical Abnormalities In FAS Children

Distinctive abnormal facial features (dysmorphism) identify children with FAS (see Figure 14.1), although not all children with these features can be presumed to have FAS. The inner corner of the eyes has a prominent fold of skin known as the *epicanthal fold*. The eyes are short from the inner to outer corners. The midface may be flat, the chin small (micrognathia), and the upper lip thin. The ears are rotated back. The philtrum (the ridges that start above the center of the upper lip and end beneath the nostrils) is indistinct and elongated. Other dysmorphic features are small teeth with poor enamel, and heart, bone, and muscle irregularities.

Figure 14.1

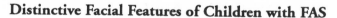

Distinctive Facial Features of Children with FAS

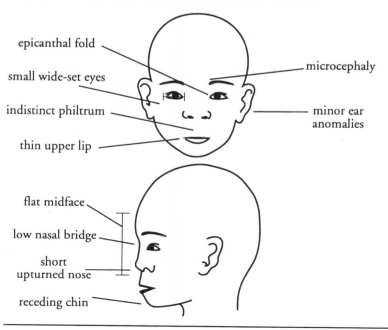

Growth deficiency is another feature of FAS and FAE. Height, weight, and head circumference are affected. The children remain small and have reduced head size (microcephaly) through childhood (Sparks, 1993). Many infants are born prematurely. Even correcting for less than nine months gestation, the infants can be underweight at birth. Studies have been reported (Fried and O'Connell, 1987; Zuckerman, 1991) that link one or two drinks daily during pregnancy to decreased infant birthweight by approximately 80–120 grams. However, associated factors including maternal nutrition, tobacco and marijuana use, and maternal health were not always considered.

FAS Infant Behavior

Infants exposed in utero to alcohol can exhibit poor arousal (the sleep patterns are irregular and fitful) and poor habituation (failure to tune out repetitive environmental stimulation or difficulty getting used to stimulation in their environment). This means that excessive motion may make the infant hyperexcitable and inconsolable. These early behaviors can develop into hyperactivity and distractability in the toddler years. The youngsters with FAS are difficult to manage and unresponsive to verbal cautions (Olson, Burgess, and Streissguth, 1992).

Infant difficulty in focusing attention to learn about the environment leads to delayed language skills in the preschool years. This critical factor can be erroneously overlooked because the small size of the youngster reduces language expectations. As speech emerges, it is characterized by sparse vocabulary and shallow word meanings. Sentence length tends to be reduced and echolalia has been noted (Streissguth, 1986b). Play routines are unimaginative and immature. Toddlers are known to be excessively friendly to strangers and fearless in new social situations. It appears as if the child does not take time to appraise new people and situations as would be expected.

The higher incidence of sensory problems associated with FAS also affects language acquisition. Church and Gerkin (1988) report sensorineural hearing loss and middle ear infection (otitis media) in children with fetal alcohol syndrome. Olson, Burgess, and Streissguth (1992) suggest visual problems that must be monitored. An insufficient sensory system and poor attending behaviors all impact on the child's ability to understand the world and other people. This affects language development, general learning, and social skills.

Behavior During the School Years

Children with FAS and FAE followed by Shaywitz, Caparulo, and Hodgson (1981) were described as hyperactive, distractable, impulsive, and forgetful by the age of five to six years. They usually were affectionate, but lacked the social skills to make friends or avoid strangers. These children failed to appreciate the communicative function of language and exhibited inappropriate spontaneous language use. The researchers reported that once the youngsters attended school, making transitions to new activities was difficult as was predicting the consequences of their behavior. This behavior was attributed to underlying conceptual confusion. The youngsters were easily terrified and bewildered by school bells and sirens. Olson, Burgess, and Streissguth (1992) report a tendency toward concrete thinking which can interfere with learning abstract concepts. These children often require simple instructions with clear consequences. The linguistic function of school-aged children with FAS and FAE is differentiated from youngsters with specific language deficits in that children with FAS and FAE seem to avoid initiating conversation in social situations (Shaywitz, Caparula, and Hodgson, 1981). Table 14.1 summarizes characteristic behaviors of children with fetal alcohol syndrome and fetal alcohol effects discussed by Sparks (1993).

Table 14.1

Characteristic Behaviors of Children and Adolescents with FAS and FAE

- Lack social skills
- Hyperactive, distractable, inattentive, impulsive
- Delayed motoric development
- Uninhibited behavior
- Lack of attachment or indiscriminate attachment
- Difficulty making transitions to new activities
- Poor judgment, poor recognition of cause-effect relationships
- Inappropriate language use in context
- Conceptual confusion
- Temper tantrums, defiance of authority

Characteristics Specific to Adolescents

- Sexual difficulties (inappropriate behaviors or easily exploited)
- Depression (due to social isolation)
- Restless
- Truant or school dropout

Dorris (1989) describes his adopted son, Adam, in *The Broken Chord* as existing in the present tense, with an occasional reference to the past. This prevented Adam from seeing future consequences. For example, he might take all three of a day's doses of medicine at once to "get them over with." The cause-effect relationship of such actions were not understood by the child. Dorris also describes poor imagination in his son. Adam did not learn to make decisions based on prior experience. He didn't understand that if you eat your lunch at 9:00 a.m., you'll be hungry in the afternoon. If his alarm clock was not set properly due to an electrical failure and the alarm sounded in the middle of the night, Adam got up and got ready for school even though it was pitch dark outside. Adam could not imagine how his behavior appeared to other people. He could not understand their responses to his actions. Therefore, following precise, trained routines was this boy's way of getting through the day. Adjustments to any unforeseen variation in the routine could not be made without external assistance.

Table 14.2

Academic Behaviors of FAS and FAE Students

Academic Difficulties in the Areas of:	Normal Academic Behavior
• Verbal comprehension	• Rote spelling
• Reading comprehension	• Word recognition
• Abstract thinking	• Concrete tasks
• Memory (especially visual/spatial)	• Penmanship
• Basic problem solving	
• Conceptualization (math and social studies) due to time and space disorientation and difficulty recognizing cause and effect relationships	

Communication Difficulties	Communication Behaviors
• Poor pragmatic language (poor judgment, impulsive behavior)	• Superficial verbal facility
• Difficulty comprehending social rules and expectations	• Talkative
• Ineffective communication— lacks substance, cohesion, meaning, and relevance	

Researchers have followed the progress of youngsters with FAS and FAE into maturity (Olson, Burgess, and Streissguth, 1992; Streissguth, Aase, Clarren, Randels, LaRue, and Smith, 1991). Adolescents usually appear at first meeting as more intelligent than their tests indicate. The average measured IQ is in the mildly mentally retarded range. However, intelligence varies from severe retardation to the normal range. Table 14.2 outlines academic performance frequently observed in FAS and FAE children. Teenagers seem to "plateau" in their daily functioning and their academic progress. Attention deficits, poor judgment, and impulsiveness make successful employment and stable living difficult. They can be socially immature and easily victimized. Alcohol abuse is a frequent adult outcome of children exposed to alcohol in utero (Olson, Burgess, and Streissguth, 1992).

THE EFFECTS OF CRACK/COCAINE ON CHILD DEVELOPMENT

In New York City, between 1985 and 1989, the state comptroller's office estimated that 22,000 infants were born who were exposed in utero to crack/cocaine (Bachrach, 1991). The long-term effects of prenatal exposure to crack/cocaine on infant development and behavior are still not fully understood. Some children appear to have mild difficulties and others have serious disorders. As recently as 1982, medical texts reported that cocaine had no harmful effects on the developing fetus (Fink, 1990). Since the mid-1980s, a number of studies (Davis, Fennoy, Laraque, Kanem, Brown, and Mitchell, 1992; Dixon, Bresnahan, and Zuckerman, 1990; Fink, 1990; Lesar, 1992; MacDonald, 1992) documented that crack and cocaine exposure places both the developing fetus and mother at risk. It also jeopardizes the baby's life during infancy. As with other substance abuse, women abusing cocaine may be polydrug users. The varying combinations of chemicals, amounts, and frequency are diverse. Furthermore, chemical substances affect the fetus during different stages of pregnancy in varying ways.

How Cocaine Affects the Fetus

Cocaine is classified as a stimulant. It causes an increase in heart rate and blood pressure in the user. Crack is cocaine that has been mixed with baking soda in a particular way. In low doses, cocaine decreases appetite. Pregnant women who ingest the drug are known to reduce nutritional intake. Cocaine can lead the user to feel a compulsive craving for the drug which leads to binges.

Fetal exposure to the drug can jeopardize developmental processes because it can cross into the placenta and produce constrictions in the circulatory system. This causes increased blood pressure, small strokes, heart attacks, and seizures. Newborns exposed to cocaine are typically of low birth weight (Sparks, 1993). This can be caused by cocaine's effect on the mother's smooth muscles, precipitating preterm labor, and by the inadequate nutritional intake of the mother. Children with lower birth weights have a higher incidence of poor health and behavior problems during early school age (McCormick, Brooks-Gunn, Workman-Daniels, Turner, and Peckham, 1992). Cocaine can also cause physical manifestations in the fetus such as small head circumference. Although a positive environment postnatally can stimulate "catch-up" head growth (Sparks, 1993), head size is considered by some researchers as an important indicator of potential mental ability.

Cocaine is believed to affect the neurotransmitters in the brain of the fetus causing excitable and depressed behaviors of the infant. Lester, Corwin, Sepkoski, Seifer, Peucker, McLaughlin, and Golub (1991) suggest that the excitable behavior patterns are caused by the direct toxic effects of cocaine on the brain pathways. Furthermore, they found that the depressed behaviors of the infants are the result of a lack of oxygen, resulting in growth retardation of the baby in utero. Over-excitability and depression in the infant affect the relationship between the caregiver and the baby which can influence the child's linguistic, social, and cognitive development.

Physical Abnormalities in Crack/Cocaine-Exposed Children

The structural defects in children exposed in utero to cocaine seem to be linked to vascular disruptions. This means that the drug interrupts the normal development of organs because of insufficient intrauterine blood supply (MacDonald, 1992). Limb reduction such as loss of fingers or arms has been documented. Urinary tract defects have also been described (Hoyme, Jones, Dixon, Jewett, Hanson, Robinson, Msall, and Allanson, 1990). The effects of cocaine on the developing central nervous system are widespread due to a restricted flow of oxygen to the fetal brain (Zuckerman and Bresnahan, 1991).

The sensory systems of these babies can show abnormalities as well. Documentation of vascular changes in the eye indicate both central and peripheral irregularities (Dixon, Bresnahan, and Zuckerman, 1990). Research has also identified very high sensitivity to sensory stimulation. Touch, lights, and movement cause severe stress in newborns who have been cocaine-exposed in utero (Lesar, 1992). While there is no greater incidence of hearing impairment from abnormalities in the ear itself, Cone-Wesson and Wu (1992) found irregularities in the auditory pathways from the inner ear to the brain. Very poor visual attention and tracking in the newborn are evident (Dixon, Coen, and Crutchfield, 1987). Visual responsiveness has also been reported to be abnormal. A somewhat higher than expected number of infants have died of sudden infant death syndrome (SIDS) as well (Zuckerman and Bresnahan, 1991).

Behavior of Crack/Cocaine-Exposed Infants

When the child exposed in utero to cocaine is born, complications are frequent. Some have suffered small strokes during gestation. Premature delivery, malnutrition of the fetus (cocaine creates decreased interest in bodily needs such as food in the drug user), and sexually transmitted disease can impact on the newborn's well-being. Some neonates exhibit poor feeding patterns and sucking, irritability, jittery and tremulous limbs and body, and hypersensitivity to stimuli. Their muscles are stiff and they cry a great deal in a high-pitched tone. Some infants have difficulty falling asleep and are easily awakened. They seem unable to calm themselves. Others retreat into a deep sleep. These babies tend to be unresponsive to the interactive efforts of their caregivers (Kronstadt, 1991; Lesar, 1992).

As seen in infants who were exposed to alcohol, babies exposed to crack/cocaine have difficulty organizing themselves in response to environmental stimuli in the neonatal period. They are hard to console and calm. The infants have limited ability to interact with caregivers because they do not maintain an alert responsive state. That is, their sensory systems are not organized enough to orient to the outside world and maintain attention (Griffith, 1988; Lesar, 1992).

The many medical complications associated with these children create prolonged hospital stays and costly intervention. One study (Phibbs, Bateman, and Schwartz, 1991) estimated neonatal hospital costs before discharge to average $5200 more for cocaine-exposed infants compared to unexposed babies. Another $3500 was spent on children remaining in the nursery for evaluation or foster care placement.

The effects of cocaine on the newborn require maximum intervention to modify their difficult behaviors. Their abrupt, inappropriate changes in behavior and their inability to tolerate even low levels of stimulation result in vacillation from agitated cry to deep sleep. The caregiver, whether a cocaine-addicted mother or an experienced professional, finds the young infant extremely difficult to manage. This places stress on the developing mother-infant bond and abusive, deficient parenting can result. Fink (1990) reports that between 1986 and 1989, New York City Family Courts saw a quadrupling of child abuse and neglect petitions that contained allegations of drug abuse. During the mid-1980s, a large number of newborns were simply abandoned in hospitals and eventually entered the foster care system (Schaffer, Yanulis, Williams, and Green, 1993). In 1989 alone, $88,000,000 was spent on foster care for these children in New York City (Bachrach, 1991).

Later Infant and Toddler Behavior

The multiple insults of cocaine on the developing fetus affect the early sensory behaviors of infants exposed in utero, which impact on developmental processes beyond infancy. An inability to focus on the environment and interact with the caregiver will influence social, language, and academic function. Information obtained from the baby's immediate world is perceived differently, thus affecting conceptual development. Deficiency in language precursors, such as gaze interaction or extended alert states for reciprocal smiles, affects later pragmatic skills. Irregular relationships sometimes result between caregiver and child. Less secure attachments between child and caregiver are indicated by the indifference of children to the caregiver's departure and return. Disorganization is present in the developmental areas of affect, attachment relationships, and cognitive skills. The children do not show the strong feelings of pleasure, anger, and distress that secure attachments generate (Howard, Beckwith, Rodning, and Kropenske, 1989; Sparks, 1993).

Play routines show striking deficits for these youngsters. There is less representational play, fantasy play, and curious exploration of toys. Unstructured free play situations which require self-organization are characterized by scattering, batting, and picking up and dropping the toys. Play events which represent typical activities of the child, such as combing hair, drinking from a cup, or putting a doll in a bed, are significantly less frequent. These behaviors suggest limited awareness of events and relationships in the child's environment. Behavior is more impulsive, less goal-directed, and more prone to temper tantrums (Howard, Beckwith, Rodning, and Kropenske, 1989).

Kronstadt (1991) discussed other developmental issues for children in preschool exposed in utero to crack/cocaine. She cites research that indicates 30% to 40% of the drug-exposed three year olds demonstrate specific problems in understanding and expressing language, focusing attention, organizing their own behavior, and being hypersensitive to the environment. Irritability, hyperactivity, aggression, poor social skills, and continued difficulty with attachment and separation are also common characteristics.

The Caregiving Environment

Cocaine-exposed children suffer a range of problems including developmental delay, delayed language development, bonding difficulties, hyperactivity, and behavioral disturbances. However, the long-range outcomes of environmental influences are unknown. Because awareness of the widespread use of cocaine, especially crack, was not prevalent until the late 1980s, it will be well into the 21st century before the children exposed in utero who are being followed reach adulthood (Antoniadis and Daulton, 1992). Nevertheless, many professionals currently contend that the caregiving environment is critically important. Researchers are now investigating the effects of environmental factors in improving the outcomes for these children.

An extensive study in New York City of 70 children between the ages of four months and seven years, who were exposed in utero to crack/cocaine, found significant problems (Schaffer, Yanulis, Williams, and Green, 1993). The youngsters resided with grandparents or with foster or adoptive parents. Many (42.4%) of the mothers were at least high school graduates. Nearly 45% of the families had incomes above $35,000. Very few of the families (5%) previously participated in foster or adoptive care although 77% had 10 or more years of parenting experience. For most of the children (52.3%), the foster or adoptive family was the first and only home placement. A total of 88% had two or fewer placements. The researchers observed satisfactory childcare and parenting in most homes. Most caregivers provided safe and predictable environments for the children. Frequent attempts to play, talk, and interact with the children were made. The study indicated that

71% of the children had already been adopted or were in the adoption process and an additional 18% lived with grandparents who were permanently committed to them.

Early intervention and special education services were being provided to 14% of the children. A majority of this select group of youngsters had been legally adopted and were referred for service by their adoptive parents. Yet, there were obvious reasons to suspect that all of the children might have significant problems. At birth, the infants remained in the hospital for an average of 28.7 days. One in five stayed more than two months. *The Infant Monitoring Questionnaire* (Squires, Bricker, and Potter, 1990) for children from 4–36 months, indicated that most of the children had some difficulty. At 24 months, 50% of them had significant problems. By age three, 67% met criteria for referral.

Overall scores from several testing instruments showed deterioration of function and behavior over time. For example, standard scores of the *Vineland Adaptive Behavior Scales* (Sparrow, Balla, and Cicchetti, 1984) decreased with age. While the mean adaptive behavior composite standard score for toddlers between the ages of 12 and 23 months was at the 21st percentile, the mean standard score for children between five and six years was at the 3rd percentile. The researchers concluded that despite competent caregiving, the children exhibited significant problems which progressively deteriorated. The researchers suggested intensive early intervention to improve the outcome.

A major finding in the Schaffer et al. (1993) study was that the children demonstrated consistently poor communication and socialization skills. The caregivers in this project were concerned that their children didn't have any friends, often not even their siblings. The crack-exposed youngsters tossed and broke their toys and did not engage in constructive or pretend play. They did not recognize emotional states such as anger or sadness in their parents or themselves. Three of the oldest children in the group were assigned to 12-month classes for children with severe emotional disturbance. Lying, stealing, and physical aggressiveness were displayed. Erratic behavior occurred which appeared to be unpredictable. The language of the children was difficult to follow and exhibited poor sentence structure. Oral communication was accompanied by excessive gesture. Danger was poorly understood as was any abstract concept.

The child who had made the most progress at the end of the study had received extensive early intervention in addition to his stable home. He was in a regular classroom but displayed extremely poor behavior. He did not interact socially with his peers. He required consistent structure to function academically. Information that most youngsters learn intuitively needed to be taught to this boy.

Schaffer et al. (1993) concluded that intensive intervention must be given to all children exposed in utero to crack/cocaine as well as to their families. The researchers also stated that the children who were given the developmental tests that are currently available demonstrated deceptively high scores, probably because the tests were administered in highly structured test situations. These individual test results did not correspond with parent reports that described what their children normally do. The researchers further reported that in school and caregiver contexts, which have less external control, the children generally do less well. For example, when the youngsters play in a room without an adult who refocuses their attention to the task at hand, they tend to exhibit poor self-regulation.

Another researcher, Sparks (1993), takes the position that with exceptional parenting and early intervention, some children exposed in utero to cocaine can expect to catch up to their nonexposed peers by age four. She observes that developmental difficulties seldom last beyond infancy. As preschoolers, language skills of these youngsters can reach normal limits. There is no greater incidence of the classic signs of learning disability. These conclusions, however, are derived from Sparks's (1993) study of two youngsters exposed in utero to crack, one of whom received extraordinary intervention from an adoptive mother, who was a professional nurse, and from intensive preschool and therapeutic services. The other child remained with his addicted mother and received no early intervention. He required intensive language stimulation when entering an elementary school.

Other professionals express the viewpoint that media coverage of this issue is exaggerated and oversimplified. Myers (1992) cites a few studies which detect no differences between cocaine-exposed and nonexposed infants. She states that the large majority of exposed infants are not premature and are not born with low birth weight. She cautions that because awareness of the problem is relatively recent, alarming accounts of crack-exposed children should be viewed in the total research context. Other professionals support the notion that developmental dysfunction may be partially or completely resolved by competent caregiving and natural brain rejuvenation (Zuckerman and Frank, 1992).

Effect of Crack/Cocaine Exposure on Language Development

Based on what is known about early language development, children exposed in utero to crack/cocaine have significant barriers to language acquisition. Prematurity, lengthy hospital stays, poor sensory systems, inability to maintain focus on the environment, and poor eye contact are characteristic features of the young crack/cocaine-exposed child. Each of these features can have an extremely negative impact on the development of communication skills.

Initial studies (Davis, Fennoy, Laraque, Kanem, Brown, and Mitchell, 1992; Rivers and Hedrick, 1992; Schaffer, Yanulis, Williams, and Green, 1993) on the effect of crack/cocaine on language indicate marked receptive and expressive language deficits. The parents of all of the children in the Schaffer et al. (1993) study found communication problems to be the first and most obvious sign of irregular development.

Rivers and Hedrick (1992) discuss characteristic behaviors by age levels. Table 14.3 displays these characteristic behaviors.

Table 14.3

Age Level Characteristics of Children Exposed in Utero to Crack/Cocaine

Age	Characteristics
Before age 2 years	• Lack of oral language abilities • Use of inappropriate gestures • Limited social interactions • Not easily comforted or consoled
2–4 years	• Inappropriate play routines • Delayed conceptual understanding • Poor pragmatic skills (e.g., turn-taking, eye contact) • Social detachment
4–6 years	• Limited vocabulary • Shallow word meanings • Inappropriate social interaction • Reduced memory skill • Language delays • Inattentiveness

Specific effects on language development, as well as a higher frequency of autism in children exposed prenatally to crack/cocaine, have been reported by Davis et al. (1992). These researchers evaluated 70 children with cocaine exposure in utero to determine whether a specific pattern of abnormalities could be discerned. They observed significant abnormalities including language delay in 94% of the children. The elevated rate of autistic disorders (11.4%) did not occur in children exposed to alcohol or opiates (e.g., heroin) alone. However, the researchers express caution in drawing conclusions, since so many women are poly-drug users which confounds the interpretation of crack/cocaine as the direct cause of autism.

The youngsters who were diagnosed as autistic did not engage in interactive activities. Characteristic difficulties included explosive behavior, uncontrollable or unprovoked laughing or crying, indiscriminate attachment to strangers, and persistent refusal to comply with simple commands. Behavioral disturbances included nonpurposeful activities such as running back and forth across the room, hyperactivity, and perseveration. The eventual course of the autistic behaviors of these children cannot be determined. Furthermore, the effect of appropriate intervention on the autistic behaviors won't be understood for quite a while. (See Chapter 11 for a more detailed discussion of autism.)

THE EFFECTS OF TOBACCO AND OTHER DRUGS ON CHILD DEVELOPMENT

Tobacco Effects

In the United States, about 14% of all preterm births are attributed to maternal smoking (ASHA, 1991). The risk of low birth weight increases over 50% for light smokers (i.e., less than one pack per day) and 130% for heavy smokers (one pack a day or more) compared to nonsmokers (ASHA, 1991). The lowered birth weight of infants whose mothers smoke during pregnancy is believed to impair the ability of the fetus to utilize nourishment in utero. Smoking during the third trimester particularly affects birth weight (Fried and O'Connell, 1987).

Bloch (1992) describes tobacco use as one of the most significant threats to fetal and infant health. She ascribes numerous complications during pregnancy including bleeding, premature rupture of membranes, premature detachment of the placenta, preterm delivery, and low birth weight. Babies born to smokers often can show decreased head circumference and birth length. Bloch (1992) also links smoking with sudden infant death syndrome. Women who smoke during pregnancy have a 25 to 50% higher rate of fetal and infant deaths compared to nonsmokers. However, quitting smoking completely in the first trimester of pregnancy appears to protect the fetus from pregnancy complications.

The behaviors of newborns who are exposed in utero to tobacco smoke and their later development have been studied. Zuckerman (1988) describes research indicating that newborns of mothers who smoke during pregnancy have greater difficulty in orienting to a voice and seem less visually alert. Tests of cognitive, fine and gross motor, and language skills indicate poorer performance among youngsters who were exposed to tobacco smoking in utero. Rush and Callahan (1989) reviewed over 30 papers on the effects of maternal smoking during pregnancy on subsequent child development. They found a consistent pattern of less advanced verbal, reading, and math skills as well as lower IQ associated with maternal smoking during pregnancy. However, tobacco smoke is one of a constellation of possible causes. Rush and Callahan (1989) believe the deficits are linked to a lack of oxygen during fetal development. They believe that the carbon monoxide in cigarette smoke impairs the flow of oxygen to the fetus. Once born, the infant's inability to function adequately has a negative impact on mother-infant interaction. This also can affect later cognitive and linguistic development.

Environmental Tobacco Smoke (ETS)

Exposure to environmental tobacco smoke (ETS) is highest among children from families with low income and less education. ETS is also known as passive or second-hand smoking and is responsible for acute and chronic respiratory disease in children younger than age 14. Although it is most hazardous during the first year of life, older children have a significantly increased risk of bronchitis, pneumonia, chronic middle ear infections, and asthma. ETS impairs postnatal lung development which could already be damaged from maternal smoking during pregnancy. Furthermore, reports indicate that children of smokers are more likely to have cognitive and behavioral deficits (Bloch, 1992; Kronstadt, 1991; Rush and Callahan, 1989).

Marijuana Effects

Unlike tobacco, research on the effects of marijuana on the fetus and newborn development is more limited and inconsistent. The small number of studies that have been reported have not always produced consistent findings regarding physical, linguistic, cognitive, or behavioral function. However, some factors have been linked to marijuana.

Neonatal testing links infant tremors, sleep disturbances, and unresponsiveness to visual stimuli when marijuana is abused by the mother during pregnancy. This can impact negatively on mother-infant interaction. The effects of prenatal exposure seem to last beyond the neonatal period. One study (Fried and Watkinson, 1990) indicated that at age four these children performed less well on the memory and verbal subscales of the *McCarthy Scales of Children's Abilities* (McCarthy, 1972) than children who are not exposed. Attention deficits are reported in children who have reached school age (Fried, Watkinson, Dillon, and Dulberg, 1987). Professionals (Zuckerman and Bresnahan, 1991) suggest that sensory difficulties may be linked to fetal lack of oxygen when the mother smoked marijuana during pregnancy. Furthermore, inadequate parenting might impact on later behavior and development of the child exposed in utero to marijuana. Zuckerman (1991) suggests that marijuana use is underreported as compared to cigarettes or alcohol because it is an illegal drug. Yet estimates of marijuana use range from 5 to 34% for mothers during pregnancy (Zuckerman and Bresnahan, 1991).

The Effects of Other Drugs

Heroin, methadone, amphetamines, phenylelidine hydrochloride (PCP) or "angel dust," as well as prescription drugs, are the other more common drugs ingested during pregnancy. Most are associated with central nervous system difficulties in newborns exposed in utero. Jitteriness, sensitivity to touch and environmental sounds, and abnormal eye movements have been noted (Van Dyke and Fox, 1990; Zuckerman and Bresnahan, 1991).

Toxic substances found in the environment, such as lead and mercury, are also associated with **microcephaly,** an abnormal smallness of the head; and with deafness; blindness; cognitive dysfunction; and mental retardation (Clark, 1989). Many children in the United States who live in dilapidated housing with peeling paint are vulnerable to lead poisoning. Fish from rivers and lakes with high concentrations of mercury can be contaminated. Children exposed to low levels of lead and mercury are at risk for intellectual impairment and behavioral problems. In addition, herbicides and pesticides used in growing the food supply are linked to respiratory difficulties and central nervous system dysfunction (ASHA, 1991). The prenatal effects of drugs on the child's brain development and function create biological vulnerability. Therefore, the postnatal environment becomes a critical component in determining the long-term development of these youngsters.

ENVIRONMENTAL FACTORS AFFECTING LANGUAGE

Prenatal drug exposure can affect an infant's development of normal communication skills. The newborn with impaired eye contact, muscle tone, and facial expression will exhibit poor precursors to language. Mutual gaze and smiles will be disturbed. Caregivers use these facial expressions to guide them in their interactions. Reduced preverbal communication can interfere with later pragmatic and social skills. Limited motor ability affects the infant's opportunities to explore and learn from the environment, which impacts on later conceptual formation. Infants with hyperirritability and unpredictable sleep patterns may develop problems in bonding with the caregiver. These factors, in combination with a higher incidence of illness and general developmental delay, place the infant at risk for delays in language development (Prizant and Meyer, 1993; Prizant and Wetherby, 1990; Sparks, 1989).

The family circumstances of mothers who ingest and abuse drugs while pregnant are often stressful and dysfunctional.

Malnourishment, poverty, child and maternal abuse, sexual abuse, violence, poor medical treatment, and continued dependence on certain substances can interfere with the ability of the caregiver to deal with the baby effectively. An unfavorable caregiving environment in combination with high perinatal stress impairs the general development and communication of the child (Fox, Long, and Langlois, 1988; Zuckerman and Bresnahan, 1991). Those youngsters who are placed in foster care often reside in multiple home placements or remain in the hospital for long periods of time. These factors affect infant bonding and successful interactive opportunities which are critical for language acquisition.

Analysis of studies of families with child neglect and abuse (Katz, 1992) indicate that the style of parent-child interaction is significantly different. **Neglect** encompasses a lack of physical caregiving and supervision and a lack of mental stimulation. Verbal harassment, rejection, and withdrawal from the child are typical parental behaviors (Skuse, 1992). The mothers tend to respond to fewer of the infants' initiatives at communication. They are less actively involved in parent-child interactions, provide less auditory stimulations such as parentese conversations, and are less involved during freeplay situations. Children are left to "go play" rather than to play with the parent and engage in naming and explaining activities. Thus, neglected children receive little environmental stimulation with less exchange of information.

Over time, maltreated children show a decline in developmental and language skills (Coster and Cicchetti, 1993; Katz, 1992). Abused infants tend to be less likely to respond when their mothers attempt to engage them in interaction. These findings raise questions as to whether the behaviors of the newborn exposed to drugs (including hyperirritability, excessive crying, disturbed sleep patterns, and poor focus for mutual gaze) can cause the parent to increase abuse, neglect, and the associated interactive patterns; or whether the parent's behavior exacerbates the child's fragile interactive abilities.

Skuse (1992) discusses the relationship of neglect and deprivation to physical growth and language development. The physical consequences among children neglected through the preschool period are poor growth in height, weight, and head circumference. Developmental delays, including exceptionally poor language skills, are predominant symptoms. Other research (Lefevre, 1975) found malnourishment affecting language development in children. However, some studies (Kronstadt, 1991; Myers, 1992) suggest that children placed in advantageous environments begin to "catch up" to their peers and display an accelerated rate of language development and physical growth. Therefore, the interventions after birth to children exposed in utero to drugs, as well as interventions for their caregivers, are critical factors in attempts to achieve optimum language and general development.

INTERVENTIONS

Children exposed to drugs in utero require early and total family intervention. Drug abuse affects the mother, the infant, and other family members. The potential for difficulties in interaction is great for a drug-abusing mother and the high-risk infant. Drug-exposed infants may need to be carefully taught how to interact with others. Yet the quality of parenting by the mother is affected by extreme stress and the naivety or irresponsibility associated with a woman's use of drugs during pregnancy (Burns and Burns, 1988). A fragile infant and the absence of a stable social support system intensify dysfunctional parenting. Often the mothers are the product of poor parenting themselves and that heritage of child-rearing is transmitted to the child.

Maternal Needs

Intervention for the mother might include drug rehabilitation, medical and nutritional service, and counseling. One study (Burns and Burns, 1988) found a cluster of tendencies in mothers who abuse drugs. They were generally immature women with a high degree of egocentrism. Because they viewed their newborn as a "gift" for themselves, they interpreted their child's communication attempts as demanding. Over half were severely depressed with mood swings. Therefore, at the time a newborn has critical needs and requires patience and encouragement to engage in social interaction, the mother sends a message of insensitivity to the needs of the infant. At best, the mothers tend to parent half-heartedly and without a genuine warmth. Often the baby is neglected and rejected. A downward spiral in development and communication results. Intensive counseling and support are required to provide more effective parent-child interaction.

Infant Intervention

Infants exposed to drugs in utero frequently are born prematurely. Often, lengthy hospital stays are indicated. In addition, the baby exposed in utero to crack/cocaine can display some of the most severe behaviors after birth. The characteristic of oversensitivity to environmental stimulation and difficulty in calming down, in addition to poor sleep/arousal regulation and interaction, make immediate intervention necessary. Comforting techniques include these:

- swaddling
- vertical rocking
- reducing environmental stimulation
- learning the early signs of overstimulation in the infant to avert inconsolable crying

Many infants cannot tolerate tactile stimulation, excessive handling, and jerky movements (MacDonald, 1992). Lewis, Bennett, and Schmeder (1989) suggest additional strategies to reduce stress and promote interaction:

- Stop activity that produces stress reaction.
- Give time-out from stressful situations.

- Provide firm, strong touch.
- Swaddle the infant with arms close to body.
- Give a warm bath.
- Adjust stimuli in response to infant cues.

Intervention should include a team of professionals. It is not unusual for speech-language intervention, occupational therapy, drug therapy, and guidance from teachers, psychologists, social workers, and physicians to be integrated for "transdisciplinary" support services. Toddlers and school-age children prenatally exposed to drugs seem to learn best in settings with a defined structure, a predictable and stable environment, and secure, nurturing attachments to adults. These protective factors should be combined with facilitation in coping skills, problem solving, self-esteem, and social interaction.

The Educational Context

The learning environment should provide consistent structure with special preparations for transitions between activities because of difficulties shifting from one activity to another. Limited materials should be provided in the room to reduce stimuli. Extended periods of play can assist the child in exploring and manipulating the environment, in expressing feelings, and in becoming a symbolic thinker. Adults participate in these play routines by sharing and encouraging. When adults respect children's work, their attempts at interaction and their feelings, positive attachments, and trust are enhanced. The adults need to develop sensitivity to the child's appropriate and inappropriate behaviors and what they mean. Mutual discussion helps the child to understand feelings, experiences, and behaviors. Verbal expression allows the child to integrate immediate feelings and experiences with prior ones. Improved verbal expression can lead to increased ability to do the following:

1. modulate behavior;
2. gain self-control; and

3. express feelings.

The effective intervention process creates a partnership between the home (parent) and school.

Language learning should provide opportunities for children to interact with significant individuals and to explore their environment. The activities should be important and interesting for the child. They must be related to everyday experiences. The children will learn by active participation. "Hands-on" activities reinforce the child's language. Eye contact and simple directions help the child comprehend expectations. Beginning attempts at verbal communication need immediate response. Negative behavior should be recognized as a signal of the child's unmet needs. Child language development depends on the ability to receive, understand, integrate, and express meaningful experiences (Los Angeles Unified School District, 1990).

EDUCATIONAL CONCERNS

The intervention process for children and their families who are exposed to drugs is intensive and costly (Rist, 1990). The cost to the medical and educational systems has increased substantially over the last few years, especially with the crack/cocaine epidemic. Several hundred thousand youngsters are born each year who were exposed in utero to drugs and have severe problems (English and Henry, 1990). Intervention includes initial hospital costs for prolonged intensive care, repeated hospitalizations during the first year for surviving children, health and education costs for the youngsters who survive the first year, maternal drug treatment and medical costs, and the cost of institutionalizing those young people who are not maintained in family settings. For example, Abel (1990) estimates that the total cost for individuals with fetal alcohol syndrome who require 24-hour residential care due to mental retardation, is $154.8 million per year.

Daunting costs, in combination with large numbers of individuals who need intervention, make the problem of adequate intervention overwhelming. Public policy perceives youngsters exposed to drugs as high-risk children. However, not all states consider high risk alone as a call for intervention. Services cannot start without an affirmation of problems. Therefore, precious time which is needed for optimum improvement is wasted. Schaffer, Yanulis, Williams, and Green (1993) report that 56 of the 70 youngsters in their study received no preschool special services. They conclude that intervention must begin immediately for all of these children so that the infant can learn to interact appropriately with the environment and can develop additional central nervous system function. Foster care agency and shelter facility workers must be trained and informed about drug-exposed babies and how to access available services for them and their families. Rist (1990) states that waiting until kindergarten age to identify and treat drug-exposed children can add substantially to overall long-term costs. Over time, the aberrant behaviors of these youngsters become more firmly entrenched and increasingly difficult to change. Sufficient funding for appropriate programs should be sought.

SUMMARY

Increasing numbers of children are being born who have been exposed in utero to drugs and toxic substances. The impact of drug abuse on the developing fetus depends on the stage during pregnancy a given substance is ingested, the dosage consumed, and the length of time the substance is abused. Many of these children exhibit low birth weight, prematurity, physical abnormalities, and abnormal behaviors associated with central nervous system dysfunction. These youngsters require longer hospital stays and additional medical intervention. Complications associated with drug use, such as AIDS and sexually transmitted diseases, compound the drug-related difficulties.

The home environment of the child can also adversely affect the child. Some youngsters are placed in multiple foster homes because the natural mothers are unable or unwilling to care for them. Others return to their natural family, which can be dysfunctional due to continued parental substance abuse. Violence, poverty, malnourishment, and neglect are frequently associated with these families. These factors have a deleterious effect on the baby's language and general development.

Newborns who have been exposed to drugs are fragile and disorganized. They have difficulty processing environmental stimulation. There is a reduced ability to maintain eye contact and to smile. These interactional skills affect future language acquisition. The caregivers are frequently untrained in effective ways to increase the baby's ability to explore the environment and interact with others. Mothers who are depressed and unstable cannot provide consistent childcare. Often mothers interpret the baby's hyperirritability and difficulty in being comforted as disinterest. Children are increasingly ignored or abused.

Studying the effects of specific drugs on the newborn is complicated by maternal polydrug ingestion and variations in the amount of each drug that is consumed. In addition, some mothers abuse drugs throughout pregnancy and some binge on drugs. The most common drugs known to affect the developing fetus are alcohol, crack/cocaine, tobacco, marijuana, heroin, PCP, amphetamines, and prescription drugs.

When language problems exist, they are related to congenital disturbances in organic development, especially in the central nervous system, and to parent-child interaction. The sensory systems are often impaired. Touch, lights, and movement cause severe stress in the newborn. Visual and auditory responsiveness are frequently disordered. These factors interfere with the young child's ability to engage in the world and to acquire information and experience. During the toddler years, play routines are particularly immature. Rather than use toys symbolically, the children frequently throw and break them. It is common for these youngsters to be aggressive or to avoid their peers. Problem solving and generalizing from past experiences are impaired.

The incidence of children born each year who were exposed in utero to drugs is estimated to be in the hundreds of thousands. Intensive, early intervention is believed to produce the best outcome for these youngsters. Effective intervention includes the entire family and a transdisciplinary team of professionals who integrate their strategies with one another. However, controversy over the long-range consequences for all children who experienced drug exposure in utero and are "at risk" for developmental difficulties causes some educational agencies to exercise restraint in providing special education services. A large group of these youngsters receive no intervention until they exhibit severe behavior problems at school or fail.

Drug exposure and its associated problems are completely preventable. By developing drug awareness and prepregnancy drug rehabilitation, the effects of prenatal drug abuse can be reduced.

SUGGESTED READINGS

Dorris, M. (1989). *The Broken Chord*. New York: Harper Perennial.

Rosetti, L. (Ed.). (1992). *Development Problems of Drug-Exposed Infants*. San Diego, CA: Singular Publishing Group. (This monograph presents relevant transdisciplinary information from various authors regarding drug-exposed infants.)

Sparks, S. (1993). *Children of Prenatal Substance Abuse*. San Diego, CA: Singular Publishing Group.

15 ISSUES IN SCHOOL-BASED INTERVENTION

Numerous appraisals of American special and regular education have reviewed the effectiveness of intervention for children with all disabilities (Audette and Algozzine, 1992; Gersten and Woodward, 1990; Miller, 1990b; Slavin, 1990). Many youngsters who receive special educational services are not progressing as expected. School systems are plagued by limited financial resources and expanding numbers of children in need of special educational services. Within this educational context, youngsters with language difficulties, as well as all students, need an education that will prepare them to function effectively and productively in society. Youngsters with language difficulties require the earliest intervention possible for optimum development. Furthermore, the language-learning process must take into account the specific biological, cognitive, emotional, social, and cultural influences on each child. The educational setting and the unique needs of the child require compatibility for successful learning.

Children who exhibit difficulty in acquiring language need intervention that utilizes meaningful interactional contexts. Language learning can be viewed in the broader context of communication skills. The **communicative competence model** characterizes the wide scope of grammatical, cognitive, social, and cultural knowledge underlying adequate language ability (Rice, 1986). The child's social and cultural environment must be considered. Parents, classroom teachers, and other members of a child's community can provide important information and language intervention.

405

Therefore, the natural, everyday environment of a youngster becomes an ideal context to develop language skill.

As professionals have become aware of the importance of language for both social and academic growth, more youngsters with communication problems have been identified. At the same time, the initiative to include children with severe disabilities into mainstream classes has intensified. These converging educational trends impact on teachers and other school personnel who often have little training and information about communication and how to work effectively with children who have language disorders. Overcrowding and budget constraints place additional burdens on professionals. These realities undermine the educational benefits afforded children with disabilities who have the opportunity to enter mainstream environments and be exposed to more typical childhood experiences.

Collaborative consultation gives the individuals working with children with disabilities the opportunity to share their expertise. This model has moved the speech-language pathologist into the classroom and home environment. It has fostered more functional language contexts during the learning process. It views language as a skill that is learned throughout a youngster's day and not a subject to be taught for two 30-minute sessions each week. However, intervention strategies that include children with disabilities in regular environments must provide support for the teacher and the parent.

With this backdrop for school-based intervention, this chapter does the following:

1. examines the federal laws and political initiatives that have affected school-based intervention as well as school personnel preparation for effective implementation of educational reform;

2. explores professional team collaboration in both the assessment and the teaching of children with language problems;

3. presents specific curricular philosophies, principles, and strategies that enhance language learning;

4. discusses the relationship of language, metalinguistic skills, and learning to read;

5. examines the critical role of parents in facilitating language learning and in assisting professionals; and

6. proposes issues requiring resolution before effective intervention programs for children with special needs will be realized.

THE IMPACT OF GOVERNMENT MANDATES

The purpose of special education law and regulation is to ensure that all children with disabilities have an equal opportunity to benefit from a free and appropriate public education. Since 1973, a series of federal legislative enactments have specified the rights and entitlements of children with disabilities. The laws have influenced the way many schools provide opportunities for children with disabilities. The laws have also shaped public awareness so more people realize that a person who is less abled is not less worthy (Turnbull, 1986).

As part of the Rehabilitation Act of 1973 (Public Law 93-112), which was the first federal civil rights law which protected individuals with disabilities, Section 504 was enacted. This ensured that qualified people with disabilities could not be excluded from or be subjected to discrimination in any activities or programs which receive federal financial assistance. The regulation applies to any state education agency, school system, college, or state vocational rehabilitation agency.

Two years later, in 1975, Public Law (PL) 94-142 was signed. Known as the Education for All Handicapped Children Act (EHA), this law attempted to correct the inconsistent and often inappropriate educational opportunities for youngsters with disabilities. In 1990, PL 94-142 was revised through the passage of PL 101-476 and was renamed IDEA (Individuals with Disabilities Education Act). The laws entitle children with disabilities to a free and appropriate public education which has been designed to meet each child's individual needs in the least restrictive environment.

Legal Provisions

Due Process

IDEA describes the "due process" procedures that provide the opportunity for advocates for the child with disabilities to challenge any aspect of education (Turnbull, 1986). **Due process** means that children with disabilities and their parents have an appeal process by which they can represent their viewpoint if they disagree with the proposed actions of the school. If there are disagreements, an impartial hearing can be arranged to resolve the differences. Parents and schools are encouraged to work together on behalf of the child with disabilities.

Least Restrictive Environment

Children with disabilities have the right to instruction in the **least restrictive environment** (LRE). This means that, to the maximum extent appropriate, they will be educated with children without disabilities. Therefore, they will be removed from the public school setting among peers without disabilities only when their needs cannot be met within the regular school setting with the use of supplementary aids and services. LRE aims for involvement with nondisabled peers, and for school programs in the child's regular school or as close to the regular school as possible. Any removal from the regular environment must be justified in terms of the special learning characteristics of the student and the potential negative effects of removal and nonremoval.

Parental Rights

The law recognizes parents as part of the educational process. Parents must be informed about the school programs and the child's rights. Parental permission is secured before formal assessments and placements are undertaken. Parental participation must be included during the assessment and development of the Individualized Education Program.

The education of every child with disabilities is individualized so that it can be appropriate and meaningful. The right to a fair evaluation so that correct educational programs and placements can be achieved is also ensured (Turnbull, 1986).

Birth Through Two Services

Congress passed an amendment to PL 94-142 in 1986 which provides service to very young children with disabilities. Part H of PL 99-457 makes funds available to states for early intervention services to infants and toddlers (ages birth through two years) with disabilities. Infants and toddlers "at risk" of developing disabilities could also be served at each state's discretion. Furthermore, all eligible children between the ages of three and five who have disabilities are entitled to receive appropriate special education services under Section 619 of the law.

Part H contains several expanded provisions for the birth to two population. First, the comprehensive, multidisciplinary evaluation assesses not only the needs of the children with disabilities but also their families. The Individualized Family Service Plan (IFSP) includes goals for the child and the family and is coordinated in a case management format so that support services for families are integrated.

Americans with Disabilities Act

The 1990 Americans with Disabilities Act (ADA) further defined the civil rights of persons with disabilities in all public accommodations, not just those receiving funds. As with Section 504, school programs, services, and activities such as after-school programs or graduation ceremonies cannot exclude qualified students with disabilities. An additional emphasis of the ADA requires that auxiliary aids to ensure effective communication are provided in public facilities. Transportation systems and buildings have physical accessibility standards. The intent of the law is to assure equal access for individuals with disabilities in all aspects of society. This corresponds with education initiatives which include youngsters with disabilities in mainstream programs.

Transition Services

The 1990 IDEA amendments mesh with the ADA requirements for equal access by adding a new emphasis on transition planning for secondary students. Schools have an obligation to prepare students to participate effectively and independently in society upon their high school graduation. This has provided a new focus for special education programs which often emphasized "academic readiness" skills throughout a student's school career. The renewed emphasis on transition to full participation in society focuses special education curriculum on functional performance in post-secondary education and community living environments.

The Team Approach

Decisions regarding a child's eligibility for special education and the type of services to be provided are made by a team of individuals. For example, IDEA regulations specify that the Individualized Education Program (IEP) planning meeting include the following participants:

1. the child's teacher (For a child with a disability who is being considered for placement in special education, the teacher could be the child's regular teacher, or a teacher qualified to provide education in the type of program in which the child may be placed, or both);

2. another representative who is qualified to provide, or supervise, the provision of special education;

3. one or both of the child's parents (who by law may opt not to participate);

4. the child, if appropriate; and

5. other individuals at the discretion of the parent or agency.

Regulations that determine the specific educational team members vary from state to state, but must at least comply with federal regulations. Furthermore, the needs and disabilities of the youngster can determine the composite of team members.

For example, a child with a language impairment would have the speech-language pathologist present or some other individual who is qualified and knowledgeable about the evaluation procedures used with the child and is familiar with the results of the evaluation. The team concept is reflected in all aspects of the child's involvement in special education. The initial assessment must be conducted by more than one person to provide a comprehensive picture of the child as well as a nondiscriminatory classification. School psychologists, physicians, social workers, teachers, speech-language pathologists, and others may gather information about the child's strengths and weaknesses and their effect on educational performance. Recommendations are made that are based on the information presented by those individuals with expertise in the child's abilities and who have knowledge about the child's progress and programs. Each state has specific time lines for completion of the initial evaluation, the placement, and the review of the program based on the federal regulations.

Program Participation

Special education is one part of the total school program. Students with disabilities have the opportunity to participate in a full range of programs and services available through regular education and special education. This *continuum of services* from less restrictive to more restrictive settings emphasizes participation in regular education classes and extracurricular activities whenever appropriate. Those children who are segregated from the regular education environment have been judged to be unable to meet the expectations of that setting. However, the goal of special education is to include students with disabilities into regular education programs as much as possible. If a particular youngster can no longer derive educational benefit from an environment in a more typical school setting, the child is moved to a more restrictive placement. For example, the child could be shifted from a regular classroom in a school with special resource room services to a special education classroom in a regular elementary school. Conversely, as the child develops skills which enable reentry into a less restrictive setting, the student is moved to the more "mainstream" environment.

In summary, there is improved access to education and heightened awareness of entitlement and due process rights. However, large-scale use of self-contained special education classes as primary educational environments is being reexamined. Many students have failed to make satisfactory progress in the segregated class format (Gartner and Lipsky, 1987). The trend in the 1990s is to include students with disabilities in regular programs wherever appropriate.

The Individualized Education Program (IEP)

Each child with disabilities has an **IEP,** which is a written statement that specifies the child's present levels of educational performance, the type of special education prescribed, the extent that the child can participate in regular educational programs, the special equipment needed, special or related services, modifications in the curriculum, and specific educational goals. It also states the projected dates for the initiation of services and the anticipated duration of the services. Appropriate criteria for determining whether the goals and objectives of the IEP are being achieved are included as well (Turnbull, 1986). The IEP is a compliance/monitoring document, which may be used to determine whether the child is actually receiving the free, appropriate education agreed to by the parents and the school. All services specified in the IEP must be provided so that the education agency is in compliance with the law. However, teachers and other school personnel are not held accountable if the child does not achieve the specific educational goals and objectives outlined in the IEP.

Parents are entitled to use due process procedures for problems related to the IEP, the school, or the teachers. This legislation has helped to define the obligations of the classroom teacher. As youngsters with disabilities participate in regular classroom activities, the classroom teacher often becomes a member of the team decision-making process.

Incidence of Language Disorders and Public Law

Speech and language programs have expanded overall since passage of PL 94-142. In the fourteenth annual report to Congress on the implementation of IDEA (U.S. Department of Education, 1992), data indicate that the children whose primary disability is labeled "speech impaired," including both speech and language impairments, account for 23.4 percent of those served. Those children who are deaf, hard of hearing, or deaf-blind comprise another 1.4 percent. When speech, language, and hearing categories are combined, the total is 24.8 percent or nearly one-fourth of all children with disabilities who receive service under IDEA. The statistics that have been obtained for the annual reports to Congress show a steady growth only since 1988 in the provision of speech and language services in schools. This contrasts with earlier decreases in the percent of children served who were identified as speech or language impaired. The report suggests that the overall decrease in the percent of students served with speech or language impairments between 1976 and 1988 can be attributed to the trend to identify students with language disorders as having specific learning disabilities rather than a speech or language impairment. Yet, a few school districts report that communication disorders comprise the majority of students classified as "handicapped" (Ehren, 1993).

The Inclusion Movement and LRE

Educators are beginning to recognize that special education is a part of the total educational continuum rather than a parallel and separate educational system. Special education and regular education need to be integrated into one educational system that provides for individual needs and differences of all children (Gloeckler, 1991). Although the intent of federal legislation (IDEA) acknowledges the importance of educating children with disabilities in the least restrictive environment (LRE), in practice the children have often been segregated more than is necessary.

Regular Education Initiative

A major influence in the impetus to reexamine the direction of special education is the *Regular Education Initiative* (Will, 1986). This document takes the position that special education programs address student failure rather than prevention, that special education is rarely connected to the regular education system, and that the result is the absence of a coherent strategy to provide service to all students who need assistance, whether they have a confirmed disability or not. Finally, those youngsters who are eligible for help through special education service are often segregated from their peers, which stigmatizes them and sometimes results in lowered academic and social expectations, poor self-esteem, and diminished performance.

A report issued from the United States Office of Special Education and Rehabilitation Services (OSERS) in the U.S. Department of Education (Will, 1986) suggested a series of reforms to assist all students in developing the skills to be independent and productive adults. First, it encouraged active parent involvement in the educational process. It also proposed early identification and intervention for learning problems. This involves curriculum-based assessment. Rather than categorizing or labeling students, each student's strengths and weaknesses would be determined for instructional planning purposes. In addition, it advised a partnership between regular and special educational systems to develop educational strategies cooperatively. It emphasized that this does not imply consolidating special education with regular education personnel. These OSERS proposals coincide with concern for improved implementation of the least restrictive environment aspect of PL 94-142. Some special educators have provided greater opportunities to include students with disabilities into mainstream environments in and out of school.

The proponents of separate special education programs argue that children with disabilities require specialized teaching methods. However, Audette and Algozzine (1992) argue that most methods textbooks used by professionals who teach students with speech-language disorders, learning disabilities, and/or cognitive disabilities use teaching methods that are extensions or refinements of general strategies rather than a new set of teaching techniques.

Professionals who oppose fundamental change in special education practices also take issue with the Regular Education Initiative (Kauffman, Gerber, and Semmel, 1988; Keogh, 1988; Shumaker and Deshler, 1988). They state that numerous national reports criticize the quality of general education and that it is illogical to assume that this system can accommodate special needs students, many of whom have previously failed in it. They also fear that the efforts to teach as many youngsters as possible in the mainstream may reduce the numbers of youngsters identified as having special needs. In addition, they are concerned about the reduction of special education services resulting from a regular education initiative. Finally, they question the ability of the system to retrain regular education teachers to accommodate youngsters with disabilities in their classrooms.

Inclusion

Paralleling the efforts to coordinate special education services with regular education and to encourage active implementation of LRE is the "inclusion movement." Gartner and Lipsky (1987) studied the overall effectiveness of PL 94-142 for all children in special education and found that the segregated special education programs that have evolved have few significant benefits for most students. Gartner and Lipsky (1987) suggest greater utilization of full- and part-time regular class placements to improve academic achievement, self-esteem, behavior, and emotional adjustment of many students who have been segregated into special placements. In most special education settings, Gartner and Lipsky (1987) found few differences from the regular education environment in curriculum adaptation, additional time on task, diverse teaching strategies, or adaptive equipment.

LRE requires a determination of educational programs and placements on a case-by-case basis for each child (Peters-Johnson, 1993). The **inclusion movement** is a belief system that goes beyond LRE. Proponents of inclusion have made the value judgment that integrated education for *all* students regardless of color, race, religion, or ability is the best and most humane system. They consider all students to be people who have equal worth and equal rights (Biklen, 1989; Stainback, Stainback, and Bunch, 1989). The inclusion movement proposes integration of students with disabilities in regular classes with adequate support and related services so that they can learn with their chronological peers. Structured opportunities are provided for interaction between the students with disabilities and their peers, including participation in all nonacademic activities of the school. The movement sets high expectations for students and emphasizes functional life skills for students with disabilities so they can learn appropriate behaviors to succeed in adulthood (Biklen, 1992).

Growth of the inclusion movement as well as the intent of LRE legislation corresponds with changing trends in language and communication intervention strategies (Locke, 1989; Shafer, Staab, and Smith, 1983; Silliman and Wilkinson, 1991; Wang, Reynolds, and

Walberg, 1988). That is, language acquisition is facilitated when there are opportunities to use language in the child's environment. Helping children to use language for a variety of functions and intentions teaches them how to communicate effectively. Separate, isolated environments with language tasks that do not relate to the child's everyday communication needs do not stimulate language growth.

Implementing Change

As youngsters with disabilities are included in regular environments, educational professionals need information and assistance in methods of delivering instruction, of effectively including all children in specific activities, and of collaborating with other special education personnel. Furthermore, the school is part of a community system. With expanded efforts to include youngsters with disabilities into regular classrooms, after-school activities, and community facilities comes the need for involving a variety of individuals including parents and nondisabled children. Participants also require adequate information and training. Only with cooperation among all children, teachers, administrators, parents, and members of the greater community can all students benefit from integration of children with disabilities into regular environments.

Children with disabilities cannot be placed into regular classrooms without adequate preparation of educational personnel. Miller (1990b) specifies that teachers who actively participate in the change process are more supportive of change. She outlines variables affecting successful change, such as leadership support from either the principal or some administrator who champions the initiative, provision of adequate resources and materials for teachers, a climate that supports change, attention to concerns of individuals involved in change, and adequate time to experiment and practice with the reforms.

Working conditions for the adults in schools are reflected in students' learning conditions. McLaughlin and Yee (1988) explored school work environments and their effect on teachers. They found that the greatest professional success occurs in educational environments with a shared sense of responsibility, provision for feedback and support, open discussion of problems, and rewards for risk-taking and experimentation. Teachers and specialists tend to perform more effectively in schools that treat them as competent professionals.

Gersten and Woodward (1990) suggest staff development programs that address changes in professional expectations in the work setting relating to the implementation of LRE and collaboration. Teachers require specific guidelines on how to translate new ideas into the realities of their classroom situations. In this context, collaboration among school professionals improves the educational environment of all students. Regular classroom teachers benefit from being sensitized to the abilities of students with special needs. In addition, the professional staff is prepared to develop awareness in the nondisabled students, parents, and community members of the feelings and characteristics of students with disabilities. Gloeckler (1991) suggests using the curriculum to provide information on disabilities in a comprehensive and consistent manner. The goal is to value and respect each child's abilities.

COLLABORATIVE LANGUAGE INTERVENTION

Since the 1970s, the concept of working with youngsters with language disabilities in their natural (or classroom) environment has gained considerable support. Research (Wilcox, Kouri, and Caswell, 1991) suggests that classroom versus individual intervention for even very young preschoolers is also preferable. The more traditional "pull-out" model for providing services has been reexamined with recent efforts to comply with the LRE mandates. Programming which promotes activities that are compatible with the child's everyday environment has focused on naturalistic settings such as the classroom. Thus, language intervention that is

integrated with classroom instruction has produced less fragmenta-
tion in learning and improved coordination of teaching.

Limitations of the "Pull-out" Model

The initiative to provide speech and language intervention in the
classroom in collaboration with the teacher and other educational
professionals is a response to the limitations of the traditional "pull-
out" model of providing service. Sending a student off to a separate
room for intervention reduces the time on task for the student,
fragments the curriculum, and minimizes the responsibility of the
classroom teacher for the student's instruction (Meyers, Gelzheiser,
and Yelich, 1991). In addition, the teachers tend to know little
about the instructional methods used with their students in the
alternate setting. Wang, Reynolds, and Walberg (1988) found that
students who received support services such as speech-language
"therapy" end up with reduced instructional time compared to students not served. The children return from their "pull-out" program
to their general class in mid-lesson, after spending time traveling to
and from the service, and are unable to benefit fully from the
remainder of the class lesson. Gersten and Woodward (1990) point
out that the materials used in a child's "pull-out" program are not
related to the core curriculum used in the classroom. Little attempt
has been made to integrate what is learned in the alternate setting to
what is taught in the classroom. Furthermore, the curriculum in the
"pull-out" setting frequently does not meet the complex academic
and social demands of the general class. The student does not
understand how to apply and generalize what was learned in the
alternate setting in the general classroom.

Language intervention in the regular classroom provides an opportunity to assess what factors in that setting contribute to a student's
problems. Programs and curriculum content can be coordinated
between the speech-language pathologist and classroom teacher.
Providing service in the classroom in collaboration with the teacher
creates a focus on specific instructional issues and the learning

environment. Collaborative meetings become more frequent. The speech-language pathologist obtains greater understanding of the child's natural environment and targets language behavior that would improve communication with adults and peers in this typical situation. Personnel other than the speech-language pathologist can become effective intervention agents. Frequently, the language specialist assumes a "modeling/consultative" role for strategies to facilitate language within the instructional context. The classroom teacher assumes a "modeling/consultative" role for strategies in classroom management and educational curriculum (Ferguson, 1992; Wilcox, Kouri, and Caswell, 1991).

Integrating Divergent Perspectives

In general, collaboration between special and regular education staff merges two perspectives on learning. Regular education is concerned about instructional curricula which have been determined as appropriate to the students in the particular school system. A specific scope and sequence is developed by teachers so that they can implement curricular objectives. Thus, the emphasis is on the prescribed curriculum, and the individual teacher has the responsibility to create an appropriate learning environment to teach it. Special education, on the other hand, focuses on the student's individual strengths and weaknesses and how they impact on learning. Intervention often emphasizes development of specific abilities of a particular student. The curriculum is secondary to the child and is used as the vehicle for solving learning problems. Since collaborative efforts have expanded, special and regular education have begun to shift their primary focus to the learning context, learning styles, policies, and attitudes. The educational process becomes the student's path toward successful integration into society.

Collaborative Models

Collaboration can be achieved in several ways. Miller (1989) proposes collaboration formats which include team teaching, consultation, and staff development. (Refer to Chapter 2 for additional discussion.) Language intervention services can be extended to the classroom to enhance communication skills and academic learning experiences. Simon and Myrold-Gunyuz (1990) describe three specific models of collaboration between the speech-language pathologist and classroom teacher to develop language skills:

1. *The Communication-Enhancement Model*—the speech-language pathologist becomes the "guest teacher" in the classroom to improve general classroom language knowledge.

2. *The Formula Model*—the classroom teacher and the speech-language pathologist are collaborative partners in teaching a supplemental language program (e.g., study skills or reading comprehension development).

3. *The Curriculum-Based Model*—the teacher presents a curricular unit and the speech-language pathologist provides additional language activities to address the language demands of the lessons.

Collaboration between the classroom teacher and speech-language pathologist links language skills to content domains. The connections between oral and written language are emphasized. Language skills are viewed as the instruments for learning to read, write, and speak throughout the school day and not skills to be drilled for two 30-minute periods per week (Achilles, Yates, and Freese, 1991; Montgomery, 1992). The speech-language pathologist provides expertise to integrate listening, reading, speaking, writing, and reasoning with the classroom curriculum in an effective and individualized format (Wadle, 1991).

Collaboration and Language Goals

When academic subjects become the framework for language intervention services, the child's language goals incorporate classroom activities. This provides opportunity throughout the day for the youngster to practice each goal in varying academic and social situations (Masterson, 1993). Wiig (1991) compares the goals generated for children in "pull-out" programs with those children whose language intervention programs are designed for participation in classroom activities. Those youngsters who do not participate in collaborative intervention tend to be given "deficit-driven" goals (e.g., *to improve auditory sequencing skills* or *to increase vocabulary*). In contrast, the language goals created for collaborative, classroom contexts tend to be curriculum-based, such as *to retell four events in correct order from a story in the reading book* or *to express thoughts in written and discussion formats using appropriate words* (Montgomery, 1992; Wiig, 1991).

The mutual deliberation between the speech-language pathologist and the classroom teacher in creating and implementing goals provides the teacher with an awareness of the impact of language on academic basic skills and social activities. Larson, McKinley, and Boley (1993) cite the definition of *basic skills* by the U.S. government. It includes reasoning skills and oral communication (i.e., listening and speaking) as well as reading, writing, and mathematics. The teacher's raised consciousness regarding the language-learning relationship benefits the basic skills and communication of all children in the classroom (Locke, 1989). For example, oral language can be utilized to compare and contrast ideas, to explain cause and effect, to report experiences, and to imagine hypothetical situations.

As students with communication problems mature, the collaboration of the speech-language pathologist with the classroom teacher can orient the teacher to the communication prerequisites for vocational contexts as well as academic areas. High school team collaboration should also include the students and their visions of what goals might provide future benefit to them (Larson, McKinley, and Boley, 1993).

Collaboration also can have a positive impact on the language development of culturally diverse populations (Wiig, 1991). Members of the school, family, and community can be consulted to develop a more accurate understanding of a child's abilities and to determine an appropriate language-learning environment.

Authors Larson, McKinley, and Boley (1993) caution that no intervention model is suitable for all students all of the time. However, intervention that promotes the most efficient process for language learning

1. is functional;

2. encourages effective communication using natural language;

3. utilizes environments where students spend a large portion of their time;

4. integrates communication skills with the curricula; and

5. bases its strategies and goals on the collective expertise of a professional team.

STRATEGIES FOR LANGUAGE INTERVENTION

Language develops best in natural contexts where it is used as a tool for communication, learning, and social interaction. Children with language disabilities benefit from interventions that are meaningful and integrate their daily experience with its corresponding language. Professionals (Duchan and Weitzner-Lin, 1987; Norris and Damico, 1990; Shafer, Staab, and Smith, 1983; Westby, 1990) have examined which skills and abilities each student requires to be an effective learner and communicator, and then they have created environments where these skills can develop. Language learning is viewed as an ongoing process that continues throughout the day, at home and at school, in all activities.

Establishing the Language Environment

Language acquisition involves the cognitive, linguistic, and social systems. Relevant language contexts engage students in natural and meaningful activities where language becomes a communication tool. Children are encouraged to observe and interact with the materials and people in the environment to obtain information and conceptual knowledge. While actively participating in their environment, children integrate language with the acquisition of world knowledge. They also develop the communicative functions of language.

When interacting with others, the language used and the way it is used produces certain effects on people. Thus, effective language learning attaches meaning and linguistic form to the child's interactions with the environment and others (Goodman, 1986; Norris and Hoffman, 1990). The teacher has the responsibility to do the following:

1. create an appropriate environment from which children can derive meaning and information;

2. facilitate the understanding and use of language as the children participate in their environment; and

3. provide responses to the child's communicative attempts.

Children learn, through meaningful language, that they are able to control and affect change in their environment and in other people.

Principles of Effective Learning

Children with language and learning difficulties can find the school environment overwhelming, confusing, distracting, and overstimulating. Therefore, it is important for the professional to consider factors which affect learning and demonstrate sensitivity to the child:

1. *Self-image*. The child's self-image is a critical factor. The learning environment should foster a positive self-image by providing activities that are designed for successful completion as well as intellectual growth. They should contain an appropriate amount of material and information which

can be completed within a manageable length of time. Self-concept is affected by interaction and reaction to other people as well. Students who have difficulty sending or receiving communications must be provided with ways to understand themselves and their place in the world.

2. *Organization of material and the context.* Order and consistency assist the child in interpreting information from the learning environment. Children with language and learning problems do not select salient information and integrate it with prior knowledge in an efficient manner. By creating a structured learning environment with consistent routines, children can begin to recognize important information to expand their knowledge base.

3. *Multiple exposures.* Repetition and reiteration of information are important for children with language impairments. The teacher should provide multiple exposures to important concepts. Specific ideas can be presented in a variety of contexts which promote a richer understanding and allow the child to generalize concepts.

The Thematic Approach

Many researchers (Ferguson, 1992; Locke, 1989; Westby and Costlow, 1991) suggest a **thematic approach** to language learning. Westby and Costlow (1991) explain how themes create semantic networks which help to relate and integrate a child's world knowledge. Activities are introduced which are concerned with a particular topic. Vocabulary and concepts are used which relate to the topic. Using an experience approach, students engage in a variety of activities that help to reinforce and generalize new ideas as well as to introduce linguistic and conceptual relationships. This new and broader conceptual knowledge is organized and stored by the child for future use in new situations. Because information understanding is expanded, the student develops improved reasoning and problem-solving skills.

For example, the theme may be *community helpers*. Students may read stories about police officers, letter carriers, and firefighters. They may have these community workers visit the classroom or they may take field trips to their workplaces. Children engage in art and music activities that are related to the theme. They might write and perform a puppet show based on firefighters or they might learn how to contact the police by telephone in case of emergency. Cooking and drawing activities as well as math, spelling, and creative writing projects all might relate to the theme. After a week or two, the children have integrated knowledge pertaining to the topic from varying contexts. This information provides the foundation for more effective interactions in the future. Norris (1992) uses the word *redundancy* to describe the repeated linguistic and conceptual encounters with a particular topic in varying contexts. Redundancy encourages gradual refinement of the child's linguistic knowledge associated with the theme.

Scaffolded Instruction

Scaffolding is a collaborative process between a teacher, parent, or speech-language pathologist and a child, which assists the youngster in communicating an effective message to a listener (Norris and Hoffman, 1990). Duchan (1988) describes scaffolding as a tool to develop conceptual understanding. The adult provides the child with a framework of basic information so that the child can search for the mental model of the concept. The new information that is presented can be attached to this prior information base. The child revises the earlier conceptual model to include the new knowledge. The basic outline or referent that the adult provides assists the child in locating and retrieving the related conceptual information.

This supportive procedure occurs as a child is engaged in routine activities. The intent is to provide assistance to the child to facilitate future independent execution of the task. A simple pragmatic example can be seen when a teacher wants the student to tell her when the instructions for solving a math problem are confusing. To provide guided practice in achieving this goal, the teacher may remind or ask the student during the first few instances to tell her whether the instructions are clear or not understood. Later, the student would be expected to initiate this process independently. Because communication is viewed as a means to enhance learning (Silliman and Wilkinson, 1991), knowledge of specific scaffolding techniques can provide the teacher with important intervention strategies. The teacher then can help the student experience the results of communication attempts and the uses of both oral and written communication.

Bruner (1978) compares scaffolding to constructing a building. Weight-bearing walls that are not secure need support with scaffolding. Once the weight-bearing walls have become structurally sound, the scaffolding can be removed. The child, like the wall, becomes more independently proficient in communication, and over time the assistance, or scaffolding, can be reduced or removed.

Scaffolding begins with infant/caretaker interactions. A mother engages in a conversation with the infant and is both the speaker and verbal responder. The infant is introduced to the notion of conversational turns. For example, the mother could say, *You're crying. Are you hungry? I know you are. I will give you some milk.* As the child begins to use verbal language, the caretaker models and expands the youngster's utterances (Silliman and Wilkinson, 1991). Preschoolers are assisted in attaching more complex language to their activities. A child may be looking at a book and say *doggie.* The adult might respond, *Yes, that's a big dog. The dog says bow-wow.* The goal is to expand the child's current level of communicative competence.

Norris and Hoffman (1990) discuss specific scaffolding strategies to assist communication:

1. ***Cloze procedure***—the child completes a statement introduced by the adult (e.g., *To brush our teeth, we need _____*);

2. *Gestures, pointing, and other nonlinguistic prompts;*

3. *Constituent questioning*—a question prompt is used to obtain a specific piece of information (e.g., *What do you need the toothpaste for?*); and

4. *Comprehension questions* (e.g., *What caused the boy to run away?*).

Reading comprehension can be improved as well through the use of scaffolding instruction. Idol (1987) outlines a *story mapping* strategy which assists the child in activating prior knowledge while reading. It makes the child aware of the relationship between what is being read and prior knowledge which promotes understanding of the material. The story map presents a framework for the basic elements of narrative stories such as setting, characters, the story problem, and the solution to the problem.

Scaffolding is the support used until the child can use a particular communication mode independently. The steps of the strategy should be clear to the child. The interaction attempt should include collaboration, active participation, practice, and appropriate adult models. Once the child has internalized the process, additional natural learning activities should be available. Scaffolding results in independent use of language which contains greater accuracy, complexity, and clarity.

Activity Presentation

An intervention strategy that is related to scaffolding is *activity presentation*. Children with a language disability sometimes have difficulty making associations between ideas, concepts, and events. They need assistance in connecting a particular activity with related prior knowledge. Therefore, activities must be presented in a format that will facilitate cognitive function (Hunter, 1986).

A specific introduction for each activity (i.e., a preparatory set) provides children with a framework to access related information from their knowledge store. It also presents a group of expectations, which assists in making the transition to a novel event. Children can orient their focus of attention to pertinent aspects of their environment. For example, children can be told that they are going to read a story. Perhaps the story is about an animal. The children can be reminded about the story they read the day before, which also concerned an animal. Do the animals have the same problem? This introduction helps to retrieve prior knowledge of a similar situation and provides a focus for the present activity, namely, finding the animal's problem in a story.

While engaging in the activity, the teacher provides ongoing opportunities for language learning by introducing related language or by encouraging the children to communicate their ideas. When the activity is completed, a review of the important concepts and events helps to reinforce them for each child. This reiteration can also be used to connect the activity with prior or future knowledge. The manner in which activities are presented influences the linguistic, cognitive, and social development of children. Isolated events that the child does not relate to a prior base of knowledge are easily forgotten.

Cooperative Learning

Cooperative learning involves interdependent learning in groups. Students work together to solve problems, discuss topics, complete assignments, and achieve common goals (Perry, 1990). Collaboration and cooperation are compatible with communication and language interaction, which also involve shared information by two or more people.

Group learning is consistent with the process of scaffolded instruction. The teacher guides the group with a conceptual framework that serves as the basis of discussion. Gersten and Domino (1989) found that low achieving students learn when they participate in cooperative learning settings that use heterogeneous groups in combination with scaffolded instruction. This finding supports the notion that ability grouping, which combines youngsters with similar strengths and achievements into one group, is not always necessary for efficient student learning. Slavin (1990) states that after material has been introduced by the teacher, students who work in small, heterogeneous learning groups improve significantly in a range of educational outcomes.

Group participation to solve problems involves speaking, listening, reasoning, and communicating on an interpersonal level. For the child with language difficulties, it provides a natural setting to practice these skills with youngsters who can serve as language models. Children can learn to request help from others to clarify their understanding of a particular concept or activity. The youngsters are actively involved in the instruction.

Peer tutoring is a facet of cooperative learning. The tutor might be an older student or a classmate. Peer tutoring provides an opportunity for two or more youngsters to work together to achieve a goal. It encourages communication between children who might not normally interact. Therefore, it is particularly beneficial in educational settings that endorse inclusion policies.

Strategies for the Older Child

As youngsters proceed through school, educational demands change and become more difficult. Textbooks use abstract terms and ideas more frequently. Students attend several daily classroom settings with different teachers. Educational teaching styles and use of language vary among the teachers. Some move around the room while speaking, some speak rapidly, and some use the chalkboard as they present material.

As students with language difficulties mature into adolescents, additional educational expectations can be overwhelming. They must develop more complex problem-solving skills. Note taking, which requires the simultaneous tasks of careful listening, extrapolation of essential information, and transposition of what is heard to written form, is routinely expected in the upper grades. Students must grasp subtle nuances of language, synthesize ideas, compare and contrast, and express thoughts in an organized format. These are difficult activities for the adolescent with language deficits.

Effective language intervention strategies for adolescents presume that the language abilities of each student are properly understood. In addition to the instructional principles outlined earlier in the chapter, Larson and McKinley (1987) describe three general procedures: mediation, bridging, and discussion.

1. *Mediation* is the intentional focus by an adult on an experience, object, or event to transmit its underlying meaning. The adolescent is guided with information as to why something exists or happens. For example, students receive an explanation of why they are being asked to do something. The explanation should relate to the adolescent's personal realm of experience and interest.

2. *Bridging* is designed to transfer newly learned information to novel situations. Adolescents bridge, or apply, new behaviors or information to other meaningful contexts. For example, a student may learn when to ask for clarification. The adolescent then offers further examples of the times that are appropriate to ask questions for clarification. The goal for the student is to understand how, when, and why to apply the new behavior in other relevant situations.

3. *Discussion* involves the conscious participation of adolescents in reflecting upon and talking about their thinking, speaking, listening, and writing (i.e., developing metalinguistic and metacognitive abilities). The students, during discussion, talk about the overall effectiveness of their communication.

The intervention strategies that have been outlined focus on lifetime adjustment as well as academic success. They relate the language and communication skills of children to effective classroom interventions. Strategies that endorse meaningful and integrated activities, collaboration, respect, and support provide the most favorable environment for language learning.

LANGUAGE AND READING

When teaching children the literate forms of language, emphasis is placed on learning to decode unknown words, recognizing commonly used words, and comprehending the information presented in the printed language. For children with language and learning difficulties, oral and written language should be presented in context. In some schools, language and reading specialists attend to specific aspects of language. The speech-language pathologist may emphasize phonemic awareness or idioms. The reading specialist may provide practice in discrete skills such as rhyming or sound-letter correspondence. All too frequently the classroom teacher, speech-language pathologist, reading specialist, and learning disabilities specialist work independently without coordination of teaching goals. The child is left to learn isolated and fragmented bits of language. Yet language is complex and the child must be capable of integrating prior knowledge with information available at any given moment.

Establishing the Reading Environment

For the child with a language disability who is learning to read, the classroom should be filled with opportunities to engage in literacy activities. Books and magazines should be available. The child should have ready access to paper, pencils, crayons, and computers. Real activities, such as reading a story in a book, provides opportunities to derive meaning and to learn specific components of the reading process such as characterization, metaphors, or sound/symbol correspondence. Norris and Hoffman (1993) describe this as a *whole-to-part* process for learning language.

For example, perhaps the child is having a birthday. The child decides to make invitations for a party. After selecting paper and markers, the child asks "How do you spell *party?*" The letters might be presented orally, one by one. Perhaps the child does not remember how to print a *y*. The teacher guides the child in this writing task. The child presents the handmade "invitation" to a friend. The writing process and the reinforcement of letter name/symbol correspondence are achieved in a context that has interest and meaning for the child. Learning is self-generated and not traditional discrete skill learning.

Discrete Skill Acquisition

In the discrete skill learning format, the letters of the alphabet and how to form them are taught to the child. The goal is to learn the alphabet. The child practices until the goal is achieved. Emphasis is on skill acquisition. An adult determines the activity and acceptable mastery of the task. The intent of discrete skill learning is to teach the individual skills required for a more complex task. The letters of the alphabet are taught for future use in reading and writing tasks.

Several problems can occur with discrete skill learning for the child with a language impairment. When isolated tasks are presented, such as learning to print the alphabet, the child may not understand the purpose of the exercise. The youngster becomes focused on duplicating "squiggles" and "marks" on the page, sometimes upside down, and sometimes backwards. After extended practice, which the child can find boring and tedious, mastery is obtained. The child may have viewed the project as a frustrating endeavor and even may have lost confidence due to the many practice sessions required.

Yet the intent of discrete skill learning is mastery of individual subskills for use in more complex tasks. For example, the child who has learned to print letters can now apply that skill in making a party invitation. However, after lengthy practice sessions, printing the letters of the alphabet may not be the child's favorite activity. The practical application of the skill is viewed as a chore. Thus, youngsters do not attach the isolated tasks to their realm of knowledge, do not always enjoy the drills, and do not acquire self-confidence due to the many trials before mastery.

Whole Language, Metalinguistics, and Reading

The whole language philosophy promotes conceptual understanding and development in children as they participate in meaningful and relevant activities. This provides a basic framework for reading comprehension. However, effective reading requires metalinguistic awareness as well as an adequate conceptual base of knowledge (Liberman and Shankweiler, 1985). Studies have documented a relationship between reading difficulties and children who lack awareness of the phonological and syllabic structure of spoken words (Chaney, 1990; Connell, 1987; Liberman and Liberman, 1990; Mann and Liberman, 1984). Those youngsters who cannot identify or generate rhyming words, or perceive the initial sound of a word, or segment words into syllables are not consciously aware of phonological structure. These metalinguistic skills are prerequisites to decoding in reading and the acquisition of literacy. Therefore, reading programs should combine language and conceptual understanding with conscious phonological manipulation.

Each child comes to a classroom with individual perceptual abilities and experiences which impact on conceptual understanding. Children possess unique sensory and neurological structures which perceive, store, associate, and integrate incoming information. Therefore, no one educational program affects children in the same way. Children with language-based learning disabilities exhibit a wide range of abilities. They need to understand what they are doing and why they are engaged in any activity. The whole language philosophy emphasizes tasks that have meaning for the child. It also assumes that the child is an active participant in the task. The information to be learned is important to the youngster. The goal is to develop written and oral language simultaneously in natural experiences. Whole language is also consistent with thematic teaching, which was discussed earlier. It integrates specific facets of language with a variety of contexts. Implementation of these philosophical guidelines can take many forms. The unique needs of each child will determine how the program is presented.

Professionals express concern for the ability to integrate metalinguistic awareness of phonological structure with the whole language philosophy in early reading. Norris and Hoffman (1993) reconcile this concern by viewing reading as a meaning-making process. The child learns the smaller parts of language such as phonemes by discovering how they function and refer to the larger activity.

Emergent Literacy

Literacy begins before the child comes to school. Daily exposure to print on food boxes, street signs, and books helps children acquire knowledge of the characteristics of letters and words in the environment. Storybook reading to very young children helps them to interpret meaning expressed in pictures and oral language. Later, children may attend to particular aspects of print or letters. Many youngsters want to write their own names. These prereading experiences teach children the conventions of the reading process such as left-to-right orientation of print in English and the relationship between print and pictures. The principles of incidental learning are seen in classrooms where written labels are affixed to objects in the room and signs such as *exit* are reviewed each time they are naturally encountered.

Early Reading

In early reading, print words parallel sounds of language in that both refer to abstract phonetic representation of words used by speakers of the language. Print requires a visual interpretation of the phoneme whereas oral sounds require an auditory interpretation. English spelling does not have uniform correspondence between each letter and phoneme. Any reader has to use cues from the preceding text and from related pictures to identify new words.

For example, the child encounters the word *was*. It is pronounced *wuz*. If each letter in this word has been taught to have a specific corresponding sound, the child may not be able to decipher *was* without considering its meaning in the context in which it appears. Phonetic rules cannot be applied consistently because the English spelling system is derived from words of other languages and dialects.

Metalinguistic Awareness

Norris and Hoffman (1993) suggest developing metalinguistic awareness by maintaining a focus on meaningful reading activities and then examining patterns in word structure that are important. For example, in developing phonological awareness of segments of words, children can clap out the syllables in their name. In another activity such as writing a recipe for cooking, the syllables of each ingredient can be determined. Each child can select a utensil needed for the cooking task such as a *pot* and try to think of words that rhyme. The teacher facilitates language learning and metalinguistic awareness using the principles of scaffolding and activity presentation. The child engages in specific tasks that are presented in the context of broader, meaningful activities. All too often, children are provided with reading worksheets to complete, and they have no knowledge of the purpose of the assignment or how it relates to reading proficiency. Meaningful and topic-related activities increase the likelihood that children will complete individual tasks with comprehension.

In summary, the components of language and metalinguistic awareness are developed during meaningful classroom activities (Norris, 1992; Norris and Hoffman, 1993; Wiig, 1991). Specific practice in a language subskill such as spelling is determined by a child's need to write real messages or stories. Reading and writing subskills have meaning for the child because they are functional tools for effective engagement in a literacy activity. Students engage in the process and meaning of activities; the mechanics of language become the means to accomplish the activity. All aspects of language are presented as an integrated system. Each activity may combine many aspects of language such as listening, reading, speaking, writing, observing, and reasoning. However, meaning and feedback are fundamental to the process (Cazden, 1988; Goodman, 1986; Norris, 1992; Shafer, Staab, and Smith, 1983).

Whole Language in the Classroom

The whole language philosophy is based on theories of language acquisition and use (Weaver, 1991). It also encompasses knowledge learned from cognitive psychology, psycholinguistics, sociolinguistics, and reading/writing research. Weaver (1991) emphasizes that whole language respects students' ability to make choices and to take responsibility for their own learning. It also views each learner as a human being. The goal is to help children to speak, listen, read, write, and think effectively so that they can function independently and successfully in the world.

The whole language philosophy has been implemented in the classroom in a variety of forms. However, whole language should not be viewed as a curriculum. Norris and Hoffman (1993) view whole language as a philosophy which promotes

1. surrounding the student with opportunities to manipulate language;

2. consciously integrating language with content areas of instruction;

3. providing language learning in meaningful contexts; and

4. providing genuine responses to a student's communicative attempts.

The specific strategies for achieving these philosophical objectives are determined by the teacher and school curricula. Insufficient training and supervision have created "whole language" classrooms that have only selected components of the philosophy. Sustained and interrelated activities are sometimes sacrificed for a 30-minute "whole language reading lesson," which is a particular teacher's program interpretation.

Language, Reading, and Linguistic Diversity

For a number of years, bilingual and foreign language educators have recognized the importance of natural language environments (Cummins, 1983b; Willig and Ortiz, 1990). These professionals claim that children who actively engage in meaningful activities use language to communicate related ideas and information. This develops proficiency and understanding of the language being acquired. Therefore, the concepts of the whole language philosophy that embrace these teaching principles have been implemented in educational settings which teach English as a second language or English as a foreign language (Norris and Damico, 1990).

Because linguistic concepts are related to the culture of the individual and the community, a student's culture becomes a resource for language learning. King and Goodman (1990) describe the importance in the whole language philosophy of valuing the language, interests, and experiences of students. Each child's special cultural knowledge is an integral part of the curriculum which helps to instill self-respect. King and Goodman (1990) report gains in linguistic and academic learning when students extend their individual cultures into the classroom to be used as a basis for language learning. In contrast, children with linguistic differences who make poor school adjustments may not have a supportive environment where language is learned in contexts that are meaningful to the child.

THE ROLE OF PARENTS

Parents of children with disabilities were a major force in the development and legislative enactment of PL 94-142 and PL 99-457. These federal mandates include parents in team decisions concerning the evaluation and education of their children. Yet researchers (Gartner and Lipsky, 1987) discuss reports on the implementation of the laws which indicate limited parental input in developing individualized education programs for their youngsters. Scanlon, Arick, and Phelps (1981) reported that only 50 percent of parents attend meetings designed to develop their child's individualized education program. These participants usually contribute little information.

When the Office of Special Education and Rehabilitation Services in the U.S. Department of Education issued its proposal for special education reform (Will, 1986), it recognized that many parents were dissatisfied with the available opportunities to participate in their children's education. Frequently, parents felt that their child's school discouraged their active participation in a cooperative, supportive partnership with teachers and other school personnel. Some parents feel intimidated by the professional team sitting opposite them, and at many conferences, it is the school personnel who determine decisions (Gartner and Lipsky, 1987). Some parents conclude that educational professionals distrust, denigrate, or dismiss their knowledge of their children. Some parents have unrealistic expectations for their children with disabilities. However, an educational process should not undervalue the knowledge that parents have and can contribute toward effective educational goals.

For children from 0–2 years of age, federal law (PL 99-457) mandates a family-centered intervention plan (IFSP). It recognizes support services for families of young children with disabilities. However, the effort to involve families in traditional service delivery models has resulted in a limited and passive role for parents in their child's assessment and intervention (Crais, 1991). Yet language learning is a continuous process that develops in functional, real situations at home and at school. Children learn language to achieve something, to understand the environment, to feel close to family members, and to obtain desired items. Therefore, active participation of family members in understanding the child with language problems and in developing effective intervention strategies is essential (MacDonald and Carroll, 1992).

Crais (1991) suggests inclusion of family members in child assessment by observing the youngster's behavior in natural family routines and by obtaining information from families regarding family strengths and needs. She also recommends applying family-centered intervention goals so that newly acquired communication skills are transferred from school to home environments. These principles of family involvement can be applied to students of all ages and special needs. The goal is to provide educational interventions that reflect the strengths and needs of the child and the child's community rather than to attempt to fit families of children with disabilities into educational plans.

Parents can be overwhelmed by the stress of parenting their child with disabilities. The degree of physical and emotional strain in each family when dealing with this unplanned situation is individual. Professionals should continually try to view the child's special needs from the parents' perspective. Honest appraisals of the child by parents should be respected. Professional jargon and terms should be clarified without being condescending when presenting information to families. It is helpful to include many significant family members at conferences, so that all pertinent viewpoints are presented and a more accurate appraisal of the child can be made. This also reduces information distortion caused by second-hand reports (Peters-Johnson, 1990).

Parents welcome resource material to help them understand and deal with their child. Some speech-language pathologists have provided parents with packets that contain computer generated information that specifically concerns their child (Masterson,

Swirbul, and Noble, 1990). Opportunities for families to observe their child in school routines help to provide constructive models for interaction with the child and to confirm educational reports regarding the child's school behavior. Parents also appreciate immediate advice regarding their child in specific situations. For example, a child may begin to bite other children. Rather than tell the parent to get the child to discontinue this behavior, the school can convene an immediate family-school consultation to review the circumstances during which this behavior occurs and, with the parent, develop specific strategies to reduce the behavior.

Although speech-language pathologists recognize the importance of family involvement in effective language intervention, its practice has been the exception rather than the rule (McDade and Varnedoe, 1987). Of those programs that include parent participation as part of the intervention strategy, the approach most frequently used is to provide handouts or to engage in occasional conferences. Instead, for preschool children, McDade and Varnedoe (1987) suggest viewing the family as the "client" so that the language intervention process includes the family in a "paraprofessional" role. Through the guidance of the professional, parents can become general language facilitators. They learn interactive styles and facilitative techniques through direct training. These strategies correspond with the approaches learned by educational professionals using collaborative consultation in the child's classroom.

Language is learned in functional contexts. It changes and develops in response to a child's needs. Children engage in interactions with others at school, at home, and in the community. By coordinating the goals of family and community members as well as educational personnel, the child can develop language skills most expediently.

Parent participation in educational planning and intervention is not always successful. Many parents work and have overwhelming family circumstances. Educational professionals have limited time designated for consultation and training. Including the parents in effective intervention programs requires the commitment of school administration and understanding of the time constraints of some families.

RESOLVING IMPLEMENTATION ISSUES

Many issues need to be researched and resolved for effective implementation of the programs outlined in this chapter:

1. Appropriate class size and sufficient support and related services for programs that include youngsters with disabilities in regular settings. The adult-child ratio must be realistic for all children to experience a positive outcome. The number of students should be reduced and qualified adult support increased, as needed, when classrooms include children with special needs.

2. Adequate training and funding for training of school personnel and family members to implement intervention goals.

3. Ample preparation and consultation time for teachers so that they can prepare stimulating language environments and can coordinate learning goals with other educational specialists and family members.

4. Schools built or remodeled to accommodate youngsters with disabilities.

5. Resolution of the problems of poverty, poor health services, and needed social service programs for the disproportionate number of children with specific needs in inner cities and other localities.

6. Collaboration among community systems for effective utilization of programs designed to prepare all children to become productive and independent adults.

SUMMARY

Federal laws have provided a framework for intervention strategies for children with disabilities. Yet the intent of the laws has not been interpreted as the legislation prescribed. In particular, provision for a continuum of services in the least restrictive environment and the active participation of families in team planning and implementation of goals have been compromised.

The U.S. Department of Education has suggested reform to rectify difficulties in applying selected aspects of the law. In particular, special education practice tends to remove youngsters from regular education programs and provide separate educational settings. This has stigmatized children with special needs and segregated them from their peers in regular classrooms. Furthermore, many education agencies have not promoted preventive programs including early intervention. Finally, parents tend to be excluded from program planning for their children. A cooperative partnership between educational professionals and the families of children with disabilities has been rare rather than typical.

Efforts to rectify these inadequacies must consider the limited financial resources in most school districts as well as the expanding numbers of children entering the special education system. Education reform proposes integrating but not combining the regular and special education systems. It encourages inclusion of youngsters with disabilities into the regular education setting with adequate support and related services wherever possible.

Children with language disabilities are appropriate candidates for regular education. The traditional "pull out" method of service delivery for these children has inhibited language intervention that focuses on natural settings such as the classroom. Placing language intervention in the classroom can integrate academic learning experiences with communication skills. Academic subjects become the basis for intervention goals. The teacher, the speech-language pathologist, and other educational professionals collaborate to combine their expertise to provide the most effective language environment for the entire class, including the child with language disorders.

Because language develops best in natural settings where it is used as a tool for learning and social interaction, strategies for language intervention must create natural communication environments. The whole language philosophy, which promotes meaningful, context-centered settings, integrates language with world knowledge and interactional skills. Children learn to create change in their environment and in others by manipulating language effectively. The whole language philosophy is particularly suited to children with different languages and cultures because activities can embrace their culture to communicate ideas. This positive reinforcement of culture instills self-respect.

The four following interventions relate to the whole language philosophy:

> *Thematic learning*—which integrates linguistic concepts in varied meaningful contexts

> *Scaffolding*—which provides a supportive framework to assist youngsters in communication

> *Appropriate presentation of activities*—which focuses on relevant introductions and review

> *Cooperative learning and peer tutoring*—which promote student collaboration to achieve a common goal

Current language assessment and intervention practices promote family participation. Language learning that occurs in the school environment can be reinforced in functional situations at home. Family members can also be the source of important information and feedback for the school concerning the child with a language disability.

School intervention strategies and reforms are most effective when consideration is given to the following:

1. appropriate class size;

2. teacher and parent training;

3. adequate funding for programs, staff, and physical accessibility; and

4. resolution of overwhelming social problems including poverty and inadequate health care.

SUGGESTED READINGS

Biklen, D. (1992). *Schooling without Labels: Parents, Educators, and Inclusive Education.* Philadelphia, PA: Temple University Press.

Gartner, A., and Lipsky, D. (1987). Beyond Special Education: Toward a Quality System for All Students. *Harvard Educational Review, 57*(4), 367–395.

Norris, J., and Hoffman, P. (1993). *Whole Language Intervention for School-age Children.* San Diego, CA: Singular Publishing Group.

GLOSSARY

ADAPTIVE BEHAVIOR. The skills that an individual acquires in the areas of social development and self-help (e.g., independent eating or washing). Also, the ability to adjust to new and novel situations.

ADULT-CONTROLLED COMMUNICATIONS. Communications in which the adult's utterances determine the topic of discussion. They are often characterized as short, literal, and concrete, with frequent questions, usually demanding short, factual answers. Children in classrooms where teachers are overcontrolling do not generate communications that involve speculation, argument, or extended narratives.

AFFECT. Emotions, feelings, or attitudes revealed through facial expressions.

AGE AT ONSET OF HEARING IMPAIRMENT. The age at which the condition causing the hearing impairment occurred.

AGE OF DIAGNOSIS OF HEARING IMPAIRMENT. The age at which the diagnosis of hearing impairment is made.

AKINESIA. A disorder resulting in the loss of movement or loss of control in the initiation, switching, or cessation of movement.

AMERICAN SIGN LANGUAGE (ASL). A manual language that has evolved naturally through use by persons who are deaf. A consistent rule-regulated language, ASL is used for communication by the Deaf community and for transmission of Deaf culture.

AMERICANS WITH DISABILITIES ACT (ADA). Federal legislation which ensures the rights of individuals with disabilities and mandates access to community facilities, programs, services, and activities.

AMPLIFICATION SYSTEMS. Electronic devices that make speech sounds louder and clearer for individuals with hearing impairment. These devices can be personal hearing aids worn by an individual, or an educational system designed to accommodate the different amplification needs of groups of children within a class. They can also be used to amplify sounds of speech or music in a large auditorium or concert hall.

ANOXIA. A loss or deprivation of oxygen, which is a potential cause of brain damage.

APHASIA. A language disorder due to brain damage or disease which affects the individual's capacity to formulate, express, and understand language.

APRAXIA. A neurological condition that prevents the individual from performing voluntary motor routines or to implement motor-planning activities in sequence even when the muscles needed to perform the movement are not weak or paralyzed.

ASSOCIATION STRATEGIES. A system used to group words or thoughts according to relationships.

AT RISK. A description of infants and children who have been exposed to environmental factors which often create learning, behavioral, and social problems. These factors which place children at risk include poverty, poor nutrition and health care, exposure in utero to harmful chemical substances, inadequate experience, and child abuse and neglect.

ATTENTION. The effort or the energy required to concentrate mentally by careful observation and listening.

ATTENTION DEFICIT/HYPERACTIVITY DISORDER (ADHD). A neurological disorder that is characterized by varying degrees of hyperactivity, distractibility, *or* impulsivity.

ATTENTION DEFICIT/HYPERACTIVITY DISORDER, COMBINED TYPE. A neurological disorder that is characterized by hyperactivity, distractibility, *and* impulsivity.

ATTENTION DEFICIT/HYPERACTIVITY DISORDER NOT OTHERWISE SPECIFIED. A disorder with the predominant symptoms of attention deficit or hyperactivity-impulsivity that does not meet the criteria for Attention Deficit/Hyperactivity Disorder delineated by the American Psychiatric Association in the *DSM-IV Draft Criteria (3/1/93).*

ATTENTION DEFICIT/HYPERACTIVITY DISORDER WITH HYPERACTIVITY, PREDOMINANTLY HYPERACTIVE-IMPULSIVE TYPE. A neurological disorder that is characterized by inability to control motor activity level; the individual cannot remain still. In addition, the individual often interrupts and intrudes on others, and is unable to reflect before acting.

ATTENTION DEFICIT/HYPERACTIVITY DISORDER WITHOUT HYPERACTIVITY, PREDOMINANTLY INATTENTIVE TYPE. A neurological disorder that is characterized by inability to sustain attention to a task. The individual is easily distracted by irrelevant stimuli. Hyperactivity is not a behavioral characteristic.

AUDITORY ACUITY. The extent to which an individual can hear auditory stimuli and discriminate individual sounds of speech without the need of amplification.

AUDITORY DISCRIMINATION. The ability to perceive differences and similarities between sounds, including phonemes. Ability to isolate a phoneme within a word in initial, medial, and final position. Ability to perceive differences in tones and inflections of the voice or sounds from the environment.

AUDITORY FIGURE-GROUND DISCRIMINATION. The ability to isolate speech sounds or a particular environmental sound from background noise.

AUDITORY INTEGRATION TRAINING (AIT). A method of retraining the ear to receive and process sound more efficiently.

AUDITORY PERCEPTION. As distinct from auditory acuity, auditory perception is the process of becoming aware of auditory stimulus and then the organizing and interpreting of all the components, including environmental sounds and speech sounds. The process is carried out in the cortex of the brain, not the ear.

AUDITORY PROCESSING. The complex organization by the brain of the details of an auditory stimulus to determine meaning, including speech sounds. The details are perceived, discriminated, combined, categorized, and related to recognizable or similar concepts that are stored in memory. The result is understanding of the auditory stimulus.

AUDITORY SEQUENCING. The ability to perceive the order or arrangement of the individual sounds within a spoken word and of the individual words within a phrase or sentence. The term also refers to the ability to remember the order of items presented orally in a sequential list.

AUDITORY SYNTHESIS. The ability to combine or blend phonemes, using silent speech, until a word is recognized.

AUGMENTATIVE COMMUNICATION SYSTEMS. Alternative systems for the communication of ideas, feelings, and knowledge when verbal language is not an efficient system. These systems can use gestures, electronic devices, or printed letters and pictures.

AURAL HABILITATION. The training of children with congenital hearing impairment, and their families, in the selection and use of hearing aids, effective use of residual hearing, auditory discrimination of speech and environmental sounds, and communication skills. Family counseling is included in the aural habilitation process with regard to options available for different communication modes (e.g., Oral Method, Manual Coded English, American Sign Language) and special education programs. *See also* AURAL REHABILITATION.

AURAL REHABILITATION. The training of children, adolescents, and adults who have lost their hearing after having acquired language. Training consists of speech-reading instruction, effective use of residual hearing, counseling with regard to selection, care, and use of hearing aids and options available for educational programs and modes of communication. *See also* AURAL HABILITATION.

AUTISM. A pervasive developmental disorder that usually appears before the age of three and affects social interaction, verbal and nonverbal communication, and movement. Children with autism often avoid other people, are affected by sensory stimulation, and whirl or shake parts of their bodies or objects.

BABBLING. The initial sound play engaged in by an infant. There is no attempt to "talk" to anyone, and there does not appear to be any relationship between the baby's vocalizing and a particular object or event.

BASIC COGNITIVE SKILLS. The mental processes which contribute to higher-level intellectual functioning (e.g., perception, attention, memory).

BICULTURAL. The equal sharing of two cultures by an individual.

BILINGUAL. The ability to speak two languages with equal skill.

BLACK ENGLISH. A language which is a variation of Standard American English that is influenced by West African and European languages and is spoken by some black people. It is also known as Ebonics or Black English Vernacular. Black English is considered to be a legitimate language.

BLIND. A condition in which individuals have only light perception or no vision.

BLISSYMBOLS. A type of augmentative communication system that uses a specific symbol system for communication. It is an international picture language presented on a grid board.

BODY IMAGE. The perception of various body parts and body boundaries. The perception of "personal space" (e.g., the position and orientation of the body in space; the feet are rooted in the ground; there is a left and right side).

BRADYKINESIA. A disorder resulting in general slowness of movement, resembling the movement of a slow motion film.

CAPACITY. The extent to which an individual has the ability to receive, store, and/or process information.

CENTRAL AUDITORY PROCESSING DISORDER. A condition which includes deficits in the perception, analysis, organization, storage, retrieval, or use of auditory information not attributable to impaired structure or functioning of the ears. These deficits are indicative of minimal damage to the cortex of the brain or the neural pathways to the brain.

CENTRAL NERVOUS SYSTEM. The neurological system related to the functioning of the brain, brain stem, and spinal cord.

CEREBRAL PALSY. A disorder occurring in the prenatal or perinatal period, characterized by brain damage that results in paralysis and problems of physical growth, movement, communication, and sensory perception.

CHILD-CENTERED LEARNING. A learning environment that is not teacher-directed but rather takes the interests of the child as the learning focus. The activities have special significance for the child and can be used as the basis for learning needed concepts and ideas.

CHILDHOOD PSYCHOSIS. A severe psychiatric condition that is characterized by personality abnormalities, difficulties relating to people, and/or problems in perceiving reality correctly.

CLOZE TASK. An activity that requires the individual to complete a phrase or sentence that has been generated by the examiner by inserting an appropriate missing word.

CLUSTERING STRATEGIES. A system used to organize and group items in order to hold the information in short-term memory.

CODE SWITCHING. The act of switching from one language to another during a conversation when an individual has some ability to speak more than one language.

COGNITION. Mental faculties that allow the individual to acquire and process knowledge including attending, perceiving, remembering, associating, recalling, and storing information.

COGNITIVE BEHAVIOR MODIFICATION. Same as METACOGNITIVE TRAINING.

COGNITIVE DISABILITIES. A current term for mental retardation, a disorder that is characterized by at least three components: significantly subaverage general intellectual functioning, with an IQ of 70 or below; depressed adaptive skills; and the existence of the condition during the developmental period.

COLLABORATIVE CONSULTATION. A teaching model in which professionals and/or parents cooperate and work together to share their expertise in an effort to provide an appropriate intervention/learning environment for children.

COMMUNICATION. The purpose and the function of language. The means by which humans can exchange information, control or influence others, and express their attitudes and feeling to others.

COMMUNICATION BOARD. A type of augmentative communication system that consists of letters, words, pictures, symbols, or photographs on a flat surface which provides the individual with a means of communicating.

COMMUNICATION DIFFERENCE/DIALECT. A variation of the symbol system used by a community of individuals that reflects and is determined by shared social and cultural variations of the symbol system. It should not be considered a disorder of speech or language.

COMMUNICATION DISORDER. An impairment in one or more of the processes of hearing, speech, or language that results in the inability to comprehend or express thoughts or concepts in oral, manual, or written form.

COMMUNICATIVE COMPETENCE. The wide scope of grammatical, cognitive, social, and cultural knowledge that underlies adequate language ability.

COMMUNICATIVE INTENT. The ability to express a range of wants and needs without necessarily using language as a means of communication. Gaze, gesture, and posture are early means of expression for very young children.

COMPLEX SENTENCE. A sentence that contains an independent clause and at least one dependent clause.

COMPOUND SENTENCE. A sentence that contains at least two independent clauses.

COMPREHENSION MONITORING. The three-step process of: 1. recognizing that a portion of the speaker's oral message has not been understood; 2. formulating a question or request for clarification; and 3. expressing the need for further information if the rephrased, confusing statement has not been sufficiently clarified.

CONCEPT. A thought, idea, or understanding that an individual derives from interaction with the people, objects, and events encountered in the environment. Concepts can change and become more complex as the individual engages in additional experiences. A concept is a perceived category of related information regarding specific objects and events.

CONDUCTIVE HEARING IMPAIRMENT. Hearing loss caused by damage to or abnormality of internal structures of the outer ear, middle ear, or ear drum (tympanic membrane). Conductive hearing loss can also be caused by fluid accumulations in the middle ear space. The nerves of the inner ear are *not* involved.

CONGENITAL DISORDER. A disorder that is present at the time of birth.

CONSTITUENT QUESTIONING. A specific strategy to assist communication in which a question prompt is used to obtain a specific piece of information.

CONTEXTUALIZED LANGUAGE. The language that concerns a shared situation between the conversational partners occurring in the here and now. It relates to the events, objects, and people in the actual environment.

CONVERSATION. An interchange between two or more people where the participants communicate ideas and emotions. A conversation requires a speaker and a listener. To engage in an effective conversation, the speaker needs to know the extent of the listener's world knowledge and the listener should be able to request clarification when the speaker is not completely understood.

CONVERSATIONAL BABBLING. Same as JARGON.

COOPERATIVE LEARNING. A learning model in which students work together to solve problems, complete assignments, discuss topics, and achieve common goals.

CUED SPEECH. A manual technique employed to help persons who are deaf discriminate speech sounds that have the same appearance on the face when spoken.

CUING ABILITY. The ability to communicate attitudes by physical indications such as eye gaze, smiles, and body positioning.

CULTURAL PLURALISM. The belief that each culture is distinct and should retain its group identity in an atmosphere of mutual respect and cooperation among all communities of people. For students of other cultures in the American schools, this ideology requires that American culture and language be added to the student's birth heritage rather than eradicating the ethnic origins.

CULTURE. The way a specific community or population of people work, behave, think, and believe at a certain time. Language affects and is affected by the experiences of a group of people and is an important aspect of culture.

DEAF. Capitalized when it refers to a community of individuals sharing a language, which is American Sign Language (ASL), and a culture. The term *deaf,* beginning with a lower case letter, refers to an audiological condition of an individual whose hearing impairment is so great, even with amplification, that vision becomes the main channel of communication.

DECIBEL (dB). The unit for measuring the relative loudness of sounds.

DECODE. The process of extracting sufficient information from a printed word to be able to recognize that it is a distinct, meaningful word.

DECONTEXTUALIZED LANGUAGE. A conversational topic that is not related to the immediate situation. It concerns events, people, or objects that are from the past or the future or are imaginary. It requires more abstract linguistic ability.

DEFERRED IMITATION. The ability to store images of people's actions and speech sounds in memory and to imitate them in a unique manner after a considerable time interval.

DEMONSTRATIVE PRONOUNS. The words *this, these, that, those.*

DESCRIPTIVE ASSESSMENT. An assessment approach to determine a child's strengths and weaknesses rather than to explore etiological factors. In a descriptive language assessment, specific linguistic characteristics are described.

DEVELOPMENTAL PERIOD. From birth to 18 years of age.

DIALECT. A variation within a specific language that is shared by a community of people.

DISTRACTIBILITY. The tendency to respond to all stimuli indiscriminately. Lack of control or ability to attend selectively to stimuli that are relevant to the task at hand.

DRUG ABUSE. Drug use which deviates from accepted medical and social practices in a given community.

DUE PROCESS. The legal process which guarantees educational rights. It is used to secure appropriate educational programs for students who have disabilities and special educational needs.

DYADIC COMMUNICATION. Communication that occurs between two people.

DYSARTHRIA. A group of motor-based speech disorders that result from damage, weakness, or lack of coordination in the central and/or peripheral nervous systems.

DYSCALCULIA. Severe deficits in mathematical concepts and the ability to acquire and perform arithmetic computational skills.

DYSFLUENCY. An interruption in the smooth, rhythmic flow of speech which is often characterized by word and sound repetitions, pauses, filler words, and other struggling behaviors as part of the speaking attempt. It may be accompanied by excessive tension and struggle behavior. Stuttering is one form of dysfluency.

DYSLEXIA. A language-based disorder manifested in severe difficulties learning to read and spell despite continuous and specifically designed instruction. The disorder is considered to be congenital and persists through adulthood. Dyslexia is also associated with brain dysfunction and neurological anomalies.

DYSMORPHISM. Impaired or abnormal structures such as those of the facial area as seen in individuals with fetal alcohol syndrome.

ECHOLALIA. Meaningless parroting or repetition of material. Immediate echolalia occurs when the individual repeats exactly what has just been heard. Delayed echolalia refers to the storage of words with repetition at a later time.

EDUCATION FOR ALL HANDICAPPED CHILDREN ACT (PL 94-142). *See* **INDIVIDUALS WITH DISABILITIES EDUCATION ACT.**

ELECTROENCEPHALOGRAM (EEG). A procedure that records the electrical activity in the brain.

ELICITED IMITATION. A task of language expression where the individual is expected to repeat a word, phrase, or sentence in the exact manner that was presented by the examiner.

EMOTIONAL DYSKINESIA. A disorder resulting in difficulty with the ability to start, execute, switch, or stop moods.

EMPATHY. The ability to put oneself in another's shoes and understand the emotions felt by another in a particular situation.

ENCODE. The translation of thought into a coded system so that it can be expressed, either by an oral or signed form of language or by a written form of language.

ENVIRONMENTAL TOBACCO SMOKE (ETS) Also known as secondhand smoke, this condition is the existence in the environment of smoke that has been exhaled by a smoker. Exposure to this smoke is known to cause respiratory complications, asthma, and middle ear infections in young children, especially during the first year of life.

EPIGLOTTIS. An elastic cartilage that is located at the root of the tongue. It serves to cover the space between the vocal cords during the act of swallowing so that food does not enter the windpipe and cause choking.

EPILEPSY. A seizure disorder that is caused by excessive electrical discharges in the brain which can result in convulsions in the body.

ETHNOGRAPHY. The investigation and study used to understand the culture of a group of people. Language and communication are aspects of the culture that are analyzed in an ethnographic study.

ETIOLOGY. The cause, origin, or reason for a disease or disability.

EXECUTIVE CONTROL. The use of inner language to plan actions prior to a problem-solving task, to evaluate effectiveness of strategies for problem solving, and to evaluate progress and outcome of strategies used for problem solving.

EXPANSION. A language facilitation technique in which a child's utterance is repeated in a longer and slightly more complex manner to expose the child to more advanced language forms.

EXPRESSIVE LANGUAGE. The symbolic language system used to convey one's thoughts, attitudes, emotions, and needs. Expressive language can be conveyed by speaking, signing, writing, and also by body positioning, gesture, tone of voice, facial expression, and forms of art.

EYE-HAND COORDINATION. The integrity and integration of motor, visual, and visual-spatial perceptual systems, which enable an individual to grasp and manipulate an object, write with a pencil, type on a keyboard, and throw and catch a ball.

FACILITATED COMMUNICATION. An alternate means of communication in which an individual gives emotional support and physical support, usually on the wrist, arm, or shoulder, to enable an individual to point to pictures, letters of the alphabet, or keys on an electronic keyboard. This form of communication is mainly used for individuals who have limited verbal language and who do not appear to have enough motor control to point independently.

FAMILY SYSTEM. The term used to describe the family of a child who is deaf. The family is considered hearing and deaf (i.e., the deafness does not belong to the child alone, but to the whole family).

FETAL ALCOHOL EFFECTS (FAE). A congenital condition characterized by some but not all of the symptoms of fetal alcohol syndrome but which is also caused by maternal ingestion of alcohol during pregnancy. *See also* FETAL ALCOHOL SYNDROME.

FETAL ALCOHOL SYNDROME (FAS). A congenital condition characterized by unusual facial formation, low infant birthweight, prematurity, growth retardation, and delayed intellectual and language development which is caused by maternal ingestion of alcohol during pregnancy.

FIGURATIVE LANGUAGE. Language that has moved beyond its concrete sense to express an imaginative or creative sense of the word. Idioms, metaphors, and proverbs are examples of figurative language.

FINE MOTOR SKILLS. The coordinated movements of the muscles, tendons, joints of the hands, fingers, and arms (e.g., writing, sewing, and sculpting are fine motor skills).

FREQUENCIES. The characteristics of sounds that are perceived as changes in pitch (e.g., high and low pitches).

FREQUENCY-MODULATED (FM) AUDITORY TRAINER. The FM auditory training system is a miniature FM radio station which broadcasts the educator's voice to each student wearing an FM hearing aid. It serves to eliminate noise and reverberation in an educational environment.

GENERALIZATION. The ability to transfer information, ideas, and words to novel situations and use them appropriately. Newly learned communication behaviors are produced in situations other than those experienced during the teaching period.

GENETIC. Relating to inherited characteristics which are transferred through the genes.

GESTALT PROCESSING. The ability to receive, integrate, and remember language and experiences as whole units rather than segmenting them into their component parts.

GESTURAL NAMING. Actions that mime an action, such as when a child drinks from an empty cup or eats from an empty spoon with a gleeful expression showing that this is a make-believe game.

GROSS MOTOR SKILLS. Skills involving the whole body and the large muscles. They include postural skills, movement, and balance.

GUSTATORY. Relating to the sense of taste.

HAPTIC PERCEPTION. The combination of tactile and kinesthetic awareness. *See also* KINESTHETIC AWARENESS and TACTILE SENSATION.

HEARING IMPAIRMENT. A generic term that includes all types and degrees of hearing loss, with mild hearing loss being the lowest degree and severe-to-profound hearing impairment being the greatest degree of hearing impairment.

HEMIPLEGIA. A motor impairment that affects either the left or right half of the body.

HIGHER-LEVEL COGNITIVE SKILLS. Ability to interpret, analyze, compare and contrast, categorize, summarize, problem solve, reason logically, make judgments, reflect on various considerations, organize, prioritize, conclude, infer, anticipate, hypothesize, and generalize.

HYDROCEPHALY. A condition in which cerebral spinal fluid pressure builds up abnormally in the brain, which can cause brain damage and/or an enlargement of the head.

HYPERACTIVITY. The inability to control gross motor activity. The individual's physical activity is haphazard, poorly organized, and not goal-directed. The youngster with hyperactivity is characterized by excessive movement, fidgeting, and running. The child is described as "motor driven." The condition is also referred to as *hyperkinesis.*

HYPERLEXIA. The unusually highly developed ability to sound out and recognize words. The corresponding ability to comprehend the words that are read is not always present.

IDIOM. A word or group of words which has special usage in a given language but which does not reflect the literal meaning or interpretation of the words. If taken literally they are meaningless (e.g., *hold your tongue*).

IF . . . THEN LINGUISTIC CONCEPTS. The contingency of an event occurring in the future based upon an action or behavior. For example, *If you finish your homework, you can watch television,* or *If Cinderella does not return by midnight, the coach will turn back into a pumpkin.*

IMAGERY. The ability to retrieve from the mind's eye, the contours, configurations, movements, colors, qualities, particular smells and sounds, and also feelings and emotions associated with specific objects, situations, and events. *See also* VISUALIZATION.

IMMERSION PROGRAM. A type of teaching strategy for second language acquisition where the individual is only taught using the second or new language.

IMPULSIVITY. The inability to reflect before acting.

INCIDENCE. The extent or frequency of occurrence of a particular disorder.

INCLUSION. A philosophy that promotes access for children with disabilities to activities, situations, and environments that are designed for individuals without disabilities by providing the support and accommodations necessary so that the child with disabilities will derive as much benefit from the experience as children without disabilities.

INCLUSION MOVEMENT. An educational and social effort to bring students with disabilities into regular classes and environments.

INDIRECT REQUEST. A request made using subtle language rather than asking directly. For example, an individual may comment that the room feels cold instead of requesting that the window be closed.

INDIVIDUALIZED EDUCATION PROGRAM (IEP). The document generated as part of the special education process which describes the program and services that a student should receive. The IEP is agreed upon by a team of professionals, with the consent of the legal guardian of the student, and contains specific educational goals and objectives.

INDIVIDUALS WITH DISABILITIES EDUCATION ACT (IDEA). Federal legislation, formerly known as the Education for All Handicapped Children Act (PL 94-142), which mandates a free and appropriate education to all eligible children with disabilities.

INDUCTION LOOP SYSTEM. A sound system that is designed to accommodate the different amplification needs of groups of children with hearing impairment within a class. It is usually installed in a small room. The educator speaks into a microphone which is connected by means of a special receiver to the student's personal hearing aids. The speaker is clearly heard without distracting background noise. There is also complete mobility by the educator and student throughout the room.

INFORMATION BASE. *See* KNOWLEDGE BASE.

INFORMATION PROCESSING. The complex organization and storage by the brain of myriad sensory stimuli. The process itself consists of identification, discrimination, and categorization of unrelated perceptions, concepts, and experiences to ensure ready accessibility and later retrieval.

INNATE. Present at birth.

INNER LANGUAGE. Speech or signs which have been internalized into thought. The language used for thinking, planning, problem solving, and self-monitoring. It is also referred to as *self-talk*.

INTELLIGENCE QUOTIENT (IQ). A statistical measure to describe how much an individual's intellectual ability deviates from the average performance of others of approximately the same chronological age.

INTENSITY. Sound which is perceived in terms of degrees of loudness.

INTERSENSORY INTEGRATION. The smooth coordination of vision, audition, motor-planning, kinesthetic, and proprioceptive abilities.

INTRUSIVE. The child does not read "privacy markers" (e.g., *Back away, You are in my private space, Leave me alone*).

IN UTERO. In the uterus.

JARGON. Also referred to as *conversational babbling* because the vocalizations sound as though the baby is actually having a conversation. They are accompanied by eye contact, gesture, facial expression, stress, and variations in pitch. However, the words are unintelligible.

KINESICS. An aspect of nonverbal communication that involves body movement (e.g., manner of walking or standing, ways the shoulders and head are held, tension of the body, gesturing, and movement of the eyes that convey meaning).

KINESTHETIC AWARENESS. The awareness of muscular tension, joint movement, and slight pressure by the muscles and tendons of the fingers and arms when exploring an object.

KNOWLEDGE BASE. The information gained from meaningful experiences that is stored in long-term memory.

LANGUAGE. A rule-regulated, code of symbols recognized by a particular community to communicate ideas, feelings, and information.

LANGUAGE DELAYED. The description of children who do not acquire language when expected and according to normal language acquisition milestones.

LANGUAGE DISORDER. A condition characterized by impaired comprehension and/or use of spoken, written and/or other symbol systems. The disorder may involve 1. the form of language (phonology, morphology, syntax), 2. the content of language (semantics), and/or 3. the function of language in communication (pragmatics).

LANGUAGE SAMPLE. A type of language measure, often informal, where language behavior under normal conditions is recorded and analyzed. It is a means of examining a person's conversational and narrative forms of language.

LARYNX. A tubelike structure in the neck containing the vocal cords which vibrate in speech production.

LEARNED HELPLESSNESS. The perception by many students with learning disabilities that they have no control over their learning and educational progress. They are convinced that their successes are not due to their ability, but to luck, to their teacher's assistance, or to some other extraneous source.

LEARNING DISABILITIES. A heterogeneous group of disorders that are intrinsic to the individual and presumed to be due to central nervous system dysfunction. These disorders are manifested in significant difficulties in the acquisition and use of listening, speaking, reading, writing, reasoning, or mathematical abilities.

LEAST RESTRICTIVE ENVIRONMENT (LRE). The appropriate educational setting that affords the student the opportunity to learn in an environment that is as close to regular education as possible and which affords the student as much interaction as possible with peers who are nondisabled.

LEXICON. Each person's individual dictionary of words and concepts. An individual's lexicon changes and grows with more experience.

LIMITED ENGLISH PROFICIENT (LEP). Limited ability to speak and use the English language by individuals whose primary language is not English.

LINGUISTIC CONCEPTS. Concepts that are understood, processed, and expressed in words or phrases of a language.

LINGUISTIC MINORITY. Those people who speak languages other than the dominant language of a culture.

LINGUISTICS. The study of the nature and structure of language and the rules that affect language structure, meaning, and use.

LITERACY. The ability to think, manipulate knowledge, and understand how language is used so that the individual can organize knowledge and to communicate effectively. It is more than the ability to read and to write.

LITERAL MEANING. An interpretation of an idea, word, or concept that has the explicit or concrete meaning and does not include any figurative or idiomatic use of the language.

LONG-TERM MEMORY. The permanent storage of information until the individual can take action to use the information in some way.

LOW VISION. A condition in which a child is still severely visually impaired even with correction, but who has significant functional vision.

MAGNETIC RESONANCE IMAGING (MRI). A nuclear imaging technique which pictures brain activity. It is used to examine brain activity to determine irregular brain function.

MALADAPTIVE BEHAVIORS. Destructive, disruptive, or violent behaviors and/or self-injurious behaviors.

MANUAL CODED ENGLISH. A manual system that has taken base signs of American Sign Language and superimposed them on English vocabulary and English sentence structure.

MATERNAL EXPRESSIVE LANGUAGE. Maternal utterances to young children that refer to persons rather than objects and that direct or regulate the child's behavior.

MATERNAL REFERENTIAL LANGUAGE. Particular characteristics of maternal utterances to young children that refer to and describe objects and people usually in view and that request and reinforce names for things.

MEAN LENGTH OF UTTERANCE (MLU). When tabulating the length of utterances in children, the morphemes are counted in each utterance. The total number of morphemes is divided by the number of utterances generated.

MEANS-ENDS BEHAVIOR. The ability to think about and anticipate results of one's actions upon objects. The attempt to solve problems encountered, such as when an infant cannot reach something, another object might be used as a tool to rake in a toy that has rolled beyond reach.

MENTAL AGE. An expression of the developmental level of an individual that is characteristic of a particular chronological age, usually a younger child.

MENTAL REPRESENTATION. The ability to picture or recreate in the mind the objects, feelings, and experiences that are no longer present.

MENTAL RETARDATION. *See* COGNITIVE DISABILITIES.

METACOGNITIVE ABILITY. The ability to deliberately think about the process of obtaining and integrating knowledge and how to solve problems.

METACOGNITIVE TRAINING. Explicit guidance in self-monitoring skills. The use of inner language to solve problems and perform a complex task. Same as COGNITIVE BEHAVIOR MODIFICATION.

METALINGUISTIC ABILITY. The ability to deliberately think about and control language, words, and sounds.

METAPHOR. A form of expression that compares the actual subject with an image of something very different (e.g., *hard as nails, soft as silk*).

METAPRAGMATIC ABILITY. The ability to deliberately reflect on the uses of language in specific contexts.

MICROCEPHALY. An abnormally small head that is also associated with impaired intellectual development.

MILD HEARING LOSS. A condition in which the person requires intensities of 25–40 decibels for most sounds to be barely detected and higher decibel levels to understand and discriminate speech.

MILD-TO-MODERATE HEARING IMPAIRMENT. A condition in which the person requires at least 40–55 decibels of intensity to detect a sound unaided.

MODALITY. Refers to the primary senses (i.e., vision, audition, touch, smell, taste).

MODELING. A language facilitation technique in which a child is provided with an example of an utterance that contains a language skill or form to be acquired by the child.

MODERATE-TO-SEVERE HEARING IMPAIRMENT. A condition in which a person requires at least 55–70 decibels of intensity for a sound to be barely detected unaided.

MONOLINGUAL. The ability to speak one language.

MORPHEME. The smallest unit of meaning in a language. One word can have more than one morpheme as in the word *boys* which has two meaning segments: young male and more than one.

MORPHOLOGICAL RULES. The rules for forming words with morphemes.

MORPHOLOGY. The study of word formation and its effect on meaning. By interchanging the morphemes within words, the speaker can form an infinite variety of meanings (e.g., rearrangement).

MOTHERESE. *See* PARENTESE; SIGNED MOTHERESE.

MOTILITY. Motor behavior and bodily motion.

MOVEMENT DISTURBANCE. The inability to organize, control, and move one's body at will.

MULTILINGUAL. The ability to speak more than two languages with equal skill.

NARRATIVE. A story or description of a real or imagined event. The ability to create a narrative is the bridge to literate thought.

NEGLECT. Also known as child neglect, it refers to the lack of physical caregiving and supervision by a child's legal guardian as well as a lack of mental stimulation.

NEONATE. Newborn infant.

NEUROLOGY. The medical study of the nervous system and its disorders.

NON-ENGLISH PROFICIENT (NEP). Virtually no ability to speak or use the English language by individuals whose primary language is not English.

NONVERBAL COMMUNICATION. Meaning transmitted by tone of voice, inflection, intensity of voice, and attitudes and emotions that are embedded within the voice itself. In addition, these attitudes, emotions, and also intentions can be transmitted by facial expression, gesture, body language, and deliberate use of posturing.

NONVERBAL INFORMATION PROCESSING DISORDER. A neurological disorder, characterized as a "right hemispheric" disorder, that is manifested by the inability to interpret paralinguistic information, such as tone of voice, inflection, intensity of voice, facial expression, body language, and the nuances of a communicative interaction. *See also* NONVERBAL PERCEPTUAL-ORGANIZATIONAL-OUTPUT DISABILITY (NPOOD).

NONVERBAL LANGUAGE. Additional information regarding meaning of a speaker's message gleaned from body and gestural language, facial expressions, and the voice (not the words) of the speaker.

NORM. The typical performance of a select group of individuals on some test or measure.

NONVERBAL PERCEPTUAL-ORGANIZATIONAL-OUTPUT DISABILITY (NPOOD). A subgroup of individuals with nonverbal information processing disorder. Refers to individuals who have well-developed, although superficial, expressive language, decoding and spelling skills. However, they exhibit serious dyscalculia and severe social interactional problems.

OBJECT CONSTANCY. The ability to perceive objects accurately even though they become distorted as they move in space or the observer moves while viewing them. *See also* SHAPE CONSTANCY.

OBJECT PERMANENCE. The ability to understand that things and places continue to exist even when they can no longer be seen.

OLFACTORY. Relating to the sense of smell.

ORAL COMMUNICATION METHOD. The use of speech, residual hearing, and speech reading as the primary means of communicating with individuals who are hearing impaired.

ORAL CONFIGURATIONS. The moving, changing shapes of the mouth, jaw, and lips when producing various speech sounds. This term usually applies to the speech-reading process.

OTITIS MEDIA WITH EFFUSION. The presence of fluid in the middle ear, sometimes following respiratory illness or symptoms of severe allergies. Fluid accumulations in the middle ear space can cause chronic middle ear disease unless treated. If bouts of otitis media with effusion occur frequently during the first three years of life, language development can be deleteriously affected.

OVEREXTENSION. The use of a label that has extracted not just one but many properties or attributes of an object and applied them to other objects that share any one of these attributes. Young children who are using one- and possibly two-word utterances will often call all men *Daddy* or a plane a *bird.*

PARALINGUISTIC CUES. Additional clues to the meaning of an oral message and the emotions contained in the message as conveyed by the tone of voice, rate of speech, volume emphasis, and pitch.

PARALLEL TALK. A language facilitation technique in which a person talks to a young child about the activities and events of the moment as the child engages in them.

PARAPLEGIA. A motor impairment that affects both legs of an individual.

PARENTESE. A current term for motherese. Adult's speech to a young infant that is characterized by exaggerated inflection, rhythm, and prosody of voice, slow and precise articulation, and simple sentence structure.

PEER TUTORING. A type of cooperative learning in which one student assists another. It provides an opportunity for two students to work together to achieve a goal.

PERCEPTION. A cognitive ability to recognize, select, interpret, and organize incoming sensory information.

PERCEPTION OF BODY SPACE. Awareness of the body in relation to other objects in space and spatial orientation.

PERCEPTION OF LOCATION IN SPACE. The perception of changes in location of an object or objects as they move from one position in space to another.

PERINATAL. Pertaining to the time of birth.

PERSEVERATION. The continued uncontrolled and repetitive execution of an action, word, or phrase beyond the period of appropriateness.

PERSONAL PRONOUN. A syntactic unit that can take the place of a noun (i.e., [subject] *I, you, he, she, it, we, they;* [object] *me, you, him, her, it, us, them*).

PERVASIVE DEVELOPMENTAL DISORDER (PDD). A disorder that usually is evident before the age of three which affects many basic areas of development simultaneously to a severe degree. Autism is recognized as the most severe form of PDD.

PHONEME. The smallest unit of sound in speech that distinguishes one utterance from another in a particular language.

PHONEME AWARENESS. Sensitivity to speech sounds of language.

PHONETIC APPROACH. The technique of decoding written words by learning the individual phonemes that are assigned to corresponding graphic symbols or letters. In the phonetic approach, the printed words are broken down into their component parts and blended together until they can be recognized as known, meaningful words.

PHONETICS. The branch of linguistics that studies the sounds of speech of a particular language and their production. Distinct symbols are used to designate sound nuances.

PHONETIC SHORT-TERM MEMORY. The ability to temporarily hold letter strings, word strings, and sentences in a phonetic representation or silent speech until they can be processed.

PHONOLOGY. The study and description of the sounds of language.

PHONOLOGICAL RULES. The rules that govern the arrangements and combinations of speech sounds (phonemes) in words.

PHONOLOGICAL MEMORY. The ability to remember spoken and written words and meaningful sentences.

PHONOLOGICAL PROCESSING. The ability to discriminate individual sounds and sound units and remember the sequences of these sound units which, when combined, comprise a word.

PIDGIN SIGN ENGLISH. A mixture of English and sign language which is used by hearing individuals who do not know enough sign language to converse fluently.

PLACE OF ARTICULATION. The positions of the lips, tongue, roof of the mouth, and throat relative to one another for producing a particular sound.

PLASTICITY. The theory that the brain has the capacity to make new neural connections and change in various ways to compensate for loss of function due to damage.

POINTS OF ARTICULATION. The movement which affects the position of the jaw, lips, tongue, soft palate, and teeth when producing various sounds.

POSTLINGUALLY DEAF. Deafened after language acquisition.

PRAGMATIC ABILITY. The ability to use language for a purpose while interacting with other human beings in different contexts.

PRAGMATICS. The appropriate use of language in specific contexts or situations.

PRAXIS. A neurological condition that affects the ability of a person to perform a motor routine or to implement motor planning.

PRECURSOR. A condition, ability, or behavior that ensures by its presence that the child will more likely progress through subsequent developmental stages, although it is not an actual requirement for such future development.

PRELINGUAL. A stage in development before the acquisition of language when the individual communicates without using verbal language.

PRELINGUALLY DEAF. Deafened before language acquisition.

PREMATURE INFANT. An infant born before the nine-month gestation period. The term also refers to a full-term infant who is born weighing less than five pounds.

PRENATAL. Pertaining to the period in utero.

PREVALENCE. The total number of cases of a disorder in a given population at a specific time.

PRENATAL MEDICAL CARE. The medical attention given to a mother and fetus during pregnancy.

PROMPTING. A language facilitation technique that elicits or requires a response from the child. Asking a question is a form of prompting.

PROPRIOCEPTIVE AWARENESS. The awareness of sensations from within the body itself, as well as an awareness of where body parts are located, general body image, and left and right orientation of the body in space.

PROSODY. The variations in rate, pitch, rhythm, stress, and intonation in continuous speech.

PROXEMICS. An aspect of nonverbal communication that refers to the purposeful use of space and distance as an individual communicates. The distance we maintain when standing or sitting next to another person expresses love, attraction, dislike, abhorrence, and clear intention.

PSYCHOLINGUISTICS. The study of language structure and meaning in relation to human development.

QUADRAPLEGIA. A motor impairment that affects all four extremities of an individual.

QUESTION PROCESSING. 1. The determination as to whether a question is clearly understood or whether more information or clarification is needed; 2. if more information is required, the ability to express an appropriately phrased question to request clarification; and 3. the determination as to whether personal knowledge is sufficient to respond to the question adequately or whether more information is needed.

REACH-ON-SIGHT. A shiny, moving, and visually attractive stimulus that motivates very young infants to reach out and attempt to grasp.

REACH-ON-SOUND. A noise-inducing stimulus that motivates very young infants to reach out and attempt to grasp.

READING COMPREHENSION. The process by which a reader understands the meaning of the entire passage, paragraph, or portion of text and can draw appropriate conclusions and inferences.

RECEPTIVE LANGUAGE. Oral speech that is perceived and processed; signed expressions that are seen and comprehended; and, printed language that is read with understanding. Receptive language also refers to the analysis and interpretation of the message expressed by dance, painting, sculpture, and music.

REFLEX. An involuntary motor response to sensory stimulation (e.g., movement near the eyes that causes an individual to blink).

REGIONAL DIALECTS. Variations within a specific language that occur when a group of people has remained socially isolated with limited exposure to the dominant language over a long period of time.

REGULAR EDUCATION INITIATIVE (REI). The document prepared by M. Will for the U.S. Office of Special Education and Rehabilitation Services, in 1986, which outlines reforms in special education including greater opportunities to include students with disabilities in regular environments.

REHEARSAL STRATEGIES. Repeating the information to oneself in silent language in order to hold the information in short-term memory.

RELIABILITY. In measures of assessment, the extent of accuracy and consistency. A test is considered reliable when various examiners obtain uniform results when the test is administered under duplicated conditions.

RESIDUAL HEARING. The hearing that is still available after sensorineural damage has occurred. The damage rarely occurs to the same degree across all intensities and all frequencies of speech.

SCAFFOLDED INSTRUCTION. An educational approach in which the teacher and student collaborate to assist the student in communicating an effective message to the listener. This supportive procedure is gradually reduced so that the student learns to execute the task independently.

SCREENING TEST. A brief evaluation procedure that attempts to determine whether or not a child might have a problem, but not necessarily meant to determine the type or scope of the problem. A screening test is usually administered before a comprehensive evaluation.

SCRIPT. A form of narrative language that is a description of common, everyday experiences.

SEIZURE. A sudden attack in which electrical activity spreads through the body resulting in petit mal or grand mal convulsions.

SELECTIVE ATTENTION. The ability to focus on some aspects of the environment for the purpose of acquiring or synthesizing information for age-appropriate periods of time. The selection of specific stimuli from an array of many stimuli for further processing.

SEMANTICS. The meaning of words in a language and the relationships between words. Semantics also relates to multiple word meanings, figurative language, and underlying meanings of words in specific contexts.

SEMILINGUAL. The limited acquisition and proficiency in a language.

SENSORINEURAL HEARING IMPAIRMENT. Hearing impairment caused by damage to the nerves in the inner ear or nerve pathways to the brain.

SENSORY INTEGRATION. The process of internalizing and organizing all the incoming visual, auditory, tactile, and kinesthetic stimuli in an efficient manner so that they can be stored in the brain for retrieval when problem solving, thinking, communicating, and learning new applications. If one modality is impaired, sensory integration has to be taught or the information about objects and events will be fragmentary.

SENSORY SYSTEM. The system of nerves and transmitters that carry sensory information from the sense organ to the brain so that the individual can obtain information using vision, hearing, smell, touch, and taste.

SEVERE-TO-PROFOUND HEARING IMPAIRMENT. A condition in which a person cannot even detect sound unless it is presented at not less than 70–90 decibels in intensity or loudness.

SHAPE CONSTANCY. The ability to recognize objects despite the fact that they are viewed from different orientations and because either the viewer or the objects move during the process. *See also* OBJECT CONSTANCY.

SHAPE AND FORM DISCRIMINATION. Ability to differentiate shapes and components of objects that are stationary and also of objects that are dynamic.

SHORT-TERM MEMORY. The temporary storage of information until the individual can take action to use the information in some way.

SIGN LANGUAGE. A manual system that is an alternative means of communication.

SIGNED MOTHERESE. The signs used by deaf mothers to their infants. Their signs are modified to be more visible and to allow the infant to observe the adult's face. The signs are accompanied by smiles and much touching. *See also* PARENTESE.

SIMULTANEOUS COMMUNICATION. A method of teaching the Total Communication philosophy. A mode of communication that incorporates the simultaneous use of oral language, speech reading, and Manual Coded English. *See also* TOTAL COMMUNICATION.

SIZE DISCRIMINATION. The ability to distinguish different sizes of objects when they are next to each other, partially occluded, far from one another, and also when they are moving apart.

SOUND/SYMBOL CORRESPONDENCE. A phoneme that is mapped onto a graphic symbol, such as a letter or combination of letters.

SPATIAL ORIENTATION. Perception of any angle, slant, or other deviation from the horizontal or the vertical. Perception of the direction an object or person is facing.

SPATIAL PERCEPTION. The estimated amount of space that separates individual objects and groups of objects, including people.

SPATIAL RELATIONSHIPS. The positions in space of two or more objects or people as they relate to each other (e.g., *on the right, on the left, in front of, in back of*).

SPECIFIC LANGUAGE DEFICIT. A category of language disorder which is known also as developmental language disorder, specific language impairment, and clinical language disorder. It is usually characterized as a language disorder which cannot be attributed to intellectual or sensory deficits but which substantially affects the child's ability to understand and express verbal and written language.

SPEECH. The motor process of orally producing the sounds and sound sequences that comprise communication.

SPEECH READING. The technique used by a hearing impaired listener to improve intelligibility of a speaker's utterance. The use of contextual clues, visually observable points of articulation, oral configurations of the speaker's mouth, gestures, and facial expressions that convey meaning.

STANDARD AMERICAN ENGLISH. The variety of English most broadly accepted in the United States.

STANDARDIZED TEST. An assessment measure that is recognized as providing information concerning the ability of the child in comparison with other children of the same specified group. A standardized test must always be administered in the same manner and under the same conditions to obtain reliability and validity. The standards of interpretation of the response behaviors are usually based on the norms of a similar population that has also completed the test.

STEREOTYPIES. A term used by psychiatrists to refer to repetitive motor movements like hand flapping, with the individual resisting change or cessation of the movement.

SUBSTANCE ABUSE. The improper use of any chemical which results in harm to the user or other individuals.

SYMBOLIC PLAY. In play, symbolic knowledge provides the child with the ability to understand and use objects in more than one way. For example, a child has the ability to pretend that a lid from a pot is a steering wheel from a car. Symbolic play allows children to transform reality to suit their own needs.

SYMBOLIC REPRESENTATION. The ability to visualize in one's mind an event, person, or object that has been previously encountered but which is no longer present.

SYMBOLIC THOUGHT. The ability to represent and manipulate ideas in the mind about real objects, people, and events.

SYNDROME. A collection of related behaviors, traits, or symptoms that are prevalent among a particular population of children or adults.

SYNESTHESIA. The intermingling of the senses. For example, certain people visualize specific colors when they hear certain sounds.

SYNTACTICAL RULES. The rules of the language that govern the arrangement and combination of words in sentences.

SYNTAX. The part of grammar which regulates the arrangement of words to form meaningful sentences.

TACTILE SENSATION. Information passively received through the skin such as that caused by wind on the face, heat or cold on the skin.

TEMPORAL CONCEPTS. Concepts pertaining to time.

TEMPORAL ORDER. Pertaining to the sequence of time. Language expression difficulties in temporal ordering can be seen when an individual utters sounds, syllables, or words out of sequence as in the word *aks* for *ask*.

TERATOGENS. A classification of drugs and substances that can cause malformations, growth deficiency, or even death in children with prenatal exposure.

THEMATIC APPROACH. An educational approach in which concepts and curriculum are integrated. When teaching language, themes create semantic networks which help to integrate and relate a student's knowledge. In this approach, a particular topic may introduce a variety of educational disciplines such as history, science, math, and language.

THRESHOLD OF COMPETENCE. A theory in second language acquisition that states that a child must reach a level of language development in the primary language before the second language can be mastered in the most advantageous manner. A child who learns an additional language either before or after this threshold of competence will expend a greater period of time working toward mastery.

TIME OUT. A behavior modification technique that removes the child who exhibits unacceptable behavior from the environment in which the behavior occurs. The goal of time out is to isolate the child for a few minutes so that the child calms down or reexamines the behavior that was considered unacceptable.

TOTAL COMMUNICATION. The philosophy or system that permits speech, sign, body language, gesture, and facial expression to be used simultaneously when conversing with a deaf child or adult. The teaching method is referred to as simultaneous communication. *See also* SIMULTANEOUS COMMUNICATION.

TRANSACTIONAL SITUATIONS. Interactions between individuals in a natural environment and in the course of natural, not contrived, activities.

TRANSDISCIPLINARY. When referring to evaluations and intervention, it integrates the expertise of a team of professionals from several disciplines.

TRANSFORMATIONAL GRAMMAR. A grammar that accounts for the construction of language by the way structures change meaning.

UNDEREXTENSIONS. Labels used by young children that are limited and inflexible. For example, the use of the word *dog* for a particular dog only but not for all canines. This tendency indicates an inadequate understanding of the range of meaning of a word.

UNDIFFERENTIATED ATTENTION DEFICIT DISORDER (UADD). The child with Attention Deficit/Hyperactivity Disorder who is not hyperactive. Now classified as Attention Deficit/Hyperactivity Disorder, Predominantly Inattentive Type.

UNVOICED SOUNDS. The speech sounds that are produced without the larynx vibrating. For example, the *s* and *f* sounds are produced without vibrating the larynx.

VALIDITY. In measures of assessment, it refers to the ability of a test to measure what it is supposed to measure. The validity of a particular test is sometimes determined by comparing the results of that test with results from a comparable test.

VESTIBULAR PERCEPTION. An awareness of motion and stabilization of balance.

VISUAL ACUITY. A person's ability to visually identify objects and symbols at a clinically measured distance. It is also defined as the ability of the eye to distinguish fine details.

VISUAL CLOSURE. The ability to recognize the identity of an object despite the fact that parts of it are distorted or hidden from view.

VISUAL FIGURE-GROUND DISCRIMINATION. The ability to distinguish an object from the background.

VISUAL IMPAIRMENT. All pathological conditions of the eye(s) or visual system that cause less than normal vision.

VISUALIZATION. The recollection of the visual details of a scene or an event, the picture in the mind's eye. When visualizing, the sounds, smells, tastes, and tactile sensations of the event are recalled, as well as the visual details. *See also* IMAGERY.

VISUAL PERCEPTION. As distinct from visual acuity, visual perception is the process of becoming aware of the visual stimulus and then organizing and interpreting all of the minute, abstract components. It is a process that is carried out in the cortex of the brain, not in the eye.

VISUAL PROCESSING. The complex organization by the brain of the details of a visual event, including lines oriented in a variety of angles, contours, shapes, and perspectives, as well as colors, shading, highlights, textures, and patterns. These details are perceived, discriminated, combined, categorized, and related to recognizable or similar concepts that are stored in memory. The result is understanding of the visual event.

VOCALIZATION. A sound that is produced by the vocal mechanism of a person but which is not necessarily speechlike.

VOICED SOUNDS. The speech sounds that are produced by vibrating the larynx. Certain sounds are formed by placing the articulators in the same position (e.g., *s* and *z*). The difference in production for these sounds depends on whether the larynx is vibrating. The *z* is voiced due to the vibrating larynx. *See also* UNVOICED SOUNDS.

WH-QUESTION TERMS. Words such as *what, who, which, where, when, why, whose* that request information.

WHOLE LANGUAGE APPROACH. A learning model in which the student learns language in realistic settings with purposeful and meaningful language-based experiences to develop listening, speaking, reading, and writing skills. It is a whole-to-part learning process where real activities such as reading the instructions and rules of a game provide the opportunities to derive meaning and learn the components of language and reading.

WORD DEFINITION TASK. An activity that requires individuals to explain a stimulus word presented to them.

WORD KNOWLEDGE. Vocabulary words in an individual's lexicon. *See also* LEXICON.

WORD RECOGNITION. The matching of a mental image of the configuration of a familiar word to a graphic or written representation of that word. At the same time, silent speech is used by most readers to say the word to themselves. The term is usually applied to sight-word vocabulary.

PROFESSIONAL ORGANIZATIONS

American Association on Mental Retardation, 1719 Kalorama Rd., N.W., Washington, DC 20009, 202-387-1968.

American Psychiatric Association, 1400 K. St., N.W., Washington, DC 20005, 202-682-6000.

American Psychological Association, 1200 17th St., N.W., Washington, DC 20036, 202-955-7600.

American Speech-Language-Hearing Association (ASHA), 10801 Rockville Pike, Rockville, MD 20852, 800-638-6868.

Association for the Education and Rehabilitation of the Blind and Visually Impaired, 206 N. Washington St., Suite 320, Alexandria, VA 22314, 703-548-1884.

Autism Society of America, 7910 Woodmont Ave., Suite 650, Bethesda, MD 20814-3015, 301-657-0881, 800-3AUTISM.

Council for Exceptional Children (CEC), 1920 Association Drive, Reston, VA 22091-1589, 703-620-3660.

International Reading Association, 800 Barksdale Road, P.O. Box 8139, Newark, DE 19714-8139, 302-731-1600.

The Learning Disabilities Association of America, 4156 Library Road, Pittsburgh, PA 15234, 412-341-1515.

National Association for the Deaf (NAD), 814 Thayer Ave., Silver Spring, MD 20910-4500, 301-587-1788.

National Education Association, 1201 16th St., N.W., Washington, DC 20036, 202-833-4000.

The Orton Dyslexia Society, 8600 La Salle Rd., Chester Bldg., Suite 382, Baltimore, MD 21286-2044, 800-222-3123.

REFERENCES

Aaron, P., Kuchta, S., and Grapethin, C. (1988). Is there a thing called dyslexia? *Annals of Dyslexia, 38,* 33–49.

Aaron, P., and Phillips, S. (1986). A decade of research with dyslexic college students. *Annals of Dyslexia, 36,* 44–68.

Abbeduto, L., and Rosenberg, S. (1980). The communicative competence of mildly retarded adults. *Applied Psycholinguistics, 1,* 405–426.

Abel, E. (1990). *Fetal alcohol syndrome.* Oradell, NJ: Medical Economics Books.

Abravanel, E., and Sigafoos, A. (1984). Exploring the presence of imitation during early infancy. *Child Development, 55,* 381–392.

Achilles, J., Yates, R., and Freese, J. (1991). Perspectives from the field: Collaborative consultation in the speech and language program of the Dallas Independent School District. *Language, Speech, and Hearing Services in Schools, 22,* 154–155.

Ackerman, P., and Dykman, R. (1982). Automatic and effortful information processing deficits in children with learning and attention disorders. *Topics in Learning Disabilities, 2,* 12–22.

Acredolo, L., and Goodwyn, S. (1985). Symbolic gesturing in language development: A case study. *Human Development, 28,* 40–49.

Adams, K., and Markham, R. (1991). Recognition of affective facial expressions by children and adolescents with and without mental retardation. *American Journal on Mental Retardation, 96*(1), 21–28.

Adamson, L., and Bakeman, R. (1985). Affect and attention: Infants observed with mothers and peers. *Child Development, 56,* 582–593.

Adelson, E. (1983). Precursors of early language development in children blind from birth. In A. Mills (Ed.), *Language acquisition in the blind child: Normal and deficient* (pp. 1–12). San Diego, CA: College-Hill Press.

Alegria, J., and Noirot, E. (1978). Neonate orientation behavior towards the human voice. *Early Human Development, 1,* 291–312.

Alley, G., and Deshler, D. (1979). *Teaching the learning disabled adolescent: Strategies and methods.* Denver, CO: Love Publishing.

American Psychiatric Association. (1987). *Diagnostic and statistical manual of mental disorders, 3rd edition, revised (DSM-III-R).* Washington, DC: Author.

American Psychiatric Association Task Force on *DSM-IV.* (1993). *DSM-IV draft criteria.* Washington, DC: Author.

American Speech-Language-Hearing Association. (1982). *Joint committee on infant hearing position statement. ASHA, 24*(12), 1017–1018.

American Speech-Language-Hearing Association. (1985). Clinical management of communicatively handicapped minority language populations. *ASHA, 27*(6), 29–32.

473

American Speech-Language-Hearing Association. (1987). *Social dialects position paper. ASHA, 29*(1), 45.

Anderson, G., and Hoshino, Y. (1987). Neurochemical studies of autism. In D. Cohen, A. Donnellan, and R. Pauls (Eds.), *Handbook of autism and pervasive developmental disorders* (pp. 166–191). New York: John Wiley and Sons.

Anderson, R., Hiebert, E., Scott, J., and Wilkinson, I. (1985). *Becoming a nation of readers: The report of the commission on reading.* Washington, DC: Department of Education.

Antoniadis, A., and Daulton, D. (1992). Meeting the needs of children in Pennsylvania who are exposed to alcohol and other drugs. In L. Rosetti (Ed.), *Developmental problems of drug exposed infants* (pp. 53–62). San Diego, CA: Singular Publishing Group.

Applebee, A. (1978). *The child's concept of story: Ages two to seventeen.* Chicago, IL: University of Chicago Press.

Aram, D. (1991). Comments on specific language impairment as a clinical category. *Language, Speech, and Hearing Services in Schools, 22,* 84–87.

Aram, D., Ekelman, B., and Nation, J. (1984). Preschoolers with language disorders: 10 years later. *Journal of Speech and Hearing Research, 27,* 232–244.

Aram, D., Morris, R., and Hall, N. (1993). Clinical and research congruence in identifying children with specific language impairment. *Journal of Speech and Hearing Research, 36*(3), 580–591.

Aram, D., and Nation, J. (1980). Preschool language disorders and subsequent language and academic difficulties. *Journal of Communication Disorders, 13,* 159–170.

ASHA Report. (March, 1989). Issues in determining eligibility for language intervention. *ASHA, 31,* 113–118.

ASHA. (1991). The prevention of communication disorders tutorial. *ASHA Supplement #6, 33*(9), 15–39.

Aslin, R., Pisoni, D., and Jusczyk, P. (1983). Auditory development and speech perception in infancy. In M. Haith and J. Campos (Eds.), *Handbook of child psychology: Vol. 2. Infancy and developmental psychology.* New York: John Wiley and Sons.

Atkins, M., Pelham, W., and Licht, M. (1985). A comparison of objective classroom measures and teacher ratings of attention deficit disorder. *Journal of Abnormal Child Psychology, 13*(1), 155–167.

Audette, B., and Algozzine, B. (1992). Free and appropriate education for all students: Total quality and the transformation of American public education. *Remedial and Special Education, 13*(6), 8–18.

Ayres, A. (1985). *Sensory integration and the child.* Los Angeles, CA: Western Psychological Services.

Bachrach, E. (1991). A preliminary analysis of the impact of prenatal exposure to crack in New York City (Report No. 22-91). New York: Office of the New York State Comptroller.

Baddeley, A. (1986). *Working memory.* New York: Oxford University Press.

Badian, N. (1986). Nonverbal disorders of learning: The reverse of dyslexia? *Annals of Dyslexia, 36,* 253–269.

Badian, N. (1992). Nonverbal learning disability, school behavior, and dyslexia. *Annals of Dyslexia, 42,* 159–178.

Baker, C. (1985). The facial behavior of deaf signers: Evidence of a complex language. *American Annals of the Deaf, 130*(4), 297–304.

Baker, L. (1982). An evaluation of the role of metacognitive deficits in learning disabilities. *Topics in Learning and Learning Disabilities, 2,* 27–36.

Baltaxe, C., and Simmons, J. (1987). Communication deficits in the adolescent with autism, schizophrenia, and language-learning disabilities. In T. Layton (Ed.), *Language and treatment of autistic and developmentally disordered children* (pp. 155–186). Springfield, IL: Charles C. Thomas.

Bamford, J., and Saunders, E. (1991). *Hearing impairment, auditory perception, and language disability.* San Diego, CA: Singular Publishing Group.

Baran, A., and van Houten, L. (1988). Lessons taught and lessons learned: A story of differential teacher adaptation of lessons for high- and low-ranked hearing impaired students. *Discourse Processes, 11,* 117–138.

Barkley, R. (1990). *Attention-deficit hyperactivity disorder: A handbook for diagnosis and treatment.* New York: Guilford.

Baron-Cohen, S. (1988). Social and pragmatic deficits in autism: Cognitive or affective? *Journal of Autism and Developmental Disorders, 18*(3), 379–402.

Barraga, N. (1983). *Visual handicaps and learning.* Austin, TX: Pro-Ed.

Barrera, M., and Maurer, D. (1981). Recognition of mother's photographed face by the 3-month-old infant. *Child Development, 52,* 714–716.

Barron, J., and Barron, S. (1992). *There's a boy in here.* New York: Simon and Schuster.

Barry, H. (1961). *The young aphasic child: Evaluation and training.* Washington, DC: Alexander Graham Bell Association for the Deaf.

Barry, H., and McGinnis, M. (1988). *Teaching aphasic children.* Austin, TX: Pro-Ed.

Bates, E. (1976). *Language and context: The acquisition of pragmatics.* New York: Academic Press.

Bates, E. (1979). *The emergence of symbols: Cognition and communication in infancy.* New York: Academic Press.

Bates, E., Bretherton, I., and Snyder, L. (1988). *From first words to grammar: Individual differences and dissociable mechanisms.* New York: Cambridge University Press.

Bates, E., O'Connell, B., and Shore, C. (1987). Language and communication in infancy. In J. Osofsky (Ed.), *Handbook of infant development* (pp. 149–203). New York: John Wiley and Sons.

Bauman, M. (1993). An interview with Dr. Margaret Bauman. *Advocate: Autism Society of America, 24*(4), 1–14.

Becker, J. (1982). Children's strategic use of requests to mark and manipulate social status. In S. Kuczaj (Ed.), *Language development: Vol 2. Language, thought, and culture.* New York: Springer.

Bedrosian, J. (1988). Adults who are mildly to moderately mentally retarded: Communicative performance, assessment, and intervention. In S. Calculator and J. Bedrosian (Eds.), *Communication assessment and intervention for adults with mental retardation* (pp. 265–308). San Diego, CA: College-Hill Press.

Bedrosian, J. (1993). Making minds meet: Assessment of conversational topic in adults with mild to moderate mental retardation. *Topics in Language Disorders, 13*(3), 36–46.

Bellugi, U. (1987). How signs express complex meanings. In C. Baker and R. Battison (Eds.), *Sign language and the Deaf community* (3rd ed.)(pp. 53–74). Silver Spring, MD: National Association of the Deaf.

Bench, R. (1992). *Communication skills in hearing impaired children.* San Diego, CA: Singular Publishing Group.

Bender, W., and Golden, L. (1990). Subtypes of students with learning disabilities as derived from cognitive, academic, behavioral, and self-concept measures. *Learning Disability Quarterly, 13,* 183–194.

Bennett, C. (1971). Communication disorders in the public schools. In L. Travis (Ed.), *Handbook of speech pathology and audiology* (pp. 963–994). New York: Appleton-Century-Crofts.

Benzaquen, S., Gagnon, R., Hunse, C., and Foreman, J. (1990). The intrauterine sound environment of the human fetus during labor. *American Journal of Obstetrics and Gynecology, 163,* 484–490.

Berard, G. (1993). *Hearing equals behavior.* New Canaan, CT: Keats.

Bergstrom, L. (1988). Infectious agents that deafen. In F. Bess (Ed.), *Hearing impairment in children* (pp. 33–56). Parkton, MD: York Press.

Bernal, E. (1983). Trends in bilingual special education. *Learning Disability Quarterly, 6,* 424–431.

Bernstein, D. (1989). Language development: The school-age years. In D. Bernstein and E. Tiegerman (Eds.), *Language and communication disorders in children* (2nd ed.) (pp. 133–156). Columbus, OH: Charles E. Merrill.

Berry, C., Shaywitz, S., and Shaywitz, B. (1985). Girls with attention deficit disorder: A silent majority? A report on behavioral and cognitive characteristics. *Pediatrics, 76,* 801–809.

Bettelheim, B. (1967). *The empty fortress: Infantile autism and the birth of self.* New York: Free Press.

Bigelow, A. (1986). Early words of blind children. *Journal of Child Language, 14,* 47–56.

Bigelow, A. (1990). Relationship between the development of language and thought in young blind children. *Journal of Visual Impairment and Blindness, 84*(8), 414–419.

Biklen, D. (1989). Making difference ordinary. In S. Stainback, W. Stainback, and M. Forest (Eds.), *Educating all students in the mainstream of regular education* (pp. 235–248). Baltimore, MD: Paul H. Brookes.

Biklen, D. (1990). Aphasia unbound: Autism and praxis. *Harvard Educational Review, 60*(3), 291–314.

Biklen, D. (1992). *Schooling without labels: Parents, educators, and inclusive education.* Philadelphia, PA: Temple University Press.

Biklen, D., Morton, M., Gold, D., Berrigan, C., and Swaminathan, S. (1992). Facilitated communication: Implications for individuals with autism. *Topics in Language Disorders, 12*(4), 1–28.

Biklen, D., and Schubert, A. (1991). New words: The communication of students with autism. *Remedial and Special Education, 12*(6), 46–57.

Billingsley, B., and Wildman, T. (1990). Facilitating reading comprehension in learning disabled students: Metacognitive goals and instructional strategies. *Remedial and Special Education, 11*(2), 18–31.

Bishop, D., and Edmundson, A. (1987). Language-impaired 4-year-olds: Distinguishing transient from persistent impairment. *Journal of Speech and Hearing Disorders, 52,* 156–173.

Blachman, B. (1991). Getting ready to read: Learning how print maps to speech. In J. Kavanagh (Ed.), *The language continuum: From infancy to literacy* (pp. 41–62). Parkton, MD: York Press.

Blake, J., and deBoysson-Bardies, B. (1992). Patterns in babbling: A cross-linguistic study. *Journal of Child Language, 19,* 51–74.

Blalock, J. (1982). Persistent auditory language deficits in adults with learning disabilities. *Journal of Learning Disabilities, 15,* 604–609.

Blank, M., Rose, S., and Berlin, L. (1978). *The language of learning: The preschool years.* New York: Grune and Stratton.

Blank, M., and White, S. (1986). Questions: A powerful but misused form of classroom exchange. *Topics in Language Disorders, 6*(2), 1–12.

Bloch, M. (1992). Tobacco control advocacy: Winning the war on tobacco. *Zero to Three, 13*(1), 29–33.

Bloom, L. (1970). *Language development: Form and function of emerging grammars.* Cambridge, MA: MIT Press.

Bloom, L. (1973). *One word at a time: The use of single word utterances before syntax.* The Hague: Mouton.

Bloom, L. (1974). Talking, understanding, and thinking. In R. Schiefelbusch and L. Lloyd (Eds.), *Language perspectives: Acquisition, retardation, and intervention.* Baltimore, MD: University Park Press.

Bloom, L., Hood, L., and Lightbown, P. (1974). Imitation in language development: If, when and why? *Cognitive Psychology, 6,* 380–420.

Bloom, L., and Lahey, M. (1978). *Language development and language disorders.* New York: Macmillan.

Bloome, D., and Knott, G. (1985). Teacher-student discourse. In N. Ripich and F. Spinelli (Eds.), *School discourse problems.* San Diego, CA: College-Hill Press.

Boder, E., and Jarrico, S. (1982). *The Boder test of reading-spelling patterns.* New York: Grune and Stratton.

Bonvillian, J., Orlansky, M., and Novak, L. (1983). Developmental milestones: Sign language acquisition and motor development. *Child Development, 54,* 1435–1445.

Borkowski, J., Johnston, M., and Reid, M. (1987). Metacognition, motivation, and controlled performance. In S. Ceci (Ed.), *Handbook of cognitive, social, and neuropsychological aspects of learning disabilities* (Vol. 2). Hillsdale, NJ: Erlbaum.

Borkowski, J., Weyhing, R., and Carr, M. (1988). Effects of attributional retraining on strategy-based reading comprehension in learning disabled students. *Journal of Educational Psychology, 80,* 46–53.

Bornstein, H., Saulnier, K., and Hamilton, L. (1980). Signed English: A first evaluation. *American Annals of the Deaf, 125*(4), 467–481.

Borod, J., Koff, E., and Caron, H. (1983). Right hemispheric specialization for the expression and appreciation of emotion: A focus on the face. In E. Perecman (Ed.), *Cognitive processing in the right hemisphere* (pp. 83–110). New York: Academic Press.

Bos, C., and Filip, D. (1982). Comprehension monitoring skills in learning disabled and average students. *Topics in Learning and Learning Disabilities, 2,* 79–86.

Bower, T. (1982). *Development in infancy* (2nd ed.). San Francisco, CA: W.H. Freeman.

Bower, T., Broughton, J., and Moore, M. (1970a). Demonstration of intention in reaching behavior of neonate humans. *Nature, 228,* 679–681.

Bower, T., Broughton, J., and Moore, M. (1970b). The coordination of visual and tactual input in infants. *Perception and Psychophysics, 8,* 51–53.

Bowerman, M. (1977). The acquisition of word meaning: An investigation of some current conflicts. In P. Johnson-Laird and P. Wason (Eds.), *Thinking: Readings in cognitive science* (pp. 239–253). New York: Cambridge University Press.

Bradley, L., and Bryant, P. (1985). *Rhyme and reason in reading and spelling.* Ann Arbor, MI: University of Michigan Press.

Brady, S., and Fowler, A. (1988). Phonological precursors to reading acquisition. In R. Masland and M. Masland (Eds.), *Preschool prevention of reading failure* (pp. 204–215). Parkton, MD: York Press.

Brady, S., and Shankweiler, D. (1991). *Phonological processes in literacy.* Hillsdale, NJ: Erlbaum.

Brady, S., Shankweiler, D., and Mann, V. (1983). Speech perception and memory coding in relation to reading ability. *Journal of Experimental Child Psychology, 35,* 345–367.

Brandes, P., and Ehinger, D. (1981). The effects of early middle ear pathology on auditory perception and academic achievement. *Journal of Speech and Hearing Disorders, 46,* 301–307.

Bretherton, I., Fritz, J., Zahn-Waxler, C., and Ridgeway, D. (1986). Learning to talk about emotions: A functionalist perspective. *Child Development, 57,* 529–548.

Bretherton, I., McNew, S., Snyder, L., and Bates, E. (1983). Individual differences at 20 months: Analytic and holistic strategies in language acquisition. *Journal of Child Language, 10,* 293–320.

Bricker, D., and Schiefelbusch, R. (1990). Infants at risk. In L. McCormick and R. Schiefelbusch (Eds.), *Early language intervention: An introduction* (2nd ed.) (pp. 334–354). New York: Charles E. Merrill.

Brinton, B., and Fujiki, M. (1982). A comparison of request response sequences in the discourse of normal and language-disordered children. *Journal of Speech and Hearing Disorders, 47,* 57–62.

Brinton, B., and Fujiki, M. (1989). *Conversational management with language-impaired children: Pragmatic assessment and intervention.* Rockville, MD: Aspen.

Britton, J. (1972). *Language and learning.* Baltimore, MD: Penguin Books.

Brown, A. (1982). Inducing strategic learning from texts by means of informed, self-control training. *Topics in Learning and Learning Disabilities, 2*(1), 1–17.

Brown, A., Day, J., and Jones, R. (1983). The development of plans for summarizing texts. *Child Development, 54,* 968–979.

Brown, R. (1973). *A first language: The early stages.* Cambridge, MA: Harvard University Press.

Bruck, M. (1982). Language-impaired children's performance in an additive bilingual education program. *Applied Psycholinguistics, 3,* 46–61.

Bruner, J. (1975). The ontogenesis of speech acts. *Journal of Child Language, 2,* 1–19.

Bruner, J. (1978). Learning how to do things with words. In J. Bruner and R. Garten (Eds.), *Human growth and development.* Oxford, UK: Oxford University Press.

Bruner, J. (1981). The social context of language acquisition. *Language and Communication, 1,* 155–178.

Bruner, J., Roy, C., and Ratner, N. (1982). The beginnings of request. In K. Nelson (Ed.), *Children's language* (Vol. 3). New York: Gardner Press.

Burger, A., Blackman, L., and Clark, H. (1981). Generalization of verbal abstraction strategies by EMR children and adolescents. *American Journal of Mental Deficiency, 85,* 611–618.

Burger, A., Blackman, L., and Tan, N. (1980). Maintenance and generalization of a sorting and retrieval strategy by EMR and nonretarded individuals. *American Journal of Mental Deficiency, 84,* 373–380.

Burke, G. (1990). Unconventional behavior: A communicative interpretation in individuals with severe disabilities. *Topics in Language Disorders, 10*(4), 75–85.

Burnham, D., Earnshaw, L., and Quinn, M. (1987). The development of categorical identification of speech. In B. McKenzie and R. Day (Eds.), *Perceptual development in early infancy: Problems and issues.* Hillsdale, NJ: Erlbaum.

Burns, W., and Burns, K. (1988). Parenting dysfunction in chemically dependent women. In I. Chasnoff (Ed.), *Drugs, alcohol, pregnancy, and parenting* (pp. 159–172). Hingham, MA: Kluwer Academic.

Butkowsky, I., and Willows, D. (1980). Cognitive motivational characteristics of children varying in reading ability: Evidence for learned helplessness in poor readers. *Journal of Educational Psychology, 72,* 408–422.

Butler, K. (1984). Language processing: Halfway up the down staircase. In G. Wallach and K.S. Butler (Eds.), *Language learning disabilities in school-age children* (pp. 60–81). Baltimore, MD: Williams and Wilkins.

Button, G., and Lee, J. (Eds.). (1987). *Talk and social organization.* Clevedon, England: Multilingual Matters.

Byrne, B. (1981). Deficient syntactic control in poor readers: Is a weak phonetic memory code responsible? *Applied Psycholinguistics, 2,* 201–212.

Cain, L., Levine, S., and Elzey, F. (1963). *Cain-Levine social competency scale.* Palo Alto, CA: Consulting Psychologists Press.

Calculator, S. (1992). Perhaps the emperor has clothes after all: A response to Biklen. *American Journal of Speech-Language Pathology, 1*(2), 18–20.

Calvert, D. (1986). Speech in perspective. In D. Luterman (Ed.), *Deafness in perspective* (pp. 167–191). San Diego, CA: College-Hill Press.

Campbell, R., and Butterworth, B. (1985). Phonological dyslexia and dysgraphia in a highly literate subject: A developmental case with associated deficits of phonemic awareness and processing. *Quarterly Journal of Experimental Psychology, 37A,* 435–475.

Campbell, S., Breaux, A., Ewing, L., and Szumowski, E. (1986). Correlates and predictors of hyperactivity and aggression: A longitudinal study of parent referred problem preschoolers. *Journal of Abnormal Child Psychology, 14,* 217–234.

Campbell, T., and Dollaghan, C. (1992). A method for obtaining listener judgments of spontaneously produced language: Social validation through direct magnitude estimation. *Topics in Language Disorders, 12*(2), 42–55.

Campos, J., and Stenberg, C. (1980). Perception, appraisal, and emotion: The onset of social referencing. In M. Lamb and L. Sherrod (Eds.), *Infant social cognition.* Hillsdale, NJ: Erlbaum.

Capute, A., Palmer, F., Shapiro, B., Wachtel, R., Schmidt, S., and Ross, A. (1986). Clinical linguistic and auditory milestone scale: Prediction of cognition in infancy. *Developmental Medicine and Child Neurology, 28,* 762–771.

Carey, A. (1992). Get involved: Multiculturally. *ASHA, 34*(5), 3–4.

Carlisle, J. (1991). Planning an assessment of listening and reading comprehension. *Topics in Language Disorders, 12*(1), 17–31.

Carr, E., and Durand, V. (1985). Reducing behavioral problems through functional communication training. *Journal of Applied Behavior Analysis, 18,* 111–126.

Carrasquillo, A. (1986). The parent factor in teaching language skills to limited English proficient learning disabled students. In A. Willig and H. Greenberg (Eds.), *Bilingualism and learning disability* (pp. 53–68). New York: American Library.

Carrow-Woolfolk, E., and Lynch, J. (1982). *An integrative approach to language disorders in children.* New York: Grune and Stratton.

Casby, M. (1992). The cognitive hypothesis and its influence on speech-language services in schools. *Language, Speech, and Hearing Services in Schools, 23*(3), 198–202.

Case, R. (1985). *Intellectual development: Birth to adulthood.* Orlando, FL: Academic Press.

Catts, H. (1989a). Phonological processing deficits and reading disabilities. In A. Kamhi and H. Catts (Eds.), *Reading disabilities: A developmental language perspective.* Boston, MA: Little, Brown and Company.

Catts, H. (1989b). Defining dyslexia as a developmental language disorder. *Annals of Dyslexia, 39,* 50–64.

Catts, H. (1991). Early identification of reading disabilities. *Topics in Language Disorders, 12*(1),1–16.

Catts, H., and Kamhi, A. (1986). The linguistic basis of reading disorders: Implications for the speech-language pathologist. *Language, Speech, and Hearing Services in Schools, 17,* 329–341.

Cazden, C. (1974). Play with language and metalinguistic awareness: One dimension of language experience. *Urban Review, 7,* 28–39.

Cazden, C. (1988). *Classroom discourse: The language of teaching and learning.* Portsmouth, NH: Heinemann.

Center for Assessment and Demographic Studies. (1993). Unpublished annual survey for hearing-impaired children and youth. Washington, DC: Gallaudet University Press.

Cesaroni, L., and Garber, M. (1991). Exploring the experience of autism through firsthand accounts. *Journal of Autism and Developmental Disorders, 21*(3), 303–313.

Champie, J. (1984). Is total communication enough? The hidden curriculum. *American Annals of the Deaf, 129,* 317–318.

Chan, L. (1991). Promoting strategy generalization through self instruction training in students with reading disabilities. *Journal of Learning Disabilities, 24*(7), 427–433.

Chaney, C. (1990). Evaluating the whole language approach to language arts: The pros and cons. *Language, Speech, and Hearing Services in Schools, 21*(4), 244–249.

Chapman, R. (1981). Exploring children's communicative intentions. In J. Miller (Ed.), *Assessing language production in children: Experimental procedures.* Baltimore, MD: University Park Press.

Cheng, L. (1987). Cross-cultural and linguistic considerations in working with Asian populations. *ASHA, 29*(6), 33–38.

Cheng, L. (1989). Service delivery to Asian/Pacific LEP children: A cross-cultural framework. *Topics in Language Disorders, 9*(3), 1–14.

Cheng, L. (1993). Deafness: An Asian/Pacific Island perspective. In K. Christensen and G. Delgado (Eds.), *Multicultural issues in deafness* (pp. 113–126). White Plains, NY: Longman.

Chomsky, N. (1957). *Syntactic structures.* The Hague: Mouton.

Chomsky, N. (1959). A review of Skinner's "Verbal Behavior." *Language, 35,* 26–58.

Chorost, S. (1988). The hearing impaired child in the mainstream: A survey of the attitudes of regular classroom teachers. *Volta Review, 90,* 7–12.

Christie, F. (1989). Language development in education. In R. Hason and J. Martin (Eds.), *Language development: Learning language, learning culture* (pp. 152–198). Norwood, NJ: Ablex.

Church, M., and Gerkin, M. (1988). Hearing disorders in children with fetal alcohol syndrome: Findings from case reports. *Pediatrics, 82,* 147–154.

Cicchetti, D., and Pogge-Hesse, R. (1980). The relation between emotion and cognition in infant development. In M. Lamb and L. Sherrod (Eds.), *Infant social cognition.* Hillsdale, NJ: Erlbaum.

Cirrin, F., and Rowland, C. (1985). Communicative assessment of nonverbal youths with severe, profound mental retardation. *Mental Retardation, 23,* 52–62.

Clark, D. (1988). Dyslexia: *Theory and practice of remedial instruction.* Parkton, MD: York Press.

Clark, D. (1989). Neonates and infants at risk for hearing and speech-language disorders. *Topics in Language Disorders, 10*(1), 1–12.

Clark, E. (1973). What's in a word? On the child's acquisition of semantics in his first language. In T. Moore (Ed.), *Cognitive development and the acquisition of language.* New York: Academic Press.

Clark, E. (1975). Knowledge, context, and strategy in the acquisition of meaning. In D. Dato (Ed.), *Developmental psycholinguistics: Theory and application.* Washington, DC: Georgetown University Press.

Clark, E. (1983). Meanings and concepts. In P. Mussen (Ed.), *Handbook of child psychology* (Vol. 3). New York: John Wiley and Sons.

Clifton, R., Morrongiello, B., Kulig, J., and Dowd, J. (1981). Developmental changes in auditory localization in infancy. In R. Aslin, J. Albert, and M. Peterson (Eds.), *Development of perception: Vol. 1. Psychobiological perspectives.* New York: Academic Press.

Coggins, T. (1991). Bringing context back into assessment. *Topics in Language Disorders, 11*(4), 43–54.

Cohen, D., Caparulo, B., and Shaywitz, B. (1985). Neurochemical and developmental models of childhood autism. In A. Donnellan (Ed.), *Classic readings in autism* (pp. 343–369). New York: Teachers College Press.

Cohen, N., Sullivan, S., Minde, K., Novak, C., and Helwig, C. (1981). Evaluation of the relative effectiveness of methylphenidate and cognitive behavior modification in the treatment of kindergarten-aged hyperactive children. *Journal of Abnormal Child Psychology, 9,* 43–54.

Cohen, O. (1993). Educational needs of African-American and Hispanic deaf children and youth. In K. Christensen and G. Delgado (Eds.), *Multicultural issues in deafness* (pp. 45–67). White Plains, NY: Longman.

Cole, K., Dale, P., and Mills, P. (1990). Defining language delay in young children by cognitive referencing: Are we saying more than we know? *Applied Psycholinguistics, 11,* 291–302.

Cole, L. (1992). Our multicultural agenda: We're serious. *ASHA, 34*(5), 38–39.

Cone, T., Wilson, L., Bradley, C., and Reese, J. (1985). Characteristics of LD students in Iowa: An empirical investigation. *Learning Disability Quarterly, 3*(3), 211–220.

Cone-Wesson, B., and Wu, P. (1992). Audiologic findings in infants born to cocaine-abusing mothers. In L. Rosetti (Ed.), *Developmental problems of drug-exposed infants* (pp. 25–34). San Diego, CA: Singular Publishing Group.

Connell, P. (1987). Teaching language form, meaning, and function to specific-language-impaired children. In S. Rosenberg (Ed.), *Advances in applied psycholinguistics: Vol. 1. Disorders of first language development* (pp. 40–75). New York: Cambridge University Press.

Connor, L. (1986). Oralism in perspective. In D. Luterman (Ed.), *Deafness in perspective* (pp. 115–129). San Diego, CA: College-Hill Press.

Conti, R. (1991). Attention disorders. In B. Wong (Ed.), *Learning about learning disabilities* (pp. 59–101). New York: Academic Press.

Cooper, D., and Anderson-Inman, L. (1988). Language and socialization. In M. Nippold (Ed.), *Later language development: Ages nine through nineteen* (pp. 228–246). Boston, MA: College-Hill Press.

Coplan, J. (1987). *Early language milestone scale.* Tulsa, OK: Modern Education.

Coplan, J., Gleason, J., Ryan, R., Burke, M., and Williams, M. (1982). Validation of early language milestone scale in a high risk population. *Pediatrics, 70,* 677–683.

Corcoran, J. (1989). The speech and language problems screening test (SLPS). In K. Mogford and J. Sadler (Eds.), *Child language disability: Implications in an educational setting* (pp. 31–39). Philadelphia, PA: Multilingual Matters.

Cornett, O. (1967). Cued speech. *American Annals of the Deaf, 112*(1), 3–13.

Coster, W., and Cicchetti, D. (1993). Research on the communicative development of maltreated children: Clinical implications. *Topics in Language Disorders, 13*(4), 25–38.

Courchesne, E. (1989). Neuroanatomical systems involved in infantile autism: The implications of cerebellar abnormalities. In G. Dawson (Ed.), *Autism: Nature, diagnosis, and treatment* (pp. 119–143). New York: Guilford Press.

Courchesne, E., Lincoln, A., Yeung-Courchesne, R., Elmasian, R., and Grillon, C. (1989). Pathophysiologic findings in nonretarded autism and receptive developmental language disorder. *Journal of Autism and Developmental Disorders, 19*(1), 1–17.

Crago, M. (1992). Ethnography and language socialization: A cross-cultural perspective. *Topics in Language Disorders, 12*(3), 28–39.

Craig, H. (1993). Social skills of children with specific language impairment: Peer relationships. *Language, Speech, and Hearing Services in Schools, 24*(4), 206–215.

Craig, H., and Evans, J. (1989). Turn exchange characteristics of SLI children's spontaneous and nonsimultaneous speech. *Journal of Speech and Hearing Disorders, 54,* 334–347.

Craig, H., and Evans, J. (1991). Turn exchange behaviors of children with normally developing language: The influence of gender. *Journal of Speech and Hearing Research, 34,* 866–878.

Crais, E. (1991). Moving from "parent involvement" to family centered services. *American Journal of Speech-Language Pathology, 1*(1), 5–8.

Crandall, K., and Albertini, J. (1980). An investigation of variables of instruction and their relation to rate of English language learning. *American Annals of the Deaf, 125,* 427–434.

Creaghead, N. (1984). Strategies for evaluation and targeting pragmatic behaviors in young children. *Seminars in Speech and Language, 5*(3), 241–252.

Crites, L., Fischer, K., McNeish-Stengel, M., and Seigel, C. (1992). Working with families of drug-exposed children: Three model programs. In L. Rosetti (Ed.), *Developmental problems of drug-exposed infants* (pp. 13–24). San Diego, CA: Singular Publishing Group.

Cromer, R. (1988). Differentiating language and cognition. In R. Schiefelbusch and L. Lloyd (Eds.), *Language perspectives: Acquisition, retardation, and intervention* (2nd ed.)(pp. 91–124). Baltimore, MD: University Park Press.

Crossley, R. (1992a). Getting the words out: Facilitated communication training. *Topics in Language Disorders, 12*(4), 46–59.

Crossley, R. (1992b). Lending a hand: A personal account of the development of facilitated communication training. *American Journal of Speech-Language Pathology, 1*(3), 15–18.

Culatta, B. (1984). A discourse-based approach to training grammatical rules. *Seminars in Speech and Language, 5*(3), 253–263.

Cummins, J. (1983a). Bilingualism and special education: Program and pedagogical issues. *Learning Disability Quarterly, 6,* 373–386.

Cummins, J. (1983b). Language proficiency and academic achievement. In J. Oller, Jr. (Ed.), *Issues in language testing research* (pp. 108–130). Rowley, MA: Newbury House.

Cummins, J. (1984). *Bilingualism and special education: Issues in assessment and pedagogy*. Austin, TX: Pro-Ed.

Cummins, J. (1989). A theoretical framework for bilingual special education. *Exceptional Children, 56*(2), 111–119.

Cunningham, C., Reuler, E., Blackwell, J., and Deck, J. (1981). Behavioral and linguistic developments in the interactions or normal and retarded children with their mothers. *Child Development, 52*, 62–70.

Currin, A., and Fitzwater, A. (1993). The body, the mind, and facilitated communication: Interventions for children with physical or sensory impairment. In D. Smukler (Ed.), *First words: Facilitated communication and the inclusion of young children* (2nd ed.) (pp. 237–268). Syracuse, NY: Jowonio School.

Curtiss, S. (1981). Dissociations between language and cognition: Cases and implications. *Journal of Autism and Developmental Disorders, 11*, 15–30.

Curtiss, S., and Tallal, P. (1991). On the nature of the impairment in language-impaired children. In J. Miller (Ed.), *Research on child language disorders: A decade of progress* (pp. 189–210). Austin, TX: Pro-Ed.

Dale, P., and Cole, K. (1991). What's normal? Specific language impairment in an individual differences perspective. *Language, Speech, and Hearing Services in Schools, 22*(2), 80–83.

Dale, P., Bates, E., Reznick, S., and Morisset, C. (1989). The validity of a parent report instrument of child language at twenty months. *Journal of Child Language, 16*, 239–250.

Damasio, A., and Maurer, R. (1985). A neurological model for childhood autism. In A. Donnellan (Ed.), *Classic readings in autism* (pp. 383–405). New York: Teachers College Press.

Damico, J. (1991). Clinical discourse analysis: A functional approach to language assessment. In C. Simon (Ed.), *Communication skills and classroom success: Assessment and therapy methodologies for language and learning disabled students* (pp. 125–150). Eau Claire, WI: Thinking Publications.

Damico, J. (1993). Language assessment in adolescents: Addressing critical issues. *Language, Speech, and Hearing Services in Schools, 24*, 29–35.

Damico, J., and Oller, J., Jr. (1980). Pragmatic verses morphological/syntactic criteria for language referrals. *Language, Speech, and Hearing Services in Schools, 9*(2), 85–94.

Damico, J., Oller, J., Jr., and Storey, M. (1983). The diagnosis of language disorders in bilingual children: Surface-oriented and pragmatic criteria. *Journal of Speech and Hearing Disorders, 48*, 385–394.

Daniloff, J., Noll, J., Fristoe, M., and Lloyd, L. (1982). Gesture recognition in patients with aphasia. *Journal of Speech and Hearing Disorders, 47*, 43–49.

Danks, J., and End, L. (1987). Processing strategies for listening and reading. In R. Horowitz and S. Samuels (Eds.), *Comprehending oral and written language*. New York: Academic Press.

Davis, E., Fennoy, I., Laraque, D., Kanem, N., Brown, G., and Mitchell, J. (1992). Autism and developmental abnormalities in children with perinatal cocaine exposure. *Journal of the National Medical Association, 84*(4), 315–319.

Dawson, G., and Lewy, A. (1989). Reciprocal subcortical-cortical influences in autism: The role of attentional mechanisms. In G. Dawson (Ed.), *Autism: Nature, diagnosis, and treatment* (pp. 144–173). New York: Guilford Press.

deBoysson-Bardies, B., Halle, P., Sagart, L., and Durand, C. (1989). A crosslinguistic investigation of vowel formants in babbling. *Journal of Child Language, 16*, 1–17.

De Casper, A., and Fifer, W. (1980). Of human bonding: Newborns prefer their mothers' voices. *Science, 208*, 1174–1176.

De Casper, A., and Spence, M. (1986). Prenatal maternal speech influences newborns' perception of speech sounds. *Infant Behavior and Development, 9*, 33–150.

DeFrancisco, V. (1992). Ethnography and gender: Learning to talk like girls and boys. *Topics in Language Disorders, 12*(3), 40–53.

DeFries, J., and Decker, S. (1982). Genetic aspects of reading disability: A family study. In R. Malatesha and P. Aarons (Eds.), *Reading disorders: Varieties and treatments* (pp. 255–280). New York: Academic Press.

Della Corte, M., Benedict, H., and Klein, D. (1983). The relationship of pragmatic dimensions of mothers' speech to the referential-expressive distinction. *Journal of Child Language, 10*, 35–44.

Dennis, R., Reichle, J., Williams, W., and Vogelsberg, R. (1982). Motoric factors influencing the selection of vocabulary for sign production programs. *Journal of the Association for the Severely Handicapped, 7, 20–32.*

de Villiers, J., and de Villiers, P. (1978). *Language acquisition.* Cambridge, MA: Harvard University Press.

Dew, N. (1984). The exceptional bilingual child: Demography. In P. Chinn (Ed.), *Education of culturally and linguistically different exceptional children.* Reston, VA: Council for Exceptional Children.

Dickinson, D., and McCabe, A. (1991). The acquisition and development of language: A social interactionist account of language and literacy development. In J. Kavanagh (Ed.), *The language continuum: From infancy to literacy* (pp. 1–40). Parkton, MD: York Press.

Diener, C., and Dweck, C. (1980). An analysis of learned helplessness: The processing of success. *Journal of Personality and Social Psychology, 39*, 940–952.

Dixon, S., Bresnahan, K., and Zuckerman, B. (1990). Cocaine babies: Meeting the challenge of management. *Contemporary Pediatrics, 9,* 70–92.

Dixon, S., Coen, R., and Crutchfield, S. (1987). Visual dysfunction in cocaine-exposed infants. *Pediatric Research, 21,* 359A.

Doehring, D., Trites, R., Patel, P., and Fiederowicz, C. (1981). *Reading disabilities: The interaction of reading, language, and neuropsychological deficits.* New York: Academic Press.

Doll, E. (1965). *Vineland social maturity scale.* Circle Pines, MN: American Guidance Service.

Dollaghan, C. (1987). Comprehension monitoring in normal and language-impaired children. *Topics in Language Disorders, 7*(2), 45–60.

Dollaghan, C., and Campbell, T. (1992). A procedure for classifying disruptions in spontaneous language samples. *Topics in Language Disorders, 12*(2), 56–68.

Dollaghan, C., and Miller, J. (1986). Observational methods in the study of communicative competence. In R. Schiefelbusch (Ed.), *Language competence: Assessment and intervention* (pp. 99–130). San Diego, CA: College-Hill Press.

Donahue, M., Pearl, R., and Bryan, T. (1983). Communicative competence in learning disabled children. In K. Gadow and I. Bialer (Eds.), *Advances in learning and behavior disabilities* (Vol. 2). Greenwich, CT: JAI Press.

Donnellan, A., Mirenda, P., Mesaros, R., and Fassbender, L. (1984). Analyzing the communicative functions of aberrant behavior. *Journal of the Association for Persons with Severe Handicaps, 9*(3), 201–212.

Donovan, E. (1993). "I NO I NOT EASY TO HELP BUT KEEP HELPING ME." Facilitated communication and behavior management. In D. Smukler (Ed.), *First words: Facilitated communication and the inclusion of young children* (2nd ed.) (pp. 269–314). Syracuse, NY: Jowonio School.

Dore, J. (1975). Holophrases, speech acts, and language universals. *Journal of Child Language, 2,* 21–40.

Dore, J. (1983). Feeling, form, and intention in the baby's transition to language. In R. Golinkoff (Ed.), *The transition from prelinguistic to linguistic communication.* Hillsdale, NJ: Erlbaum.

Dore, J. (1986). The development of conversational competence. In R. Schiefelbusch (Ed.), *Language competence: Assessment and intervention.* San Diego, CA: College-Hill Press.

Dorris, M. (1989). *The broken chord.* New York: Harper Perennial.

Down, M. (1980). The hearing of Down's individuals. *Seminars in Speech and Language, 1,* 24–38.

Duchan, J. (1983). Language processing and geodesic domes. In T. Gallagher, and C. Prutting (Eds.), *Pragmatic assessment and intervention issues in language* (pp. 83–100). San Diego, CA: College-Hill Press.

Duchan, J. (1988). Assessment principles and procedures. In N. Lass, L. McReynolds, J. Northern, and D. Yoder (Eds.), *Handbook of speech-language pathology and audiology* (pp. 356–376). Philadelphia, PA: B.C. Decker.

Duchan, J., and Weitzner-Lin, B. (1987). Nurturant naturalistic intervention for language-impaired children: Implications for planning lessons and tracking progress. *American Speech-Language-Hearing Association, 29*(7), 45–49.

Duncan, D. (1989). *Working with bilingual language disability.* London: Chapman and Hall.

Dunlea, A. (1984). The relationship between concept formation and semantic roles: some evidence from the blind. In L. Feagans, C. Garvey, and R. Golinkoff (Eds.), *The origins and growth of communication* (pp. 224–244). Norwood, NJ: Ablex.

Dunlea, A. (1989). *Vision and the emergence of meaning: Blind and sighted children's early language.* New York: Cambridge University Press.

Dunn, J., Bretherton, I., and Munn, P. (1987). Conversations about feeling states between mothers and their young children. *Developmental Psychology, 23,* 132–139.

Durning, A. (1992). Life on the brink. In G. Albee, L. Bond, T. Cook-Monsey (Eds.), *Improving children's lives: Global perspectives on prevention* (pp. 37–48). Newbury Park, CA: Sage Publications.

Dweck, C., and Licht, B. (1980). Learned helplessness and intellectual achievement. In J. Gerber and M. Seligman (Eds.), *Human helplessness: Theory and application.* New York: Academic Press.

Dyslexia's cause is reportedly found. (1987, January 13). *New York Times.*

Edwards, M., and Shriberg, L. (1983). *Phonology: Applications in communicative disorders.* San Diego, CA: College-Hill Press.

Ehren, T. (1993). Tests: A significant difference? *American Journal of Speech-Language Pathology, 2*(1), 17–19.

Eimas, P., and Clarkson, R. (1986). Speech perception in children: Are there effects of otitis media? In J. Kavanaugh (Ed.), *Otitis media and child development* (pp. 139–159). Parkton, MD: York Press.

Eisenson, J. (1972). *Aphasia in children.* New York: Harper and Row.

Elliott, J. and Connolly, K. (1984). A classification of manipulative hand movements. *Developmental Medicine and Child Neurology, 26*(3), 283–295.

Elstner, W. (1983). Abnormalities in the verbal communication of visually impaired children. In A. Mills (Ed.), *Language acquisition in the blind child: Normal and deficient* (pp. 18–41). San Diego, CA: College-Hill Press.

English, A., and Henry, M. (1990). Legal issues affecting drug exposed infants. *Youth Law News, 11*(1), 1–33.

Ensher, G. (1989). The first three years: Special education perspectives on assessment and intervention. *Topics in Language Disorders, 10*(1), 80–90.

Epstein, K. (1985). Analysis: Measurement of cognitive potential in learning impaired learners. In D. Martin (Ed.), *Cognition, education, and deafness: Directions for research and instruction* (pp. 156–164). Washington, DC: Gallaudet University Press.

Erickson, J., and Iglesias, A. (1986). Speech and language disorders in Hispanics. In O. Taylor (Ed.), *Nature of communication disorders in culturally and linguistically diverse populations* (pp. 181–218). San Diego, CA: College-Hill Press.

Erickson, J., and Walker, C. (1983). Bilingual exceptional children: What are the issues? In D. Omark and J. Erickson (Eds.), *The bilingual exceptional child* (pp. 3–23). San Diego, CA: College-Hill Press.

Erickson, M. (1978). *Child psychopathology.* Englewood Cliffs, NJ: Prentice-Hall.

Erin, J. (1990). Language samples from visually impaired four and five year olds. *Journal of Childhood Communication Disorders, 13*(2), 181–191.

Erting, C., Prezioso, C., and Hynes, M. (1990). The interactional context of deaf mother-infant communication. In V. Volterra and C. Erting (Eds.), *From gesture to language in hearing and deaf children.* Berlin: Springer-Verlag.

Estrin, E., and Chaney, C. (1988). Developing a concept of the word. *Childhood Education, 43,* 78–82.

Fantini, M. (1972). Beyond cultural deprivation and compensatory education. In R. Abrahams and R. Troike (Eds.), *Language and cultural diversity in American education* (pp. 16–19). Englewood Cliffs, NJ: Prentice-Hall.

Faye, E. (Ed.). (1976). *Clinical low vision.* New York: Little, Brown and Company.

Feagans, L. (1986). Otitis media: A model for long-term effects with implications for intervention. In J. Kavanaugh (Ed.), *Otitis media and child development* (pp. 192–208). Parkton, MD: York Press.

Feagans, L., Blood, I., and Tubman, J. (1988). Otitis media: Models of effects and implications for intervention. In F. Bess (Ed.), *Hearing impairment in children* (pp. 347–374). Parkton, MD: York Press.

Feagans, L., Garvey, C., and Golinkoff, R. (Eds.). (1984). *The origin and growth of communication.* New York: Academic Press.

Ferguson, M. (1991). Collaborative/consultative service delivery: An introduction. *Language, Speech, and Hearing Services in Schools, 22*(3), 147.

Ferguson, M. (1992). Clinical forum: Implementing collaborative consultation. The transition to collaborative teaching. *Language, Speech, and Hearing Services in Schools, 23,* 371–372.

Fernald, A. (1984). The perceptual and affective salience of mother's speech to infants. In L. Feagans, C. Garvey, and R. Golinkoff (Eds.), *The origin and growth of communication.* New York: Academic Press.

Fernald, A. (1985). Four-month-old infants prefer to listen to motherese. *Infant Behavior and Development, 8,* 181–195.

Fernald, A. (1991). Prosody and focus in speech to infants and adults. *Developmental Psychology, 27,* 209–221.

Fernald, A., and Kuhl, P. (1987). Acoustic determinants of infants' preference for motherese speech. *Infant Behavior and Development, 10,* 279–293.

Field, D., Muir, D., Pilon, R., Sinclair, M., and Dodwell, P. (1980). Infants' orientation to lateral sounds from birth to 3 months. *Child Development, 50,* 295–298.

Field, T., and Fox, N. (Eds.). (1985). *Social perception in infants.* Norwood, NJ: Ablex.

Field, T., Woodson, R., Cohen, D., Greenberg, R., Garcia, R., and Collins, K. (1983). Discrimination and imitation of facial expressions by term and preterm neonates. *Infant Behavior and Development, 6,* 485–490.

Field, T., Woodson, R., Greenberg, R., and Cohen, D. (1982). Discrimination and imitation of facial expressions by neonates. *Science, 218,* 179–181.

Fink, J. (1990). Reported effects of crack and cocaine on infants. *Youth Law News: Special Issue,* 37–39.

Fiore, T., Becker, E., and Nero, R. (1993). Educational interventions for students with attention deficit disorder. *Exceptional Children, 60*(2), 163–173.

Fischler, R. (1988). The pediatrician's role in early identification. In E. Cherow, N. Matkin, and R. Trybus (Eds.), *Hearing impaired children and youth with developmental disabilities* (pp. 101–121). Washington, DC: Gallaudet University Press.

Fisher, A., Murray, E., and Bundy, A. (1991). *Sensory integration: Theory and practice.* Philadelphia, PA: F.A. Davis.

Fletcher, P., and Hall, D. (Eds.). (1992). *Specific speech and language disorders in children.* San Diego, CA: Singular Publishing Group.

Fontaine, R. (1984). Imitative skills between birth and 6 months. *Infant Behavior and Development, 7,* 323–333.

Ford, A., and Mirenda, P. (1984). Community instruction: A natural cues and corrections decision model. *Journal of the Association for Persons with Severe Handicaps, 9,* 79–88.

Forrell, E., and Hood, J. (1985). A longitudinal study of two groups of children with early reading problems. *Annals of Dyslexia, 35,* 97–116.

Foss, J. (1991). Nonverbal learning disabilities and remedial intervention. *Annals of Dyslexia, 41,* 128–140.

Foster, S. (1985). The development of discourse topic skills by infants and young children. *Topics in Language Disorders, 5,* 31–45.

Fox, B., and Routh, D. (1980). Phonemic analysis and severe reading disability in children. *Journal of Psycholinguistic Research, 9,* 115–119.

Fox, B., and Routh, D. (1983). Reading disability, phonemic analysis, and dysphonetic spelling: A follow-up study. *Journal of Clinical Child Psychology, 12,* 28–32.

Fox, L., Long, S., and Langlois, A. (1988). Patterns of language comprehension deficit in abused and neglected children. *Journal of Speech and Hearing Disorders, 53*(3), 239–244.

Fraiberg, S. (1974). Blind infants and their mothers: An examination of the sign system. In M. Lewis and A. Rosenblum (Eds.), *The effects of the infant on its caregiver* (pp. 215–232). New York: John Wiley and Sons.

Fraiberg, S. (1977). *Insights from the blind: Comparative studies of blind and sighted infants.* New York: Basic Books.

Fraiberg, S., and Adelson, E. (1975). Self-representation in young blind children. In E. Lenneberg and E. Lenneberg (Eds.), *Foundations of language development: A multidisciplinary approach* (Vol. 2, pp. 177–192). New York: Academic Press.

Frauenheim, J., and Heckerl, J. (1983). A longitudinal study of psychological and achievement test performance in severe dyslexic adults. *Journal of Learning Disabilities, 16,* 339–47.

Freeman, N., Lloyd, S., and Sinha, C. (1980). Infant search tasks reveal early concepts of containment and canonical usage of objects. *Cognition, 8,* 243–262.

Fried, P., and O'Connell, C. (1987). A comparison of the effects of prenatal exposure to tobacco, alcohol, cannabis, and caffeine on birth size and subsequent growth. *Neurotoxicology and Teratology, 9,* 79–85.

Fried, P., and Watkinson, B. (1990). 36- and 48-month neurobehavioral follow-up of children prenatally exposed to marihuana, cigarettes, and alcohol. *Journal of Developmental Behavior in Pediatrics, 11,* 4958.

Fried, P., Watkinson, B., Dillon, R., and Dulberg, E. (1987). Neonatal neurological status in a low-risk population after prenatal exposure to cigarettes, marijuana, and alcohol. *Journal of Developmental and Behavioral Pediatrics, 8,* 318–326.

Frith, U. (1993). Autism. *Scientific American, 268*(6), 108–114.

Fujiki, M., and Brinton, B. (1987). Elicited imitation revisited: A comparison with spontaneous language production. *Language, Speech, and Hearing Services in Schools, 18*(4), 301–311.

Gaddes, W. (1985). *Learning disabilities and brain function: A neurological approach* (2nd ed.). New York: Springer-Verlag.

Galaburda, A. (1983). Developmental dyslexia: Current anatomical research. *Annals of Dyslexia, 33,* 41–54.

Galaburda, A. (1985). Developmental dyslexia: A review of biological interactions. *Annals of Dyslexia, 35,* 21–34.

Galaburda, A. (1989). Ordinary and extraordinary brain development: Anatomical variation in developmental dyslexia. *Annals of Dyslexia, 39,* 67–80.

Ganschow, L. (1984). Analysis of written language of a language learning disabled (dyslexic) college student and instructional implications. *Annals of Dyslexia, 34,* 271–284.

Garcia, G. (1992). Ethnography and classroom communication: Taking an "emic" perspective. *Topics in Language Disorders, 12* (3), 54–66.

Gardner, H. (1983). *Frames of mind.* New York: Basic Books.

Gartner, A., and Lipsky, D. (1987). Beyond special education: Toward a quality system for all students. *Harvard Educational Review, 57*(4), 367–395.

Garvey, C. (1990). *Play.* Cambridge, MA: Harvard University Press.

Gavelek, J., and Raphael, T. (1982). Instructing metacognitive awareness of question-answer relationships: Implications for the learning disabled. *Topics in Learning and Learning Disabilities, 2*(1), 69–77.

Geers, A., Moog, J., and Schick, B. (1984). Acquisition of spoken and signed English by profoundly deaf children. *Journal of Speech and Hearing Disorders, 49,* 378–388.

Gerber, A. (1991). *Language-related learning disabilities: Their nature and treatment.* Baltimore, MD: Paul H. Brookes.

Gerhardt, J. (1982). The development of object play and classification skills in a blind child. *Journal of Visual Impairment and Blindness, 76,* 219–223.

Gerner de Garcia, B. (1993). Addressing the needs of Hispanic deaf children. In K. Christensen and G. Delgado (Eds.), *Multicultural issues in deafness* (pp. 69–90). White Plains, NY: Longman.

Gersten, R., and Domino, J. (1989). Teaching literature to at risk students. *Educational Leadership, 46*(5), 53–58.

Gersten, R., and Woodward, J. (1990). Rethinking the regular education initiative: Focus on the classroom teacher. *Remedial and Special Education, 11*(3), 7–16.

Giangreco, C., and Giangreco, M. (1980). Reverse mainstreaming: A different approach. *American Annals of the Deaf, 125*(4), 491–494.

Gibson, E., and Spelke, E.(1983). The development of perception. In J. Flavell and E. Markman (Eds.), *Handbook of child psychology: Vol. 3. Cognitive development* (pp. 1–76). New York: John Wiley and Sons.

Glasscock, M., McKennan, K., and Levine, S. (1988). Differential diagnosis of sensorineural hearing loss in children. In F. Bess (Ed.), *Hearing impairment in children* (pp. 1–14). Parkton, MD: York Press.

Gleason, J. (1989). *The development of language* (2nd ed.). New York: Macmillan.

Gloeckler, L. (1991). Fostering integration through curriculum development. *Teaching Exceptional Children, 23*(3), 52–53.

Godfrey, J., Syrdal-Lasky, A., Millaj, K., and Knox, C. (1981). Performance of dyslexic children on speech perception tests. *Journal of Experimental Child Psychology, 32,* 401–424.

Gold, S., and Sherry, L. (1984). Hyperactivity, learning disabilities, and alcohol. *Journal of Learning Disabilities, 17*(1), 3–6.

Goldberg, S. (1982). Some biological aspects of early parent infant interaction. In S. Moore and C. Cooper (Eds.), *The young child: Reviews of research.* Washington, DC: National Association for the Education of Young Children.

Goldfield, B. (1985/86). Referential and expressive language: A study of two mother-child dyads. *First Language, 6,* 119–131.

Goldfield, B. (1987). The contributions of child and caregiver to referential and expressive language. *Applied Psycholinguistics, 8,* 267–280.

Goldfield, B., and Snow, C. (1989). Individual differences in language acquisition. In J. Gleason (Ed.), *The development of language* (2nd ed.) (pp. 303–325). New York: Charles E. Merrill.

Golinkoff, R. (Ed.). (1983). *The transition from prelinguistic to linguistic communication.* Hillsdale, NJ: Erlbaum.

Golinkoff, R., and Gordon, L.(1988). What makes communication run?: Characteristics of immediate successes. *First Language, 8,* 103–124.

Goodman, K. (1986). *What's whole in whole language?* Portsmouth, NH: Heinemann.

Gopnik, A., and Meltzoff, A. (1984). Semantic and cognitive development in 15–21 month old children. *Journal of Child Language, 11*, 495–513.

Gopnik, A., and Meltzoff, A. (1987a). Early semantic developments and their relation to object permanence, means-ends understanding, and categorization. In K. Nelson and A. van Kleeck (Eds.), *Children's language* (Vol. 6, pp. 191–212). Hillsdale, NJ: Erlbaum.

Gopnik, A., and Meltzoff, A. (1987b). The development of categorization in the second year and its relation to other cognitive and linguistic developments. *Child Development, 58,* 1523–1531.

Graham, S., and Harris, K. (1989a). Components analysis of cognitive strategy instruction: Effects on learning disabled students' compositions and self-efficacy. *Journal of Educational Psychology, 81,* 353–361.

Graham, S., and Harris, K. (1989b). Cognitive training: Implications for written language. In J. Hughes and R. Hall (Eds.), *Cognitive behavioral psychology in the schools: A comprehensive handbook* (pp. 247–279). New York: Guilford.

Greenfield, P. (1980). Toward an operational and logical analysis of intentionality: The use of discourse in early child language. In D. Olson (Ed.), *The social foundations of language and thought.* New York: Norton.

Greenspan, S. (1992). Reconsidering the diagnosis and treatment of very young children with autistic spectrum or pervasive developmental disorder. *Zero to Three, 13*(2), 1–9.

Gregory, S., and Mogford, K. (1981). Early language development in deaf children. In B. Woll, J. Kyle, and Deuchar, M. (Eds.), *Perspectives on British Sign Language and deafness* (pp. 218–237). London, England: Croom Helm.

Griffith, D. (1988). The effects of perinatal cocaine exposure on infant neurobehavior and early maternal-infant interactions. In I. Chasnoff (Ed.), *Drugs, alcohol, pregnancy and parenting* (pp. 105–113). Hingham, MA: Kluwer Academic.

Grimes, L. (1981). Learned helplessness and attribution theory: Redefining children's learning problems. *Learning Disability Quarterly, 4,* 91–100.

Grossen, B. (1991). The fundamental skills of higher order thinking. *Journal of Learning Disabilities, 24*(6), 343–353.

Grossman, H., (Ed.). (1983). *Classification in mental retardation.* Washington, DC: American Association on Mental Deficiency.

Gustason, G. (1983). Where do we go from here? In J. Kyle and B. Woll (Eds.), *Language in sign: An international perspective on sign language.* London, England: Croom Helm.

Gustason, G., Pfetzing, D., and Zawolkow, E. (1980). *Signing exact english.* Rossmoor, CA: Modern Signs Press.

Gutowski, W., and Chechile, R. (1987). Encoding, storage, and retrieval components of associative memory deficits of mildly mentally retarded adults. *American Journal of Mental Deficiency, 92,* 85–93.

Hall, A. (1981). Mental images and cognitive development of the congenitally blind. *Journal of Visual Impairment and Blindness, 76,* 281–285.

Hallahan, D. (1992). Some thoughts on why the prevalence of learning disabilities has increased. *Journal of Learning Disabilities, 25*(8), 523–528.

Hallahan, D., and Bryan, T. (1981). Learning disabilities. In J. Kauffman and D. Hallahan (Eds.), *Handbook of special education.* Englewood Cliffs, NJ: Prentice-Hall.

Halle, J. (1984). Arranging the natural environment to occasion language: Giving severely language-delayed children reasons to communicate. *Seminars in Speech and Language, 5*(3), 185–198.

Halliday, M. (1975). *Learning how to mean: Explorations in the development of language.* New York: Edward Arnold.

Hammill, D. (1990). On defining learning disabilities: An emerging consensus. *Journal of Learning Disabilities, 23*(2), 74–84.

Hammond, S., and Meiners, L. (1993). American Indian deaf children and youth. In K. Christensen and G. Delgado (Eds.), *Multicultural issues in deafness* (pp. 143–166). White Plains, NY: Longman.

Harding, C. (1983). Setting the stage for language acquisition: Communication development in the first year. In R. Golinkoff (Ed.), *The transition from prelinguistic to linguistic communication*. Hillsdale, NJ: Erlbaum.

Harris, K. (1991). An expanded view on consultation competencies for educators serving culturally and linguistically diverse exceptional students. *Teacher Education and Special Education, 14*(1), 25–29.

Harris, M., Barrett, M., Jones, D., and Brooks, S. (1988). Linguistic input and early word meanings. *Journal of Child Language, 15*, 77–94.

Hart, B. (1981). Pragmatics: How language is used. *Analysis and Intervention in Developmental Disabilities, 1*, 299–313.

Hasan, R., and Martin, J. (Eds.). (1989). *Language development: Learning language, learning culture*. Norwood, NJ: Ablex.

Hegde, M. (1991). *Introduction to communication disorders*. Austin, TX: Pro-Ed.

Heimann, M., and Schaller, J. (1985). Imitative reactions among 14–21-day-old infants. *Infant Mental Health Journal, 6*, 31–39.

Henderson, D., and Hendershott, A. (1991). ASL and the family system. *American Annals of the Deaf, 136*(4), 325–329.

Hill, D., and Leary, M. (1993). *Movement disturbance: A clue to hidden competencies in persons diagnosed with autism and other developmental disabilities*. Madison, WI: DRI Press.

Hirsh-Pasek, K., Treiman, R., and Schneiderman, M. (1984). Brown and Hamlon revisited: Mother's sensitivity to ungrammatical forms. *Journal of Child Language, 11*, 81–88.

Hodson, B., and Paden, E. (1983). *Targeting intelligible speech*. San Diego, CA: College-Hill Press.

Hoffmeister, R. (1982). Acquisition of signed languages by deaf children. In H. Holman and R. Wilbur (Eds.), *Communication in two societies* (pp. 165–205). Washington, DC: Gallaudet University Press.

Holmes, K., and Holmes, D. (1980). Signed and spoken language development in a hearing child of hearing parents. *Sign Language Studies, 28*, 239–254.

Holmes, A., and Weitzner, L. (1990). Communication characteristics and strategies for intervention. *Outreach, 6*(2), 1–13.

Hoover, J., and Collier, C. (1991). Teacher preparation for educating culturally and linguistically diverse exceptional learners. *Teacher Education and Special Education, 14*(1), 3–4.

Horner, R., Sprague, J., and Wilcox, B. (1982). General case programming for community activities. In B. Wilcox and G. Bellamy (Eds.), *Design of high school programs for severely handicapped students* (pp. 61–98). Baltimore, MD: Paul H.Brookes.

Howard, J., Beckwith, L., Rodning, C., and Kropenske, V. (1989). The development of young children of substance-abusing parents: Insights from seven years of intervention and research. *Zero to Three, 9*(5), 8–12.

Hoyme, H., Jones, K., Dixon, S., Jewett, T., Hanson, J., Robinson, L., Msall, L., and Allanson, J. (1990). Prenatal cocaine exposure and fetal vascular disruption. *Pediatrics, 85*, 743–747.

Hull, R., and Dilka, K. (1984). *The hearing impaired child in school*. Orlando, FL: Grune and Stratton.

Hulme, C. (1981). The effects of manual training on memory in normal and retarded readers: Some implications for multisensory teaching. *Psychological Research, 43*, 179–191.

Humphries, T. (1993). Deaf culture and cultures. In K. Christensen and G. Delgado (Eds.), *Multicultural issues in deafness* (pp. 3–15). White Plains, NY: Longman.

Hunter, M. (1986). Knowing teaching and supervising. In P. Hosford (Ed.), *Using what we know about teaching*. Alexandria, VA: ASCD.

Hynd, G., and Semrud-Clikeman, M. (1989). Dyslexia and neurodevelopmental pathology: Relationship to cognition, intelligence and reading skill acquisition. *Journal of Learning Disabilities, 22*(4), 204–216.

Idol, L. (1987). Group story mapping: A comprehension strategy for both skilled and unskilled readers. *Journal of Learning Disabilities, 20*(4), 196–205.

Izard, C., Huebner, R., Risser, D., McGuiness, G., and Dougherty, L. (1980). The young infants' ability to produce discrete emotion expressions. *Developmental Psychology, 16*(2), 132–140.

Jackson-Maldonado, D. (1993). Mexico and the United States: A cross-cultural perspective on the education of deaf children. In K. Christensen and G. Delgado (Eds.), *Multicultural issues in deafness* (pp. 91–112). White Plains, NY: Longman.

Jacobson, J. (1982). Problem behavior and psychiatric impairment with a developmentally disabled population: I. Behavior frequency. *Applied Research in Mental Retardation, 3,* 121–139.

Jacobson, S. (1979). Matching behavior in the young infant. *Child Development, 50,* 425–430.

James, S. (1989). Assessing children with language disorders. In D. Bernstein and E. Tiegerman (Eds.), *Language and communication disorders in children* (2nd ed.) (pp.157–207). Columbus, OH: Charles E. Merrill.

Jerger, S., Jerger, J., Alford, B., and Abrams, S. (1983). Development of speech intelligibility in children with recurrent otitis media. *Ear and Hearing, 4*(3), 138–145.

Johnson, D. (1985). Using reading and writing to improve oral language skills. *Topics in Language Disorders, 5*(3), 55–69.

Johnson, D. (1988). Review of research on specific reading, writing, and mathematics disorders. In J. Kavanagh and T. Truss, Jr. (Eds.), *Learning disabilities: Proceedings of the national conference.* Parkton, MD: York Press.

Johnson, D., and Myklebust, H. (1967). *Learning disabilities: Educational principles and practices.* New York: Grune and Stratton.

Johnson, D., and Whitehead, R. (1989). Effect of maternal rubella on hearing and vision: A twenty year post-epidemic study. *American Annals of the Deaf, 134*(3), 232–242.

Johnston, J. (1988). Specific language disorders in the child. In N. Lass, L. McReynolds, J. Northern, and D. Yoder (Eds.), *Handbook of speech-language pathology and audiology* (pp. 685–715). Philadelphia, PA: B.C. Decker.

Johnston, J. (1991). The continuing relevance of cause: A reply to Leonard's "specific language impairment as a clinical category," *Language, Speech, and Hearing Services in Schools, 22,* 75–79.

Jones, K., and Smith, D. (1973). Recognition of the fetal alcohol syndrome in early infancy. *Lancet, 2,* 999–1001.

Kaiser, A., and Warren, S. (1988). Pragmatics and generalization. In R. Schiefelbusch and L. Lloyd (Eds.), *Language perspectives: Acquisition, retardation, and intervention* (2nd ed.)(pp. 393–442). Baltimore, MD: University Park Press.

Kaitz, M., Meschulach-Sarfaty, O., Auerbach, J., and Eidelman, A.(1988). A reexamination of newborn's ability to imitate facial expressions. *Developmental Psychology, 24,* 3–7.

Kalmanson, B. (1992). Diagnosis and treatment of infants and young children with pervasive developmental disorders. *Zero to Three, 13*(2), 21–26.

Kamhi, A., and Johnston, J. (1982). Toward an understanding of retarded children's linguistic deficiencies. *Journal of Speech and Hearing Research, 25,* 435–445.

Kamhi, A., and Koenig, L. (1985). Metalinguistic awareness in normal and language-disordered children. *Language, Speech, and Hearing Services in Schools, 16,* 199–210.

Kamhi, A., and Masterson, J. (1989). Language and cognition in the mentally handicapped: Last rites for the difference-delay controversy. In B. Beveridge, G. Conti-Ramsden, and I. Leudar (Eds.), *Language and communication in mentally handicapped children.* London: Routledge, Chapman, and Hall.

Kanner, L. (1943). Autistic disturbances of affective contact. *Nervous Child, 2,* 217–250.

Kanner, L. (1985a). Autistic disturbances of affective contact. In A. Donnellan (Ed.), *Classic readings in autism* (pp. 11–50). New York: Teachers College Press.

Kanner, L. (1985b). Follow-up study of eleven autistic children originally reported in 1943. In A. Donnellan (Ed.), *Classic readings in autism* (pp. 223–234). New York: Teachers College Press.

Kantor, R. (1982). Communicative interaction: Mother modification and child acquisition of American Sign Language. *Sign Language Studies, 36,* 233–282.

Karchmer, M. (1985). A demographic perspective. In E. Cherow, N. Matkin, and R. Trybus (Eds.), *Hearing-impaired children and youth with developmental disabilities* (pp. 36–56). Washington, DC: Gallaudet University Press.

Karlan, G., and Lloyd, L. (1983). Consideration in the planning of communication intervention: I. Selecting the lexicon. *Journal of the Association for Severely Handicapped, 8,* 13–25.

Katz, K. (1992). Communication problems in maltreated children: A tutorial. *Journal of Childhood Communication Disorders, 14*(2), 147–163.

Katz, R., Shankweiler, D., and Liberman, I. (1981). Memory for item order and phonetic recoding in the beginning reader. *Journal of Experimental Child Psychology, 32,* 474–484.

Kauffman, J., Gerber, M., and Semmel, M. (1988). Arguable assumptions underlying the regular education initiative. *Journal of Learning Disabilities, 21*(1), 6–11.

Kavanagh, J., and Truss, T., Jr. (Eds.). (1988). *Learning disabilities: Proceedings of the national conference.* Parkton, MD: York Press.

Kaye, K., and Charney, R. (1981). Conversational asymmetry between mothers and children. *Journal of Child Language, 8,* 35–49.

Kayser, H. (1989). Speech and language assessment of Spanish English speaking children. *Language, Speech, and Hearing Services in Schools, 20*(3), 226–244.

Kelly, D., Forney, J., Parker-Fisher, S., and Jones, M. (1993a). The challenge of attention deficit disorder in children who are deaf or hard of hearing. *American Annals of the Deaf, 138*(4), 343–348.

Kelly, D., Forney, J., Parker-Fisher, S., and Jones, M. (1993b). Evaluating and managing attention deficit disorder in children who are deaf or hard of hearing. *American Annals of the Deaf, 138*(4), 349–357.

Kelly, D., Kelly, B., Jones, M., Moulton, N., Verhulst, S., and Bell, S. (1993). Attention deficits in children and adolescents with hearing loss: A survey. *American Journal of Diseases of Children, 147*(7), 737.

Keogh, B. (1988). Improving services for problem learners: Rethinking and restructuring. *Journal of Learning Disabilities, 21*(1), 19–22.

Kernan, K., and Sabsay, S. (1989). Communication in social interactions: Aspects of an ethnography of mildly mentally handicapped adults. In M. Beveridge, G. Conti-Ramsden, and I. Leudar (Eds.), *Language and communication in mentally handicapped people* (pp. 229–253). London: Routledge, Chapman and Hall.

King, C. (1984). National survey of language methods used with hearing impaired students in the United States. *American Annals of the Deaf, 129,* 311–316.

King, D., and Goodman, K. (1990). Whole language: Cherishing learners and their language. *Language, Speech, and Hearing Services in Schools, 21*(4), 221–227.

King, R., Jones, D., and Lasky, E. (1982). In retrospect: A 15 year follow-up of speech-language disordered children. *Language, Speech, and Hearing Services in Schools, 13,* 24–32.

Kirchner, C., and Peterson, R. (1980). Multiple impairments among non-institutionalized blind and visually impaired persons. *Journal of Visual Impairment and Blindness, 74,* 42–44.

Kitz, W., and Tarver, S. (1989). Comparison of dyslexic and nondyslexic adults on decoding and phonemic awareness tasks. *Annals of Dyslexia, 39,* 196–205.

Klecan-Aker, J., and Kelty, K. (1990). An investigation of the oral narratives of normal and language-learning disabled children. *Journal of Childhood Communication Disorders, 13*(2), 207–216.

Klee, T. (1985). Role of inversion in children's question development. *Journal of Speech and Hearing Research, 28*(2), 225–232.

Klee, T. (1992). Developmental and diagnostic characteristics of quantitative measures of children's language production. *Topics in Language Disorders, 12*(2), 28–41.

Klein, J. (1986). Risk factors for otitis media in children. In J. Kavanagh (Ed.), *Otitis media and child development* (pp. 45–51). Parkton, MD: York Press.

Klima, E., and Bellugi, U. (1979). *The signs of language.* Cambridge, MA: Harvard University Press.

Klink, M., Gerstman, L., Raphael, L., Schlanger, B., and Newsome, L. (1986). Phonological process usage by young EMR children and nonretarded preschool children. *American Journal of Mental Deficiency, 91,* 190–195.

Kluwin, T. (1983). Discourse in deaf classrooms: The structure of teaching episodes. *Discourse Processes, 6,* 275–293.

Knell, S., and Klonoff, E. (1983). Language sampling in deaf children: A comparison of oral and signed communication modes. *Journal of Communication Disorders, 16,* 435–447.

Kolb, B., and Whishaw, I. (1985). *Fundamentals of human neuro-psychology* (2nd ed.). San Francisco, CA: W.H. Freeman and Company.

Kolligian, K., and Sternberg, R. (1987). Intelligence, information processing, and specific learning disabilities: A triarchic synthesis. *Journal of Learning Disabilities, 20,* 8–17.

Korhonen, T. (1991). Neuropsychological stability and prognosis of subgroups of children with learning disabilities. *Journal of Learning Disabilities, 24,* 48–52.

Kretschmer, R., and Kretschmer, L. (Eds.). (1988). Communication assessment of hearing impaired children: From conversation to classroom. *Journal of the Academy for Rehabilitative Audiology Monograph Supplement, 21.*

Kretschmer, R., and Kretschmer, L. (1989). Communication competence: Impact of the pragmatics revolution on education of hearing impaired individuals. *Topics in Language Disorders, 9*(4) 1–16.

Kronick, D. (1981). *Social development of learning disabled persons.* San Francisco, CA: Jossey-Bass.

Kronstadt, D. (1991). Complex developmental issues of prenatal drug exposure. *The Future of Children, 1*(1), 36–49.

Kuczaj, S. (1987). Deferred imitation and the acquisition of novel lexical items. *First Language, 7,* 177–182.

Kuhl, P., and Meltzoff, A. (1982). A bimodal perception of speech in infancy. *Science, 218,* 1138–1141.

Kuhl, P., and Meltzoff, A. (1988). Speech as an intermodal object of perception. In A. Yonas (Ed.), *Perceptual development in infancy: Vol. 20. Minnesota symposia on child psychology* (pp. 235–266). Hillsdale, NJ: Erlbaum.

Kysela, G., Holdgrafer, G., McCarthy, C., and Stewart, T. (1990). Turn taking and pragmatic language skills of developmentally delayed children: A research note. *Journal of Communication Disorders, 23,* 135–149.

Lahey, M. (1988). *Language disorders and language development.* New York: Macmillan.

Lahey, M. (1990). Who shall be called language disordered? Some reflections and one perspective. *Journal of Speech and Hearing Disorders, 55*(4), 612–620.

Landau, B., and Gleitman, L. (1985). *Language and experience: Evidence from the blind child.* Cambridge, MA: Harvard University Press.

Langdon, H. (1983). Assessment and intervention strategies for the bilingual language disordered student. *Exceptional Children, 50,* 37–45.

Langdon, H. (1989). Language disorder or difference? Assessing the language skills of Hispanic students. *Exceptional Children, 56*(2), 160–167.

Larson, V., and McKinley, N. (1987). *Communication assessment and intervention strategies for adolescents.* Eau Claire, WI: Thinking Publications.

Larson, V., McKinley, N., and Boley, D. (1993). Service delivery models for adolescents with language disorders. *Language, Speech, and Hearing Services in Schools, 24*(1), 36–42.

La Sasso, C. (1987). Survey of reading instruction for hearing impaired students in the United States. *Volta Review, 89,* 85–98.

La Vigna, G. (1987). Non-aversive strategies for managing behavior problems. In D. Cohen and A. Donnellan (Eds.) *Handbook of autism and pervasive developmental disorder.* New York: John Wiley and Sons.

Leary, M. (1992, October). *A speech pathologist's point of view on autism and communication.* Presentation at the Geneva Centre Conference, Toronto, Canada.

Leary, W. (1993, March 10). U.S. panel backs testing all babies to uncover hearing losses early. *The New York Times,* p. C12.

Lee, L. (1974). *Developmental sentence analysis.* Evanston, IL: Northwestern University Press.

Lefevre, A. (1975). Language development in malnourished children. In E. H. Lenneberg and E. Lenneberg (Eds.), *Foundations of language development: Vol. 2. A multidisciplinary approach* (pp. 279–295). New York: Academic Press.

Leiter, R. (1979). *Leiter international performance scale.* Chicago, IL: Stoelting.

Lemoine, P., Harousseau, H., Bortenyu, J., and Menuet, J. (1968). Les enfants de parents alcololiques: Anamalies observée à propos de 127 cas. (The children of alcoholic parents: Anomalies observed in 127 cases.), *Quest Medicale, 21,* 476–482.

Leonard, L. (1990). Language disorders in preschool children. In G. Shames and E. H. Wiig (Eds.), *Human communication disorders: An introduction* (3rd ed.) (pp. 159–192). New York: Charles E. Merrill.

Leonard, L. (1991). Specific language impairment as a clinical category. *Language, Speech, and Hearing Services in Schools, 22,* 66–68.

Leonard, L., and Reid, L. (1979). Children's judgments of utterance appropriateness. *Journal of Speech and Hearing Research, 22,* 500–515.

Lerner, J. (1985). *Learning disabilities: Theories, diagnosis, and teaching strategies* (4th ed.). Dallas, TX: Houghton Mifflin.

Lesar, S. (1992). Prenatal cocaine exposure: The challenge to education. In L. Rosetti (Ed.), *Developmental problems of drug-exposed infants* (pp. 35–52). San Diego, CA: Singular Publishing Group.

Lester, B. (1984). Infant crying and the development of communication. In N. Fox and R. Davidson (Eds.), *The psychobiology of affective development* (pp. 231–258). Hillsdale, NJ: Erlbaum.

Lester, B., Corwin, J., Sepkoski, C., Seifer, R., Peucker, M., McLaughlin, S., and Golub, H. (1991). Neurobehavioral syndromes in cocaine-exposed newborn infants. *Child Development, 62,* 694–705.

Lester, B., and Zeskind, P. (1982). A biobehavioral perspective on crying in early infancy. In H. Fitzgerald, B. Lester, and M. Yogman (Eds.), *Theory and research in behavioral pediatrics* (Vol. 1). New York: Plenum.

Levitt, A., and Aydelott-Utman, J. (1992). From babbling towards sound systems of English and French: A longitudinal two-case study. *Journal of Child Language, 19*, 19–49.

Lewis, K., Bennett, B., and Schmeder, N. (1989). The care of infants menaced by cocaine abuse. *Maternal Child Nursing, 14*(5), 324–329.

Lewitter, F., DeFries, J., and Elston, R. (1980). Genetic models of reading disability. *Behavior Genetics, 10*(1), 9–30.

Liberman, I. (1983). A language-oriented view of reading and its disabilities. In H. Myklebust (Ed.), *Progress in learning disabilities* (Vol. 5, pp. 81–101). New York: Grune and Stratton.

Liberman, I., and Liberman, A. (1990). Whole language versus code emphasis: Underlying assumptions and their implications for reading instruction. *Annals of Dyslexia, 40*, 51–76.

Liberman, I., Mann, V., Shankweiler, D., and Werfelman, M. (1982). Children's memory for recurring linguistic and nonlinguistic material in relation to reading ability. *Cortex, 18*, 367–375.

Liberman, I. Rubin, H., Duques, S., and Carlisle, J. (1985). Linguistic abilities and spelling proficiency in kindergartners and adult poor spellers. In D. Gray and J. Kavanagh (Eds.), *Biobehavioral measures of dyslexia*. Parkton, MD: York Press.

Liberman, I., and Shankweiler, D. (1985). Phonology and the problems of learning to read and write. *Remedial and Special Education, 6*(6), 8–17.

Lieven, E. (1984). Interactional style and children's language learning. *Topics in Language Disorders, 4*(4), 15–23.

Light, R. (1972). On language arts and minority group children. In R. Abrahams and R. Troike (Eds.), *Language and cultural diversity in American education* (pp. 9–15). Englewood Cliffs, NJ: Prentice-Hall.

Lindamood, P., Bell, N., and Lindamood, P. (1992). Issues in phonological awareness assessment. *Annals of Dyslexia, 42*, 242–259.

Lindfors, J. (1987). *Children's language and learning* (2nd ed.). Englewood Cliffs, NJ: Prentice-Hall.

Little, R., and Wendt, J. (1991). The effects of maternal drinking in the reproductive period: An epidemiologic review. *Journal of Substance Abuse, 3*, 187–204.

Lobato, D., Barrera, R., and Feldman, R. (1981). Sensorimotor functioning and prelinguistic communication of severely and profoundly retarded individuals. *American Journal of Mental Deficiency, 85*, 489–496.

Locke, A. (1989). Screening and intervention with children with speech and language difficulties in mainstream schools. In K. Mogford and J. Sadler (Eds.), *Child language disability: Implications in an educational setting* (pp. 40–51). Philadelphia, PA: Multilingual Matters.

Locke, J. (1993). *The child's path to spoken language*. Cambridge, MA: Harvard University Press.

Lorch, R. (1982). Priming and search processes in semantic memory: A test of three models of spreading activity. *Journal of Verbal Learning and Verbal Behavior, 21*, 468–492.

Lord, C. (1985). Contribution of behavioral approaches to the language and communication of persons with autism. In E. Schopler and G. Mesibov (Eds.), *Communication problems in autism* (pp. 59–68). New York: Plenum Press.

Lorsbach, T. (1982). Individual differences in semantic encoding processes. *Journal of Learning Disabilities, 15*, 476–480.

Los Angeles Unified School District. (1990). *Today's challenge: Teaching strategies for working with young children pre-natally exposed to drugs/alcohol.* Los Angeles, CA: Pre-natally Exposed to Drugs (PED) Program.

Lotter, V. (1985). Epidemiology of autistic conditions in young children: Part I. Prevalence. In A. Donnellan (Ed.), *Classic readings in autism* (pp. 223–234). New York: Teachers College Press.

Lucas, C., and Valli, C. (1989). Language contact in the American Deaf community. In C. Lucas (Ed.), *The sociolinguistics of the Deaf community*. San Diego, CA: Academic Press.

Luckner, J. (1991). Mainstreaming hearing impaired students: Perceptions of regular educators. *Language, Speech, and Hearing Services in Schools, 22,* 302–307.

Lund, N., and Duchan, J. F. (1988). *Assessing children's language in naturalistic contexts* (2nd ed.). Englewood Cliffs, NJ: Prentice-Hall.

Lyon, G., Newby, R., Recht, D., and Caldwell, J. (1991). Neuropsychology and learning disabilities. In B. Wong (Ed.), *Learning about learning disabilities* (pp. 375–406). New York: Academic Press.

MacArthur, C., and Graham, S. (1988). Learning disabled students composing under three methods of text production: Handwriting, word processing, and dictation. *The Journal of Special Education, 21,* 22–42.

Macchello, R. (1986). Language and autistic children. In V. Reed (Ed.), *An introduction to children with language disorders* (pp. 128–156). New York: Macmillan.

MacDonald, C. (1992). Perinatal cocaine exposure: Predictor of an endangered generation. In L. Rossetti (Ed.), *Developmental problems of drug-exposed infants* (pp. 1–12). San Diego, CA: Singular Publishing Group.

MacDonald, J., and Carroll, J. (1992). A social partnership model for assessing early communication development: An intervention model for preconversational children. *Language, Speech, and Hearing Services in Schools, 23,* 113–124.

Mahoney, G., Glover, A., and Finger, I. (1981). Relationship between language and sensorimotor development of Down syndrome and nonretarded children. *American Journal of Mental Deficiency, 86,* 21–27.

Malatesta, C. (1982). The expression and regulation of emotion: A lifespan perspective. In T. Field and A. Fogel (Eds.), *Emotion and interaction.* Hillsdale, NJ: Erlbaum.

Malatesta, C., and Haviland, J. (1982). Learning display rules: The socialization of emotion expression in infancy. *Child Development, 53,* 991–1003.

Malatesta, C., and Izard, C. (1984). The ontogenesis of human social signals: From biological imperatives to symbol utilization. In N. Fox and R. Davidson (Eds.), *The psychology of affective development* (pp. 161–206). Hillsdale, NJ: Erlbaum.

Maldonado-Colon, E. (1986). Assessment: Considerations upon interpreting data of linguistically/culturally different students referred for disabilities or disorders. In A. Willig and H. Greenberg (Eds.), *Bilingualism and learning disability.* (pp. 69–80). New York: American Library.

Mann, V. (1991). Language problems: A key to early reading problems. In Wong, B. (Ed.), *Learning about learning disabilities* (pp. 129–162). New York: Academic Press.

Mann, V. (1993). Phoneme awareness and future reading ability. *Journal of Learning Disabilities, 26*(4), 259–269.

Mann, V., and Brady, S. (1988). Reading disability: The role of language deficiencies. *Journal of Consulting and Clinical Psychology, 56,* 811–816.

Mann, V., Cowin, E., and Schoenheimer, J. (1989). Phonological processing, language comprehension, and reading ability. *Journal of Learning Disabilities, 22*(2), 76–89.

Mann, V., and Liberman, I. (1984). Phonological awareness and verbal short-term memory: Can they presage early reading success? *Journal of Learning Disabilities, 17,* 592–598.

Marcell, M., and Jett, D. (1985). Identification of vocally expressed emotions by mentally retarded and nonretarded individuals. *American Journal of Mental Deficiency, 89,* 537–545.

Marchant, C., Shurin, P., Turczyk, V. Wasikowski, D., Tutihasi, M., and Kinney, S. (1984). Course and outcome of otitis media in early infancy: A prospective study. *Journal of Pediatrics, 104,* 826–831.

Maria, K. (1990). *Reading comprehension instruction: Issues and strategies.* Parkton, MD: York Press.

Maria, K., and MacGinitie, W. (1982). Reading comprehension disabilities: Knowledge structures and nonaccommodating text processing strategies. *Annals of Dyslexia, 32,* 33–59.

Markman, E., and Gorin, L. (1981). Children's ability to adjust their standards for evaluating comprehension. *Journal of Educational Psychology, 73*, 320–325.

Martin, F., Bernstein, M., Daly, J., and Cody, J. (1988). Classroom teachers' knowledge of hearing disorders and attitudes about mainstreaming hard-of-hearing children. *Language, Speech, and Hearing Services in Schools, 19*, 83–95.

Masi, W., and Scott, K. (1983). Preterm and full term infants' visual responses to mothers' and strangers' faces. In T. Field and A. Sostek (Eds.), *Infants born at risk: Perceptual and physiological processes*. New York: Grune and Stratton.

Maskarinec, A., Cairns, G., Butterfield, E., and Weamer, D. (1981). Longitudinal observations of individual infants' vocalizations. *Journal of Speech and Hearing Disorders, 46*, 267–273.

Masterson, J. (1993). Classroom-based phonological intervention. *American Journal of Speech-Language Pathology, 2*(1), 5–9.

Masterson, J., Swirbul, T., and Noble, D. (1990). Computer generated information packets for parents. *Language, Speech, and Hearing Services in Schools, 21*(2), 114–115.

Masur, E., and Gleason, J. (1980). Parent-child interaction and the acquisition of lexical information during play. *Developmental Psychology, 16*, 404–409.

Matsuda, M. (1989). Working with parents: Some communication strategies. *Topics in Language Disorders, 9*(3), 45–53.

Maurer, H., and Newbrough, J. (1987). Facial expressions by mentally retarded and nonretarded children: Recognition by mentally retarded and nonretarded adults. *American Journal of Mental Deficiency, 91*, 505–510.

Maurer, R., and Damasio, A. (1982). Childhood autism from the point of view of behavioral neurology. *Journal of Autism and Developmental Disorders, 12*(2), 195–205.

Maxwell, M. (1986). Beginning reading and deaf children. *American Annals of the Deaf, 131*(1), 14–20.

Maxwell, S., and Wallach, G. (1984). The language-learning disabilities connection: Symptoms of early language disability change over time. In G. Wallach and K. Butler (Eds.), *Language learning disabilities in school-age children* (pp. 13–34). Baltimore, MD: Williams and Wilkins.

Mayer, P., and Lowenbraun, S. (1990). Total communication use among elementary teachers of hearing impaired children. *American Annals of the Deaf, 135*, 257–263.

McCarthy, D. (1972). *McCarthy Scales of Children's Abilities*. San Antonio, TX: The Psychological Corporation.

McCauley, R., and Swisher, L. (1984a). Psychometric review of language and articulation tests for preschool children. *Journal of Speech and Hearing Disorders, 49*, 34–42.

McCauley, R., and Swisher, L. (1984b). Use and misuse of norm-referenced tests in clinical assessment: Hypothetical case. *Journal of Speech and Hearing Disorders, 49*, 338–348.

McCormick, L. (1990). Sequence of language and communication development. In L. McCormick and R. Schiefelbusch (Eds.), *Early language intervention: An introduction* (2nd ed.) (pp.71–105). New York: Charles E. Merrill.

McCormick, M., Brooks-Gunn, J., Workman-Daniels, K., Turner, J., and Peckham, G. (1992). The health and developmental status of very low-birth weight children at school age. *Journal of the American Medical Association, 267*(16), 2204–2208.

McCormick, L., and Schiefelbusch, R. (Eds.). (1990). *Early language intervention: An introduction* (2nd ed.). New York: Charles E. Merrill.

McCune-Nicolich, L., and Carroll, S. (1981). Development of symbolic play: Implications for the language specialist. *Topics in Language Disorders, 2*(1), 1–15.

McDade, H., and Varnedoe, D. (1987). Training parents to be language facilitators. *Topics in Language Disorders, 7*(3), 19–30.

McGurk, H. (1983). Effectance motivation and the development of communicative competence in blind and sighted children. In A. Mills (Ed.), *Language acquisition in the blind child: Normal and deficient* (pp. 108–113). San Diego, CA: College-Hill Press.

McKean, T. (1993). An insiders look at auditory training. *Advocate: Autism Society of America, 25*(1), 13–15.

McLaughlin, M., and Yee, S. (1988). School as a place to have a career. In A. Lieberman (Ed.), *Building a professional culture in schools* (pp. 23–44). New York: Teachers College Press.

McLean, J., and Snyder-McLean, L. (1984a). Strategies of facilitating language development in clinics, schools, and homes. *Seminars in Speech and Language, 5*(3), 213–228.

McLean, J., and Snyder-McLean, L. (1984b). Recent developments in pragmatics: Remedial implications. In D. Muller (Ed.), *Remediating children's language* (pp. 55–82). San Diego, CA: College-Hill Press.

McLean, J., and Snyder-McLean, L. (1988). Applications of pragmatics to severely mentally retarded children and youth. In R. Schiefelbusch and L. Lloyd (Eds.), *Language perspectives: Acquisition, retardation, and intervention* (pp. 255–288). Austin, TX: Pro-Ed.

McLeavey, B., Toomey, J., and Dempsey, P. (1982). Nonretarded and mentally retarded children's control over syntactic structures. *American Journal of Mental Deficiency, 86*, 485–494.

McNaughton, S. (1975). *Symbol secrets.* Ontario: University of Toronto Press.

McTear, M., and Conti-Ramsden, G. (1992). *Pragmatic disability in children.* San Diego, CA: Singular Publishing Group.

Meador, D. (1984). Effects of color on visual discrimination of geometric symbols by severely and profoundly mentally retarded individuals. *American Journal of Mental Deficiency, 89*, 275–286.

Meadow, K. (1980). *Deafness and child development.* Berkeley, CA: University of California Press.

Meadow, K., Greenberg, M., Erting, C., and Carmichael, H. (1981). Interactions of deaf mothers and deaf preschool children: Comparisons with three other groups of deaf and hearing dyads. *American Annals of the Deaf, 126*, 454–468.

Mehler, J. (1985). Language related dispositions in early infancy. In J. Mehler and R. Fox (Eds.), *Neonate cognition: Beyond the blooming, buzzing confusion* (pp. 7–28). Hillsdale, NJ: Erlbaum.

Meier, R., and Newport, E. (1990). Out of the hands of babes: On a possible sign advantage in language acquisition. *Language, 66*, 1–23.

Meltzoff, A. (1985a). The roots of social and cognitive development: Model of man's original nature. In T. Field and N. Fox (Eds.), *Social perception in infants* (pp. 1–30). Norwood, NJ: Ablex.

Meltzoff, A. (1985b). Immediate and deferred imitation in fourteen and twenty-four-month-old infants. *Child Development, 56*, 62–72.

Meltzoff, A. (1988a). Infant imitation and memory. Nine-month-olds in immediate and deferred tests. *Child Development, 59*, 217–225.

Meltzoff, A. (1988b). Infant imitation after a 1-week delay: Long-term memory for novel acts and multiple stimuli. *Developmental Psychology, 24*, 470–476.

Meltzoff, A., and Gopnik, A. (1989). On linking nonverbal imitation representation and language learning in the first two years of life. In G. Speidel and K. Nelson (Eds.), *The many faces of imitation in language learning* (pp. 23–51). New York: Springer-Verlag.

Meltzoff, A., and Kuhl, P. (1989). Infants' perception of faces and speech sounds: Challenges to developmental theory. In P. Zelazo and R. Barr (Eds.), *Challenges to developmental paradigms.* Hillsdale, NJ: Erlbaum.

Meltzoff, A., and Moore, M. (1977). Imitation of facial and manual gestures by human neonates. *Science, 198,* 75–78.

Meltzoff, A., and Moore, M. (1983a). Newborn infants imitate adult facial gestures. *Child Development, 54,* 702–709.

Meltzoff, A., and Moore, M. (1983b). The origins of imitation in infancy: Paradigm, phenomena, and theories. In L. Lipsitt (Ed.), *Advances in infancy research* (Vol.2, pp. 265–301). Norwood, NJ: Ablex.

Meltzoff, A., and Moore, M. (1985). Cognitive foundations and social functions of imitation and intermodal representation in infancy. In J. Mehler and R. Fox (Eds.), *Neonate cognition: Beyond the blooming, buzzing confusion* (pp.139–156). Hillsdale, NJ: Erlbaum.

Menn, L. (1989). Phonological development: Learning sounds and sound patterns. In J. Gleason (Ed.), *The development of language* (2nd ed.). (pp. 59–100). New York: Charles E. Merrill.

Menyuk, P. (1986). Predicting speech and language problems with persistent otitis media. In J. Kavanaugh (Ed.), *Otitis media and child development* (pp. 83–96). Parkton, MD: York Press.

Menyuk, P. (1988). Language development and reading. In M. Nippold (Ed.), *Later language development: Ages nine through nineteen* (pp. 151–170). Boston, MA: College-Hill Press.

Menyuk, P., and Flood, J. (1981). Linguistic competence, reading, writing problems and remediation. *Bulletin of the Orton Society, 31,* 13–28.

Merrill, E. (1985). Differences in semantic processing speed of mentally retarded and nonretarded persons. *American Journal of Mental Deficiency, 90,* 71–80.

Mesibov, G. (1991). Learning styles of students with autism. *Advocate: Autism Society of America, 22*(4), 12–14.

Meyers, J., Gelzheiser, L., and Yelich, G. (1991). Do pull-in programs foster teacher collaboration? *Remedial and Special Education, 12*(2), 7–15.

Miller, C., and Byrne, J. (1984). The role of temporal cues in the development of language and communication. In L. Feagans, C. Garvey, and R. Golinkoff (Eds.), *The origins and growth of communication.* New York: Academic Press.

Miller, J. (1981a). *Assessing language production in children: Experimental procedures.* Baltimore, MD: University Park Press.

Miller, J. (1981b). Early psycholinguistic acquisition. In R. Schiefelbusch and D. Bricker (Eds.), *Early language: Acquisition and intervention.* Baltimore, MD: University Park Press.

Miller, J. (1983). Identifying children with language disorders and describing their language performance. In J. Miller, D. Yoder, and R. Schiefelbusch (Eds.), *Contemporary issues in language intervention* (pp. 61–74). Rockville, MD: American Speech-Language-Hearing Association.

Miller, J. (1991). Quantifying productive language disorders. In J. Miller (Ed.), *Research on child language disorders: A decade of progress* (pp. 211–220). Austin, TX: Pro-Ed.

Miller, L. (1978). Pragmatics and early childhood language disorders: Communicative interactions in a half-hour sample. *Journal of Speech and Hearing Disorders, 43*(4), 419–436.

Miller, L. (1989). Classroom-based language intervention. *Language, Speech, and Hearing Services in Schools, 20*(2), 153–169.

Miller, L. (1990a). The roles of language and learning in the development of literacy. *Topics in Language Disorders, 10*(2), 1–24.

Miller, L. (1990b). The regular education initiative and school reform: Lessons from the mainstream. *Remedial and Special Education, 11*(3), 17–22.

Miller, L. (1993). *What we call smart: A new narrative for intelligence and learning.* San Diego, CA: Singular Publishing Group.

Miller, M. (1985). Experimental use of signed presentations of the verbal scale of the WISC-R with profoundly deaf children: A preliminary report. In D. Martin (Ed.), *Cognition, education, and deafness: Directions for research and instruction* (pp. 134–136). Washington, DC: Gallaudet University Press.

Miller, N. (1984). *Bilingualism and language disability: Assessment and remediation.* San Diego, CA: College-Hill Press.

Montague, M., Maddux, C., and Dereshiwsky, M. (1990). Story grammar and comprehension and production of narrative prose by students with learning disabilities. *Journal of Learning Disabilities, 23,* 190–197.

Montgomery, J. (1992). Perspectives from the field: Language, speech, and hearing services in schools. *Language, Speech, and Hearing Services in Schools, 23*(4), 363–364.

Moon, C., and Fifer, W. (1990). Syllables as signals for 2-day old infants. *Infant Behavior and Development, 13,* 377–390.

Moore-Brown, B. (1991). Moving in the direction of change: Thoughts for administrators and speech-language pathologists. *Language, Speech, and Hearing Services in Schools, 22,* 148–149.

Moores, D. (1987). *Educating the deaf: Psychology, principles and practices* (3rd ed.). Dallas, TX: Houghton Mifflin.

Moores, D., and Kluwin, T. (1986). Issues in school placement. In A. Schildroth and M. Karchmer (Eds.), *Deaf children in America* (pp. 105–123). San Diego, CA: College-Hill Press.

Moran, M. (1988). Reading and writing disorders in the learning disabled student. In N. Lass, L. McReynolds, J. Northern, and D. Yoder (Eds.), *Handbook of speech-language pathology and audiology.* Philadelphia, PA: B.C. Decker.

Moran, M., Money, S., and Leonard, D. (1984). Phonological process analysis of the speech of mentally retarded adults. *American Journal of Mental Deficiency, 89,* 304–306.

Mulford, R. (1983). Referential development in blind children. In A. Mills (Ed.), *Language acquisition in the blind child* (pp. 89–107). London: Croom Helm.

Mulford, R. (1986). First words in the blind child. In M. Smith and J. Locke (Eds.), *The emergent lexicon: The child's development of a linguistic vocabulary* (pp. 293–338). New York: Academic Press.

Muma, J. (1983). Speech-language pathology: Emerging clinical expertise in language. In T. Gallagher and C. Prutting (Eds.), *Pragmatic assessment and intervention issues in language* (pp. 195–214). San Diego, CA: College-Hill Press.

Murray, L., and Trevarthen, C. (1987). Emotional regulation of interactions between 2-month-olds and their mothers. In T. Field and N. Fox (Eds.), *Social perception in infants* (pp. 101–125). Norwood, NJ: Ablex.

Musselman, C., and Churchill, A. (1991). Conversation control in mother-child dyads: Auditory-oral versus total communication. *American Annals of the Deaf, 136*(1), 5–16.

Myers, B. (1992). Cocaine-exposed infants: Myths and misunderstandings. *Zero to Three, 13*(1), 1–5.

Myklebust, H. (1954). *Auditory disorders in children.* New York: Grune and Stratton.

Myklebust, H. (1971). Childhood aphasia: An evolving concept. In L. Travis (Ed.), *Handbook of speech pathology and audiology* (pp. 1181–1202). New York: Appleton-Century-Crofts.

National Accreditation Council. (1981). *Low vision services.* New York: Author.

Nelson, K. (1973). Some evidence for the cognitive primacy of categorization and its functional basis. *Merrill-Palmer Quarterly Journal of Behavior and Development, 19,* 21–39.

Nelson, K. (1974a). Concept, word, and sentence: Interrelations in acquisition and development. *Psychological Review, 81,* 267–285.

Nelson, K. (1974b). Variations in children's concepts by age and category. *Child Development, 45,* 577–584.

Nelson, K. (1981a). Individual differences in language development: Implications for development and language. *Developmental Psychology, 17,* 170–187.

Nelson, K. (1981b). Social cognition in a script framework. In J. Flavell and L. Ross (Eds.), *Social cognitive development.* New York: Cambridge University Press.

Nelson, K. (1985). *Making sense: The acquisition of shared meaning.* New York: Academic Press.

Nelson, N. (1986). Individual processing in classroom settings. *Topics in Language Disorders, 6*(2), 13–27.

Nelson, N. (1988). The nature of literacy. In M. Nippold (Ed.), *Later language development: Ages nine through nineteen* (pp. 11–28). Boston, MA: College-Hill Press.

Newell, W., Stinson, M., Castle, D., Mallery-Ruganis, D., and Holcomb, B. (1990). Simultaneous communication: A description by deaf professionals working in an educational setting. *Sign Language Studies, 69,* 391–414.

Newport, E., and Meier, R. (1985). Acquisition of American Sign Language. In D. Slobin (Ed.), *The cross-linguistic study of language acquisition* (Vol. 1, pp. 881–938). Hillsdale, NJ: Erlbaum.

Nicolich, L. (1977). Beyond sensorimotor intelligence: Assessment of symbolic maturity through analysis of pretend play. *Merrill-Palmer Quarterly, 23*(2), 89–101.

Niedelman, M. (1991). Problem solving and transfer. *Journal of Learning Disabilities, 24*(6), 322–329.

Nihira, K., Foster, R., Shellhaas, M., and Leland, H. (1974). *AAMD Adaptive Behavior Scale.* Washington, DC: American Association on Mental Deficiency.

Ninio, A. (1980). Picture book reading in mother-infant dyads belonging to two subgroups in Israel. *Child Development, 51,* 587–590.

Ninio, A. (1983). Joint book reading as a multiple vocabulary acquisition device. *Developmental Psychology, 19,* 445–451.

Ninio, A. (1992). The relation of children's single word utterances to single word utterances in the input. *Journal of Child Language, 19,* 87–110.

Ninio, A., and Bruner, J. (1978). The achievement and antecedents of labeling. *Journal of Child Language, 5,* 1–15.

Nippold, M. (1985). Comprehension of figurative language in youth. *Topics in Language Disorders, 5*(3), 1–20.

Nippold, M. (Ed.). (1988). *Later language development: Ages nine through nineteen.* Boston, MA: College-Hill Press.

NJCLD Memorandum. (1988). Letter to National Joint Committee on Learning Disabilities member organizations.

Noonan, M., and Siegel-Causey, E. (1990). Special needs of students with severe handicaps. In L. McCormick and R. Schiefelbusch (Eds.). *Early language intervention: An introduction* (2nd ed.)(pp. 384–425). New York: Macmillan.

Norris, J. (1992). Some questions and answers about whole language. *American Journal of Speech-Language Pathology, 1*(4), 11–14.

Norris, J., and Damico, J. (1990). Whole language in theory and practice: Implications for language intervention. *Language, Speech, and Hearing Services in Schools, 21*(4), 212–220.

Norris, J., and Hoffman, P. (1990). Language intervention within naturalistic environments. *Language, Speech, and Hearing Services in Schools, 21*(2), 72–84.

Norris, J., and Hoffman, P. (1993). *Whole language intervention for school-age children.* San Diego, CA: Singular Publishing Group.

Norton, D. (1989). *The effective teaching of the language arts* (3rd ed.). Columbus, OH: Charles E. Merrill.

Nye, C., and Montgomery, J. (1989). Identification criteria for language disordered children: A national survey. *Hearsay: The Journal of the Ohio Speech and Hearing Association,* Spring, 26–33.

O'Brien, M., and Nagle, K. (1987). Parents' speech to toddlers: The effect of play context. *Child Language, 14,* 269–279.

Ochoa, A., Pacheco, R., and Omark, D. (1983). Addressing the learning disability needs of limited-English proficient students: Beyond language and race issues. *Learning Disability Quarterly, 6,* 416–423.

Ogura, T. (1991). A longitudinal study of the relationship between early language development and play development. *Journal of Child Language, 18,* 273–294.

Olsen-Fulero, L. (1982). Style and stability in mother conversational behavior: A study of individual differences. *Journal of Child Language, 9,* 543–564.

Olson, H., Burgess, D., and Streissguth, A. (1992). Fetal alcohol syndrome (FAS) and fetal alcohol effects (FAE): A lifespan view, with implications for early intervention. *Zero to Three, 13*(1), 29–33.

Omark, D., and Erickson, J. (Eds.). (1983). *The bilingual exceptional child.* San Diego, CA: College-Hill Press.

Orlansky, M., and Bonvillian, J. (1988). Early sign language acquisition. In M. Smith and J. Locke (Eds.), *The emergent lexicon: The child's development of a linguistic vocabulary* (pp. 263–292). New York: Academic Press.

Ornitz, E. (1989). Autism at the interface between sensory and information processing. In G. Dawson (Ed.), *Autism: Nature, diagnosis, and treatment* (pp. 174–207). New York: Guilford Press.

Osberger, M. (1990). Audition. *Volta Review, 92,* 34–53.

Owens, R. (1988). *Language development. An introduction* (2nd ed.). Columbus, OH: Charles E. Merrill.

Owens, R. (1989). Mental retardation: Difference or delay. In D. Bernstein and E. Tiegerman (Eds.), *Language and communication disorders in children* (2nd ed.)(pp. 229–297). Columbus, OH: Charles E. Merrill.

Owens, R. (1991). *Language disorders: A functional approach to assessment and intervention.* New York: Charles E. Merrill.

Owens, R. (1992). *Language development: An introduction* (3rd ed.). New York: Charles E. Merrill.

Owens, R., and MacDonald, J. (1982). Communicative uses of the early speech of nondelayed and Down syndrome children. *American Journal of Mental Deficiency, 86,* 503–510.

Ozols, E., and Rourke, B. (1985). Dimensions of social sensitivity in two types of learning disabled children. In B. Rourke (Ed.), *Neuropsychology of learning disabilities.* New York: Guilford Press.

Pace, A. (1980, April). *Further explorations of young children's sensitivity to world knowledge-story information discrepancies.* Paper presented at the meeting of the Southeastern Conference on Human Development, Alexandria, VA.

Pacheco, R. (1983). Bilingual mentally retarded children: Language confusion or real deficits? In D. Omark and J. Erickson (Eds.), *The bilingual exceptional child.* San Diego, CA: College-Hill Press.

Padden, C. (1980). The Deaf community and the culture of Deaf people. In C. Baker and R. Battison (Eds.), *Sign language and the deaf community: Essays in honor of William C. Stokoe.* Silver Spring, MD: National Association of the Deaf.

Padden, C., and Humphries, T. (1988). *Deaf in America: Voices from a culture.* Cambridge, MA: Harvard University Press.

Papousek, M., and Papousek, H. (1981). Musical elements in infants' vocalization: Their significance for communication, cognition, and creativity. In L. Lipsitt and C. Rovee-Collier (Eds.), *Advances in infancy research* (Vol. 1, pp. 163–224). Norwood, NJ: Ablex.

Papousek, H., and Papousek, M. (1987). Intuitive parenting: A didactic counterpart to the infant's integrative competence. In J. Osofsky (Ed.), *Handbook of infant development* (2nd ed.) (pp. 669–720). New York: John Wiley and Sons.

Paradise, J. (1980). Otitis media in infants and children. *Pediatrics, 65,* 917–943.

Paris, S. (1991). Assessment and remediation of metacognitive aspects of children's reading comprehension. *Topics in Language Disorders, 12*(1), 32–50.

Parnell, M., Amerman, J., and Harting, R. (1986). Responses of language disordered children to wh-questions. *Language, Speech, and Hearing Services in Schools, 17,* 95–106.

Paterson, M. (1986). Maximizing the use of residual hearing with school-age hearing impaired students: A perspective. *Volta Review, 88,* 93–106.

Patton, M., and Westby, C. (1992). Ethnography and research: A qualitative view. *Topics in Language Disorders, 12*(3), 1–14.

Paul, R. (1987). Communication. In D. Cohen, A. Donnellan, and R. Paul (Eds.), *Handbook of autism and pervasive developmental disorders* (pp. 61–84). New York: John Wiley and Sons.

Paul, R. (1991). Profiles of toddlers with slow expressive language development. *Topics in Language Disorders, 11*(4), 1–13.

Payne, K. (1986). Cultural and linguistic groups in the United States. In O. Taylor (Ed.), *Nature of communication disorders in culturally and linguistically diverse populations* (pp. 19–46). San Diego, CA: College-Hill Press.

Pearl, R., Bryan, T., and Donahue, M. (1980). Learning disabled children's attributions for success and failure. *Learning Disability Quarterly, 3,* 3–9.

Pease, D., and Gleason, J. (1985). Gaining meaning: Semantic development. In J. Gleason (Ed.), *The development of language* (pp. 103–138). Columbus, OH: Charles E. Merrill.

Pease, D., Gleason, J., and Pan, B. (1989). Gaining meaning: Semantic development. In J. Gleason (Ed.), *The development of language* (2nd ed.) (pp. 101–134). New York: Charles E. Merrill.

Pellegrini, A., and Galda, L. (1990). Children's play, language and early literacy. *Topics in Language Disorders, 10*(3), 76–88.

Pembrey, M. (1992). Genetics and language disorder. In P. Fletcher and D. Hall, (Eds.), *Specific speech and language disorders in children* (pp. 51–62). San Diego, CA: Singular Publishing Group.

Perfetti, C. (1985). *Reading skill.* Hillsdale, NJ: Erlbaum.

Perfetti, C., and Roth, S. (1981). Some of the interactive processes in reading and their role in reading skill. In A. Lesgold and C. Perfetti (Eds.), *Interactive processes in reading.* Hillsdale, NJ: Erlbaum.

Perner, J., Frith, M., Leslie, A., and Leekam, S. (1989). Exploration of the autistic child's theory of mind: Knowledge, belief, and communication. *Child Development, 60,* 689–700.

Perry, T. (1990). Cooperative learning = effective therapy. *Language, Speech, and Hearing Services in Schools, 21*(2), 120.

Peters-Johnson, C. (1990). Action: School services. *Language, Speech, and Hearing Services in Schools, 21*(4), 250–252.

Peters-Johnson, C. (1993). Action: School services. *Language, Speech, and Hearing Services in Schools, 24*(3), 188–191.

Petersen, G., and Sherrod, K. (1982). Relationship of maternal language to language development and language delay in children. *American Journal of Mental Deficiency, 86,* 391–398.

Petitto, L., and Marentette, P. (1991). Babbling in manual mode: Evidence of ontogeny of language. *Science, 251,* 1493–1496.

Phibbs, C., Bateman, D., and Schwartz, R. (1991). The neonatal costs of maternal cocaine use. *Journal of the American Medical Association, 266,* 1521–1526.

Piaget, J. (1950). *The psychology of intelligence.* London: Routledge and Kegan Paul.

Piaget, J. (1952). *The origins of intelligence in children.* New York: International Universities Press.

Piaget, J. (1954). *The construction of reality in the child.* New York: Basic Books.

Piaget, J. (1955). *The language and thought of the child.* Cleveland, OH: World.

Piaget, J. (1962). *Play, dreams, and imitation in childhood.* New York: W.W. Norton.

Piaget, J., and Inhelder, B. (1969). *The psychology of the child.* New York: Basic Books.

Piaget, J., and Inhelder, B. (1971). *Mental imagery in the child.* New York: Basic Books.

Poole, I. (1934). Genetic development of articulation of consonant sounds in speech. *Elementary English Review, 11,* 159–161.

Poplin, M., and Wright, P. (1983). The concept of cultural pluralism: Issues in special education. *Learning Disability Quarterly, 6,* 367–371.

Prather, E. (1984). Developmental language disorders: Adolescents. In A. Holland (Ed.), *Language disorders in children: Recent advances* (pp. 159–172). San Diego, CA: College-Hill Press.

Prather, E., Hedrick, D., and Kern, C. (1975). Articulation development in children aged two to four years. *Journal of Speech and Hearing Disorders, 40,* 179–191.

Pratt, A., and Brady, S. (1988). Relation of phonological awareness to reading disability in children and adults. *Journal of Educational Psychology, 80,* 319–323.

Prickett, H., and Prickett, J. (1992). Vision problems among students in schools and programs for deaf children. *American Annals of the Deaf, 137*(1), 56–60.

Prizant, B. (1987). Theoretical and clinical implications of echolalic behavior in autism. In T. Layton (Ed.), *Language and treatment of autistic and developmentally disordered children* (pp. 65–88). Springfield, IL: Charles C. Thomas.

Prizant, B., and Meyer, E. (1993). Socioemotional aspects of language and social-communication disorders in young children and their families. *American Journal of Speech-Language Pathology, 2*(3), 56–71.

Prizant, B., and Schuler, A. (1987). Facilitating communication: Theoretical foundations. In D. Cohen, A. Donnellan, and R. Pauls (Eds.), *Handbook of autism and pervasive developmental disorders* (pp. 289–300). New York: John Wiley and Sons.

Prizant, B., and Wetherby, A. (1985). Intentional communicative behavior of children with autism: Theoretical and practical issues. *Australian Journal of Human Communication Disorders, 13,* 21–59.

Prizant, B., and Wetherby, A. (1987). Communicative intent: A framework for understanding social-communicative behavior in autism. *Journal of the American Academy of Child Psychiatry, 26,* 472–479.

Prizant, B., and Wetherby, A. (1990). Toward an integrated view of early language and communication development and socioemotional development. *Topics in Language Disorders, 10*(4), 1–16.

Proctor, A. (1989). Stages of normal noncry vocal development in infancy: A protocol for assessment. *Topics in Language Disorders, 10*(1), 26–42.

Prutting, C., and Connolly, J. (1976). Imitation: A closer look. *Journal of Speech and Hearing Disorders, 41,* 412–422.

Prutting, C., and Kirchner, D. (1987). A clinical appraisal of the pragmatic aspects of language. *Journal of Speech and Hearing Disorders, 52*(2), 105–119.

Quenin, C., and Blood, I. (1989). A national survey of cued speech programs. *Volta Review, 91,* 283–289.

Quigley, S., and King, C. (Eds.). (1982). *Reading milestones, Level 5.* Beaverton, OR: Dormac.

Quigley, S., and Kretschmer, R. (1982). *The education of deaf children: Issues, theory and practice.* Baltimore, MD: University Park Press.

Quigley, S., and Paul, P. (1990). *Language and deafness* (2nd ed.). San Diego, CA: Singular Publishing Group.

Quina, K., Wingard, J. and Bates, H. (1987). Language style and gender stereotypes in person perception. *Psychology of Women Quarterly, 11,* 111–122.

Rakow, L. (1986). Rethinking gender research in communication. *Journal of Communication, 36,* 11–26.

Rapin, I. (1991). Autistic children: Diagnosis and clinical features. *Pediatrics, 87,* 751–760.

Ratner, N. (1989). Atypical language development. In J. Berko Gleason (Ed.), *The development of language* (2nd ed.)(pp. 369–406). New York: Macmillan.

Ratner, V. (1985). Spatial relationship deficits in deaf children: The effect on communication and classroom performance. *American Annals of the Deaf, 130*(3), 250–254.

Ratner, V. (1988a). New tests for identifying hearing impaired students with visual perceptual deficits: Relationship between deficits and ability to comprehend sign language. *American Annals of the Deaf, 133*(5), 336–343.

Ratner, V. (1988b). *Test of visual perceptual abilities (TVPA): Version for hearing impaired.* New York: Visual Perception.

Ratner, V. (1988c). *Test of spatial perception in sign language (TSPSL).* New York: Visual Perception.

Ratner, V. (1988d). An additional handicap: Visual perceptual learning disabilities in deaf children. *Proceedings of the 8th Southeast Region Conference,* Cave Spring, GA.

Ratner, V. (1990). Contribution of learning disabilities to emotional disturbance among hearing impaired individuals. *Proceedings of the International Congress on Education of the Deaf,* Rochester, NY.

Ratner, V. (1991). Nonverbal learning disabilities and concomitant emotional disorders among deaf individuals. *Proceedings of the CAID/CEASD Convention,* (pp. 372–373). New Orleans, LA.

Ratner, V. (1993). *Standardization of test of visual perceptual abilities on children with hearing impairment: Test of Visual Perceptual Abilities (TVPA), Revised.* New York: Visual Perception.

Raven, J. (1956). *Standard progressive matrices.* Cleveland, OH: Psychological Corporation.

Rea, C., Bonvillian, J., and Richards, H. (1988). Mother-infant interactive behaviors: Impact of maternal deafness. *American Annals of the Deaf, 133*(5), 317–324.

Read, C., and Ruyter, L. (1985). Reading and spelling skills in adults of low literacy. *Remedial and Special Education, 6,* 43–52.

Read, C., Zhang, Y., Nie, H., and Ding, B. (1986). The ability to manipulate speech sounds depends on knowing alphabetic writing. *Cognition, 24,* 31–44.

Reed, V. (1986). *An introduction to children with language disorders.* New York: Macmillan.

Reich, P. (1986). *Language development.* Englewood Cliffs, NJ: Prentice-Hall.

Reich, R. (1978). Gestural facilitation of expressive language in moderately/severely retarded preschoolers. *Mental Retardation, 24,* 87–92.

Reichle, J., Williams, W., and Ryan, S. (1981). Selecting signs for the formulation of an augmentative communication modality. *The Journal of the Association for Severely Handicapped, 6,* 48–56.

Reid, G. (1980). Overt and covert rehearsal in short-term motor memory of mentally retarded and nonretarded persons. *American Journal of Mental Deficiency, 85,* 69–77.

Rescorla, L. (1989). The language development survey: A screening tool for delayed language in toddlers. *Journal of Speech and Hearing Disorders, 54,* 587–599.

Rescorla, L. (1991). Identifying expressive language delay at age two. *Topics in Language Disorders, 11*(4), 14–20.

Resnick, T., Allen, D., and Rapin, I. (1984). Disorders of language development: Diagnosis and intervention. *Pediatrics in Review, 6,* 85–92.

Reznick, J., and Kagan, J. (1983). Category detection in infancy. In L. Lipsitt and C. Rovee-Collier (Eds.), *Advances in infancy research* (Vol. 2). Norwood, NJ: Ablex.

Rice, M. (1983). Contemporary accounts of the cognition/language relationship: Implications for speech-language clinicians. *Journal of Speech and Hearing Disorders, 48*(4), 347–359.

Rice, M. (1986). Mismatched premises of the communicative competence model and language intervention. In R. Schiefelbusch (Ed.), *Language competence: Assessment and intervention* (pp. 261–280). San Diego, CA: College-Hill Press.

Rice, M., and Kemper, S. (1984). *Child language and cognition.* Baltimore, MD: University Park Press.

Richman, N., Stevenson, J., and Graham, P. (1982). *Preschool to school: A behavioral study.* New York: Academic Press.

Rimland, B. (1964). *Infantile autism.* New York: Appleton-Century-Crofts.

Rimland, B. (1985). The etiology of infantile autism: The problem of biological versus psychological causation. In A. Donnellan (Ed.), *Classic readings in autism* (pp. 84–103). New York: Teachers College Press.

Rimland, B., Callaway, E., and Dreyfus, P. (1985). The effect of high doses of vitamin B6 on autistic children: A double-blind crossover study. In A. Donnellan (Ed.), *Classic readings in autism* (pp. 408–414). New York: Teachers College Press.

Rist, M. (1990). "Crack babies" in school. *Educational Digest, 55,* 30–33.

Rivers, K., and Hedrick, D. (1992). Language and behavioral concerns for drug-exposed infants and toddlers. In L. Rosetti (Ed.), *Developmental problems of drug-exposed infants* (pp. 63–73). San Diego, CA: Singular Publishing Group.

Rogers, D. (1992). *Motor disorder in psychiatry: Towards a neurological psychiatry.* New York: John Wiley and Sons.

Rogers, S. and Puchalski, C. (1984). Development of symbolic play in visually impaired young children. *Topics in Early Childhood Special Education, 3*(4), 57–63.

Rogow, S. (1987). The ways of the hand: Hand function in blind, visually impaired, and visually impaired multihandicapped children. *British Journal of Visual Impairment, 5*(2), 59–62.

Rogow, S. (1988). *Helping the visually impaired child with developmental problems.* New York: Teachers College Press.

Romski, M., Sevcik, R., and Rumbaugh, D. (1985). Retention of symbolic communication in five severely retarded persons. *American Journal of Mental Deficiency, 89,* 441–444.

Rosenberg, S. (1982). The language of the mentally retarded. In S. Rosenberg (Ed.), *Handbook of applied psycholinguistics: Major thrusts of research and theory.* Hillsdale, NJ: Erlbaum.

Rosetti, L. (Ed.). (1992). *Development problems of drug-exposed infants.* San Diego, CA: Singular Publishing Group.

Ross, B., and Berg, C. (1990). Individual differences in script reports: Implications for language assessment. *Topics in Language Disorders, 10*(3), 30–44.

Ross, D., and Ross, S. (1982). *Hyperactivity: Research, theory, and action.* New York: John Wiley and Sons.

Ross, G. (1980). Concept categorization in one-to-two-year-olds. *Developmental Psychology, 16,* 391–396.

Ross, G., Nelson, K., Wetstone, H., and Tanouye, E. (1986). Acquisition and generalization of novel object concepts by young language learners. *Journal of Child Language, 13,* 67–83.

Roth, F., and Spekman, N. (1984a). Assessing the pragmatic abilities of children: Part 1. Organizational framework and assessment parameters. *Journal of Speech and Hearing Disorders, 49*, 2–11.

Roth, F., and Spekman, N. (1984b). Assessing the pragmatic abilities of children: Part 2. Guidelines, considerations, and specific evaluation procedures. *Journal of Speech and Hearing Disorders, 49*, 12–17.

Roth, F., and Spekman, N. (1986). Narrative discourse: Spontaneously generated stories of learning disabled and normally achieving students. *Journal of Speech and Hearing Disorders, 51*, 8–23.

Rourke, B. (1982). Central processing deficiencies in children: Toward a developmental neuropsychological model. *Journal of Clinical Neuropsychology, 4*, 1–18.

Rourke, B. (1989). *Nonverbal learning disabilities.* New York: Guilford Press.

Rourke, B., and Strang, J. (1983). Subtypes of reading and arithmetic disabilities: A neuropsychological analysis. In M. Rutter (Ed.), *Developmental neuropsychiatry.* New York: Guilford Press.

Rourke, B., Young, G., and Leenaars, A. (1989). A childhood learning disability that predisposes those afflicted to adolescent and adult depression and suicide risk. *Journal of Learning Disabilities, 22*, 169–175.

Rowland, C. (1983). Patterns of interaction between three blind infants and their mothers. In A. Mills (Ed.), *Language acquisition in the blind child* (pp. 114–132). San Diego, CA: College-Hill Press.

Rowland, C. (1984). Preverbal communication of blind infants and their mothers. *Journal of Visual Impairment and Blindness, 78*(7), 297–302.

Ruiz, N. (1989). An optimal learning environment for Rosemary. *Exceptional Children, 56*(2), 130–144.

Rumsey, J. (1985). Commentary. In A. Donnellan (Ed.), *Classic readings in autism* (p. 134). New York: Teachers College Press.

Rush, D., and Callahan, K. (1989). Exposure to passive cigarette smoking and child development. *Annals of New York Academy of Sciences, 562*, 74–100.

Rutter, M. (1983). Cognitive deficits in pathogenesis of autism. *Journal of Child Psychology and Psychiatry, 24*(5), 513–531.

Rutter, M. (1985). Concepts of autism: A review of research. In A. Donnellan (Ed.), *Classic readings in autism* (pp. 179–208). New York: Teachers College Press.

Ryan, E., Ledger, G., Short, E., and Weed, K. (1982). Promoting the use of active comprehension strategies by poor readers. *Topics in Learning and Learning Disabilities, 2*(1), 53–60.

Sabsay, S., and Kernan, K. (1993). On the nature of language impairment in Down Syndrome. *Topics in Language Disorders, 13*(3), 20–35.

Sachs, J. (1984a). Children's play and communicative development. In R. Schiefelbusch and J. Pickar (Eds.), *The acquisition of communicative competence* (pp. 109–140). Baltimore, MD: University Park Press.

Sachs, J. (1984b). Talking about the there and then: The emergence of displaced reference in parent-child discourse. In K. Nelson (Ed.), *Children's language* (Vol. 4). Hillsdale, NJ: Erlbaum.

Sachs, J. (1989). Communication development in infancy. In J. Gleason (Ed.), *The development of language* (2nd ed.) (pp. 35–57). San Francisco, CA: Charles E. Merrill.

Sacks, O. (1989). *Seeing voices: A journey into the world of the deaf.* Berkeley, CA: University of California Press.

Sacks, O. (1990). *Awakenings.* New York: Harper Perennial.

Sak, R., and Ruben, R. (1981). Recurrent middle ear effusion in childhood: Implications of temporary auditory deprivation for language and learning. *Annals of Otology, Rhinology, and Laryngology, 90*, 546–551.

Salomon, G., and Perkins, D. (1987). Transfer of cognitive skills from programming: When and how? *Journal of Educational Computing Research, 3*(2), 149–169.

Samuda, R. (1975). *Psychological testing of American minorities.* Issues and consequences. New York: Harper and Row.

Samuels, S. (1987). Information processing abilities and reading. *Journal of Learning Disabilities, 20*(1), 18–22.

Samuels, S., and Peterson, E. (1986). *Toward a theory of word recognition: Integrative data from subjects, materials, task, and context.* Washington, DC: National Institutes of Education.

Sander, E. (1972). When are speech sounds learned? *Journal of Speech and Hearing Disorders, 37,* 55–63.

Sanders, D. (1982). *Aural rehabilitation* (2nd ed.). Englewood Cliffs, NJ: Prentice-Hall.

Sandoval, J., and Lambert, N. (1984). Hyperactive and learning disabled children: Who gets help? *Journal of Special Education, 18,* 495–503.

Saville-Troike, L. (1986). Anthropological considerations in the study of communication. In O. Taylor (Ed.), *Nature of communication disorders in culturally and linguistically diverse populations* (pp. 47–72). San Diego, CA: College-Hill Press.

Saville-Troike, M. (1982). *The ethnography of communication: An introduction.* Baltimore, MD: University Park Press.

Saville-Troike, M. (1989). *The ethnography of communication: An introduction* (2nd ed.). Oxford, England: Blackwell.

Scanlon, C., Arick, J., and Phelps, N. (1981). Participation in the development of the IEP: Parents' perspective. *Exceptional Children, 47,* 373.

Schaffer, J., Yanulis, M., Williams, B., and Green, B. (1993). When love is not enough: The children of crack cocaine. Unpublished raw data.

Schein, J. (1984). *Speaking the language of sign.* Garden City, NY: Doubleday.

Schein, J. (1989). *At home among strangers.* Washington, DC: Gallaudet University Press.

Schery, T., and O'Connor, L. (1992). The effectiveness of school-based computer language intervention with severely handicapped children. *Language, Speech, and Hearing Services in Schools, 23*(1), 43–47.

Schiefelbusch, R. (1993). Communication in adults with mental retardation. *Topics in Language Disorders, 13*(3), 1–8.

Schiefelbusch, R., and Lloyd, L. (Eds.). (1988). *Language perspectives: Acquisition, retardation, and intervention* (2nd ed.). Austin, TX: Pro-Ed.

Schieffelin, B. (1986). *How Kaluli children learn what to say, what to do, and how to feel.* New York: Cambridge University Press.

Schiff-Myers, N. (1992). Considering arrested language development and language loss in the assessment of second language learners. *Language, Speech, and Hearing Services in Schools, 23,* 28–33.

Schildroth, A., Rawlings, B., and Allen, T. (1989). Hearing impaired children under age 6: A demographic analysis. *American Annals of the Deaf, 134*(2), 63–69.

Schlesinger, H. (1986). Total communication in perspective. In D. Luterman (Ed.), *Deafness in perspective* (pp. 87–116). San Diego, CA: College-Hill Press.

Schopler, E., and Mesibov, G. (1985). Introduction to communication problems in autism. In E. Schopler and G. Mesibov (Eds.), *Communication problems in autism* (pp. 3–16). New York: Plenum Press.

Schwartz, L., and McKinley, N. (1984). *Daily communication.* Eau Claire, WI: Thinking Publications.

Schwartz, R., Stool, S., Rodriguez, W., and Grundfast, K. (1981). Acute otitis media: Toward a more precise definition. *Clinical Pediatrics, 20*(9), 549–554.

Schwartz, S., and Heller-Miller, J. (1988). *The language of toys.* Rockville, MD: Woodbine House.

Scollon, S., and Scollon, S. (1981). *Narrative, literacy and face in interethnic communication.* Norwood, NJ: Ablex.

Scott, K. (1980). Learning theory, intelligence, and mental development. *American Journal of Mental Deficiency,* *82,* 325–336.

Scoville, R. (1983). Development of the intention to communicate: The eye of the beholder. In I. Feagans, C. Garvey, and R. Golinkoff (Eds.), *The origins and growth of communication.* Norwood, NJ: Ablex.

Semrud-Clikeman, M., and Hynd, G. (1990). Right hemispheric dysfunction in nonverbal learning disabilities: Social, academic, and adaptive functioning in adults and children. *Psychological Bulletin, 107*(2), 196–209.

Sever, J. (1986). Perinatal infections and damage to the central nervous system. In M. Lewis (Ed.), *Learning disabilities and prenatal risk* (pp. 194–209). Chicago, IL: University of Illinois Press.

Shafer, R., Staab, C., and Smith, K. (1983). *Language functions and school success.* Glenview, IL: Scott Foresman.

Shane, H. (1985). Selection of augmentative communication systems. In E. Cherow, N. Matkin, and R. Trybus (Eds.), *Hearing impaired children and youth with developmental disabilities* (pp. 270–292). Washington, DC: Gallaudet University Press.

Shanok, R. (1992). Simon: Intensive, multi-faceted therapy with a developmentally delayed little boy. *Zero to Three, 13*(2), 16–36.

Shaw, M. (1982). Attending to multiple sources of information: The integration of information in decision making. *Cognitive Psychology, 14,* 353–409.

Shaywitz, S., Caparulo, B., and Hodgson, E. (1981). Developmental language disability as a consequence of prenatal exposure to ethanol. *Pediatrics, 68*(6), 850–855.

Shaywitz, S., and Shaywitz, B. (1988). Attention deficit disorder: Current perspectives. In J. Kavanagh and T. Truss, Jr. (Eds.), *Learning disabilities: Proceedings of the national conference* (pp. 369–523). Parkton, MD: York Press.

Shaywitz, S., and Shaywitz, B. (1991). Introduction to the special series on attention deficit disorder. *Journal of Learning Disabilities, 24*(2), 68–71.

Sherrod, L. (1981). Issues in cognitive-perceptual development: The special case of social stimuli. In M. Lamb and L. Sherrod (Eds.), *Infant social cognition.* Hillsdale, NJ: Erlbaum.

Shiffrin, R., and Schneider, W. (1984). Automatic and controlled processing revisited. *Psychological Review, 91,* 269–276.

Shumaker, J., and Deshler, D. (1988). Implementing the regular education initiative in secondary schools: A different ball game. *Journal of Learning Disabilities, 21*(1), 36–42.

Siegel, L., and Ryan, E. (1984). Reading disability as a language disorder. *Remedial and Special Education, 5,* 28–33.

Silberberg, N., and Silberberg, M. (1967). Hyperlexia: Specific word recognition skills in young children. *Exceptional Children, 34,* 41–42.

Silberman-Miller, M. (1981). A model for providing comprehensive speech services within a total communication program for the deaf. *American Annals of the Deaf, 126*(7), 803–805.

Silliman, E. (1984). Interactional competencies in the instructional context: The role of teaching discourse in learning. In G. Wallach and K. Butler (Eds.), *Language learning disabilities in school-age children* (pp. 288–317). Baltimore, MD: Williams and Wilkins.

Silliman, E. (1992). Three perspectives of facilitated communication: Unexpected literacy, clever Hans, or enigma? *Topics in Language Disorders, 12*(4), 60–68.

Silliman, E., and Wilkinson, L. (1991). *Communicating for learning: Classroom observation and collaboration.* Gaithersburg, MD: Aspen.

Silver, L. (1990). Attention deficit hyperactivity disorder: Is it a learning disability or a related disorder? *Journal of Learning Disabilities, 23*(7), 394–397.

Silverman, F. (1980). *Communication for the speechless.* Englewood Cliffs, NJ: Prentice-Hall.

Simon, C. (1991). (Ed.). *Communication skills and classroom success: Assessment and therapy methodologies for language and learning disabled students.* Eau Claire, WI: Thinking Publications.

Simon, C., and Myrold-Gunyuz, P. (1990). *Into the classroom: The SLP in the collaborative role.* Tucson, AR: Communication Skill Builders.

Sinatra, G. (1990). Convergence of listening and reading processing. *Reading Research Quarterly, 15,* 115–130.

Skinner, B. (1957). *Verbal behavior.* New York: Appleton-Century-Crofts.

Skuse, D. (1992). The relationship between deprivation, physical growth and the impaired development of language. In P. Fletcher, and D. Hall (Eds.), *Specific speech and language disorders in children* (pp. 29–50). San Diego, CA: Singular Publishing Group.

Skutnabb-Kangas, T., and Toukomaa, P. (1976). Teaching migrant children's mother tongue and learning the language of the host country in the context of the sociocultural situation of the migrant family. Helsinki: The Finnish National Commission for UNESCO.

Slavin, R. (1990). General education under the regular education initiative: How must it change? *Remedial and Special Education, 11*(3), 40–50.

Slobin, D. (1978a). A case study of early language awareness. In A. Sinclair, R. Jarvella, and W. Levelt (Eds.), *The child's conception of language* (pp. 45–54) New York: Springer-Verlag.

Slobin, D. (1978b). Cognitive prerequisites for the development of grammar. In L. Bloom (Ed.), *Readings in language development* (pp. 407–432). New York: John Wiley and Sons.

Smith, C. (1983). *Learning disabilities: The interaction of learner, task, and setting.* Boston, MA: Little, Brown and Company.

Smith, M. (1933). Grammatical errors in the speech of preschool children. *Child Development, 4,* 183–190.

Smith, M. (1985). Managing the aggressive and self-injurious behavior of adults disabled by autism. *Journal of the Association for Persons with Severe Handicaps, 10,* 228–232.

Smith, M., and Richards, S. (1990). Some essential aspects of effective audiological management programme for school age hearing impaired children. *Journal of the British Association of Teachers of the Deaf, 14,* 104–113.

Snow, C. (1981). Social interaction and language acquisition. In P. Dale and D. Ingram (Eds.), *Child language: An international perspective* (pp. 195–214). Baltimore, MD: University Park Press.

Snow, C. (1983). Literacy and language: Relations during the preschool years. *Harvard Educational Review, 53,* 165–189.

Snyder, L. (1984). Developmental language disorders: Elementary school age. In A. Holland (Ed.), *Language disorders in children: Recent advances* (pp. 129–158). San Diego, CA: Singular Publishing Group.

Snyder, L., Bates, E., and Bretherton, I. (1981). Content and context in early lexical development. *Journal of Child Language, 8,* 565–582.

Snyder, L., and Godley, D. (1992). Assessment of word-finding disorders in children and adolescents. *Topics in Language Disorders, 13*(1), 15–32.

Snyder, L., and Silverstein, J. (1988). Pragmatics and child language disorders. In R. Schiefelbusch and L. Lloyd (Eds.), *Language perspectives: Acquisition, retardation and intervention* (pp. 189–222). Austin, TX: Pro-Ed.

Snyder-McLean, L., Solomonson, B., McLean, J., and Sack, S. (1984). Structuring joint action routines: A strategy for facilitating communication and language development in the classroom. *Seminars in Speech and Language, 5*(3), 213–228.

Sorsby, A., and Martlew, M. (1991). Representational demands in mothers' talk to preschool children in two contexts: Picture book reading and a modelling task. *Journal of Child Language, 18,* 373–395.

Sparks, S. (1989). Assessment and intervention with at-risk infants and toddlers. Guidelines for the speech-language pathologist. *Topics in Language Disorders, 10*(1), 43–56.

Sparks, S. (1993). *Children of prenatal substance abuse.* San Diego, CA: Singular Publishing Group.

Sparrow, S., Balla, D., and Cicchetti, D. (1984). *Vineland Adaptive Behavior Scales.* Circle Pines, MN: American Guidance Service.

Spear, L., and Sternberg, R. (1986). An information-processing framework for understanding learning disabilities. In S. Ceci (Ed.), *Handbook of cognitive, social, and neuropsychological aspects of learning disabilities* (Vol. 2, pp. 2–30). Hillsdale, NJ: Erlbaum.

Spence, M., and De Casper, A. (1982). *Human fetuses perceive maternal speech.* Paper presented at the International Conference on Infant Studies, Austin, TX.

Spence, M., and De Casper, A. (1987). Prenatal experience with low-frequency maternal voice sounds influence neonatal perception of maternal voice samples. *Infant Behavior and Development, 10*, 133–142.

Spencer, P. (1993). The expressive communication of hearing mothers to deaf infants. *American Annals of the Deaf, 138*(3), 275–283.

Spender, D. (1980). *Man made language.* London: Routledge and Kegan Paul.

Spohr, H., and Steinhausen, H. (1987). Follow-up studies of children with fetal alcohol syndrome. *Neuropediatrics, 18*, 13–17.

Squires, J., Bricker, D., and Potter, L. (1990). *Infant/child monitoring questionnaires procedures.* Eugene, OR: University of Oregon Center on Human Development.

Stainback, W., Stainback, S., and Bunch, G. (1989). Introduction and historical background. In S. Stainback, W. Stainback, and M. Forest (Eds.), *Educating all students in the mainstream of regular education* (pp. 3–15). Baltimore, MD: Paul H. Brookes.

Stanovich, K. (1985). Explaining the variance in reading ability in terms of psychological processes: What have we learned? *Annals of Dyslexia, 35*, 67–96.

Stanovich, K., Cunningham, A., and Freeman, D. (1984). Intelligence, cognitive skills, and early reading progress. *Reading Research Quarterly, 14*, 279–303.

Stark, R., and Tallal, P. (1981). Selection of children with specific language deficits. *Journal of Speech and Hearing Disorders, 46*(2), 114–122.

Stehli, A. (1992). *The sound of a miracle.* New York: Avon Books.

Stein, N. (1983). On the goals, functions, and knowledge of reading and writing. *Contemporary Educational Psychology, 8*, 261–292.

Stein, R. (1983). Hispanic parents' perspective and participation in their children's special education program: Comparisons by program and race. *Learning Disability Quarterly, 6*, 432–439.

Stephens, B. and Grube, C. (1982). Development of Piagetian reasoning in congenitally blind children. *Journal of Visual Impairment and Blindness, 76*(4), 133–143.

Stephens, M. (1988). Pragmatics. In M. Nippold, (Ed.), *Later language development: Ages nine through nineteen* (pp. 247–262). Boston, MA: College-Hill Press.

Stern, D. (1985). *The interpersonal world of the infant: A view from psychoanalysis and developmental psychology.* New York: Basic Books.

Sternberg, R. (1984). Toward a triarchic theory of human intelligence. *Behavioral and Brain Sciences, 7*, 269–315.

Sternberg, R. (1985). *Beyond IQ: A triarchic theory of human intelligence.* New York: Cambridge University Press.

Sternberg, R., and Wagner, R. (1982). Automatization failure in learning disabilities. *Topics in Learning and Learning Disabilities, 2*, 1–11.

Stevens, R. (1987). Education in schools for deaf children. In C. Baker and R. Battison (Eds.), *Sign language and the Deaf community: Essays in honor of William C. Stokoe* (3rd ed.) (pp. 177–191). Silver Spring, MD: National Association of the Deaf.

Stockman, I. (1986). Language acquisition in culturally diverse populations: The black child as a case study. In O. Taylor (Ed.), *Nature of communication disorders in culturally and linguistically diverse populations* (pp. 117–155). San Diego, CA: College-Hill Press.

Stoel-Gammon, C. (1987). Phonological skills of two-year-olds. *Language, Speech, and Hearing Services in Schools, 18*(4), 323–329.

Stoel-Gammon, C. (1991). Normal and disordered phonology in two-year-olds. *Topics in Language Disorders, 11*(4), 21–32.

Stoel-Gammon, C., and Cooper, J. (1984). Patterns of early lexical and phonological development. *Journal of Child Language, 11*, 247–271.

Stokoe, W. (1960). Sign language structure: An outline of the visual communication systems of the American deaf. *University of Buffalo Occasional Papers, 8* (revised 1978). Silver Spring, MD: Linstock Press.

Stokoe, W., Casterline, D., and Croneberg, G. (1965). *A dictionary of American Sign Language on linguistic principles.* Silver Spring, MD: Linstock Press.

Stone, C. (1989). Improving the effectiveness of strategy training for learning disabled students: The role of communication dynamics. *Remedial and Special Education, 10*(1), 35–42.

Strang, J., and Rourke, B. (1983). Concept formation/nonverbal reasoning abilities of children who exhibit specific academic problems with arithmetic. *Journal of Clinical Child Psychology, 12*, 33–39.

Strang, J., and Rourke, B. (1985). Adaptive behavior of children who exhibit specific arithmetic disabilities and associated neuropsychological abilities and deficits. In B. Rourke (Ed.), *Neuropsychology of learning disabilities.* New York: Guilford Press.

Streissguth, A. (1983). Smoking and drinking. In C. Brown (Ed.), *Childhood learning disabilities and prenatal risk: An inter-disciplinary data review for health care professionals and parents* (pp. 49–56). Skillman, NJ: Johnson and Johnson.

Streissguth, A. (1986a). Smoking and drinking during pregnancy and offspring learning disabilities: A review of the literature and development of a research strategy. In M. Lewis (Ed.), *Learning disabilities and prenatal risk* (pp. 28–67). Champaign, IL: University of Illinois Press.

Streissguth, A. (1986b). The behavioral teratology of alcohol: Performance, behavioral, and intellectual deficits in prenatally exposed children. In J. West (Ed.), *Alcohol and brain development* (pp. 3–44). New York: Oxford University Press.

Streissguth, A., Aase, J., Clarren, S., Randels, S., LaRue, R., and Smith, D. (1991). Fetal alcohol syndrome in adolescents and adults. *Journal of the American Medical Association, 265*, 1961–1967.

Streissguth, A., Clarren, S., and Jones, K. (1985). Natural history of the fetal alcohol syndrome: A 10-year follow-up of eleven patients. *Lancet, 2*, 5–91.

Studdert-Kennedy, M. (1986). Development of the speech-perceptuo-motor system. In B. Lindblom and R. Zetterstrom (Eds.), *Precursors of early speech* (pp 205–217). New York: Stockton.

Study links dyslexia to brain flaw affecting vision. (1991, September 15). *The New York Times.*

Sugarman, S. (1981). The cognitive basis of classification in very young children: An analysis of object ordering trends. *Child Development, 52*, 1172–1178.

Sugarman, S. (1983). *Children's early thought: Developments in classification.* New York: Cambridge University Press.

Sutton-Smith, B. (1986). The development of fictional narratives. *Topics in Language Disorders, 7*(1), 1–10.

Swanson, L. (1983). A study of nonstrategic linguistic coding on visual recall of learning disabled readers. *Journal of Learning Disabilities, 16*, 209–216.

Swisher, L. (1985). Language disorders in children. In J. Darby (Ed.), *Speech and language evaluation in neurology: childhood disorders* (pp. 33–97). New York: Grune and Stratton.

Tager-Flusberg, H. (1985). Putting words together: Morphology and syntax in the preschool years. In J. Gleason (Ed.), *The development of language* (pp. 139–171). Columbus, OH: Charles E. Merrill.

Tager-Flusberg, H. (1989). Putting words together: Morphology and syntax in the preschool years. In J. Gleason (Ed.), *The development of language* (2nd ed., pp.135–165). New York: Charles E. Merrill.

Tallal, P. (1988). Developmental language disorders. In J. Kavanagh and T. Truss, Jr. (Eds.), *Learning disabilities: Proceedings of the national conference* (pp. 182–272). Parkton, MD: York Press.

Tallal, P., Ross, R., and Curtiss, S. (1989). Familial aggregation in specific language impairment. *Journal of Speech and Hearing Disorders, 54*, 167–173.

Tapp, K., Wilhelm, J., and Loveless, L. (Eds.). (1991). *A guide to curriculum planning for visually impaired children*. Madison, WI: Wisconsin Department of Public Instruction.

Taylor, O. (1986). *Nature of communication disorders in culturally and linguistically diverse populations*. San Diego, CA: College-Hill Press.

Taylor, O. (1992). Hold fast to dreams. *ASHA, 34*(5), 53.

Teele, D., Klein, J., and Rosner, B. (1984). Otitis media with effusion during first three years of life and development of speech and language. *Pediatrics, 74*, 282–287.

Templin, M. (1957). *Certain language skills in children: Their development and interrelationships* (Institute of Child Welfare, Monograph 26). Minneapolis, MN: University of Minnesota Press.

Terman, L., and Merrill, M. (1973). *Stanford-Binet intelligence scale*. Chicago, IL: Riverside.

Thompson, M., and Swisher, M. (1985). Acquiring language through total communication. *Ear and Hearing, 6*, 29–32.

Thompson, O. (1985). The nonverbal dilemma. *Journal of Learning Disabilities*, 18, 400–402.

Thomson, M., and Watkins, E. (1990). *Dyslexia: A teaching handbook*. London: Whurr Publishers.

Tomasello, M., and Todd, J. (1983). Joint attention and lexical acquisition style. *First Language, 4*, 197–212.

Tomblin, J. (1989). Familial concentration of developmental language impairment. *Journal of Speech and Hearing Disorders, 54*, 287–295.

Tomblin, J. (1991). Examining the cause of specific language impairment. *Language, Speech, and Hearing Services in Schools, 22*, 69–74.

Torgesen, J. (1980). Conceptual and educational implications of the use of efficient task strategies by learning disabled children. *Journal of Learning Disabilities, 13*(7), 19–26.

Torgesen, J. (1985). Memory processes in reading disabled children. *Journal of Learning Disabilities, 18*, 350–357.

Torgesen, J. (1988). Studies of learning disabled children who perform poorly on memory span tasks. *Journal of Learning Disabilities, 21*, 605–612.

Trevarthen, C. (1983a). Emotions in infancy: Regulators of contacts and relationships with persons. In K. Scherer and P. Ekman (Eds.), *Approaches to emotion*. Hillsdale, NJ: Erlbaum.

Trevarthen, C. (1983b). Interpersonal abilities of infant as generators for transmission of language and culture. In A. Oliverio and M. Zappella (Eds.), *The behavior of human infants*. New York: Plenum.

Tronick, E., Als, H., and Brazelton, T. (1980). Monadic phases: A structural descriptive analysis of infant-mother face-to-face interaction. *Merrill-Palmer Quarterly, 26*, 3–24.

Tunmer, W., and Bowey, J. (1983). Metalinguistic awareness and reading acquisition. In W. Tunmer, C. Pratt, and M. Herriman (Eds.), *Metalinguistic awareness in children: Theory, research, and implications.* New York: Springer-Verlag.

Tunmer, W., and Cole, P. (1991). Learning to read: A metalinguistic act. In C. Simon (Ed.), *Communication skills and classroom success: Assessment and therapy methodologies for language and learning disabled students* (pp. 386–402). Eau Claire, WI: Thinking Publications.

Turnbull, H., III. (1986). *Free appropriate public education: The law and children with disabilities.* Denver, CO: Love Publishing.

Turner, L., and Bray, N. (1985). Spontaneous rehearsal by mildly mentally retarded children and adolescents. *American Journal of Mental Deficiency, 90,* 57–63.

U.S. Department of Education. (1992). Fourteenth annual report to Congress on the implementation of the individuals with disabilities education act. Washington, DC: U.S. Government Printing Office.

U.S. Department of Education. (1991). *Policy memorandum.* Washington, DC: Author.

U.S. Office of Education. (1977). *Federal Register, Part III. Education of handicapped children: Assistance to states. Procedures for evaluating specific learning disabilities.* (pp. 42478, 52404) Washington, DC: Department of Health, Education, and Welfare.

Urwin, C. (1983). Dialogue and cognitive functioning in the early language development of three blind children. In A. Mills (Ed.), *Language acquisition in the blind child: Normal and deficient* (pp. 142–161). San Diego, CA: College-Hill Press.

Valletutti, P., and Dummett, L. (1992). *Cognitive development: A functional approach.* San Diego, CA: Singular Publishing Group.

Van der Geest, T. (1983). Cognition, interaction, and development, with special reference to education of the handicapped child. In A. Mills (Ed.), *Language acquisition in the blind child: Normal and deficient* (pp. 133–141). San Diego, CA: College-Hill Press.

Van der Vlugt, H. (1991). Neuropsychological validation studies of learning disability subtypes: Verbal, visual-spatial, and psychomotor abilities. In B. Rourke (Ed.), *Neuropsychological validation of learning disability subtypes* (pp. 140–159). New York: Guilford.

Van Dyke, D., and Fox, A. (1990). Fetal drug exposure and its possible implications for learning in the preschool and school-age population. *Journal of Learning Disabilities, 23*(3), 160–163.

van Kleeck, A. (1984a). Metalinguistic skills: Cutting across spoken and written language and problem-solving abilities. In G. Wallach and K. Butler (Eds.), *Language learning disabilities in school-age children* (pp. 128–153). Baltimore, MD: Williams and Wilkins.

van Kleeck, A. (1984b). Assessment and intervention: Does "meta" matter? In G. Wallach and K. Butler (Eds.), *Language learning disabilities in school-age children* (pp. 179–198). Baltimore, MD: Williams and Wilkins.

Vellutino, F., and Denkla, M. (1990). Cognitive and neuro-psychological foundations of word identification. In R. Barr, M. Kamil, P. Mosenthal, and P. Pearson (Eds.), *Handbook of reading research* (Vol. 2, pp. 571–608). New York: Longman.

Vellutino, F., and Scanlon, D. (1986). Linguistic coding and metalinguistic awareness: Their relationship to verbal memory and code acquisition in poor and normal readers. In D. Yaden and S. Templeton (Eds.), *Metalinguistic awareness and beginning literacy.* Portsmouth, NH: Heinemann.

Vellutino, F., and Scanlon, D. (1988). Phonological coding, phonological awareness, and reading ability: Evidence from a longitudinal and experimental study. In K. Stanovich (Ed.), *Children's reading and the development of phonological awareness.* Detroit, MI: Wayne State University Press.

Vihman, M., and Greenlee, M. (1987). Individual differences in phonological development: Ages one and three years. *Journal of Speech and Hearing Research, 30,* 503–521.

Vihman, M., Macken, M., Miller, R., Simmons, H., and Miller, J. (1985). From babbling to speech: A re-assessment of the continuity issue. *Language, 61*, 397–445.

Vinter, A. (1986). The role of movement in eliciting early imitations. *Child Development, 57*, 66–71.

Volkmar, F. (1987). Social development. In D. Cohen, A. Donnellan, and R. Paul (Eds.), *Handbook of autism and pervasive developmental disorders* (pp. 41–60). New York: John Wiley and Sons.

Vygotsky, L. (1962). *Thought and Language.* Cambridge, MA: MIT Press.

Wadle, S. (1991). Why speech-language clinicians should be in the classroom. *Language, Speech, and Hearing Services in Schools, 22*(4), 277.

Wagner, R., and Torgesen, J. (1987). The nature of phonological processing and its causal role in the acquisition of reading skills. *Psychological Bulletin, 101*, 192–212.

Walden, T., and Field, T. (1982). Discrimination of facial expressions by preschool children. *Child Development, 53*, 1312–1319.

Wallach, G., and Butler, K. (Eds.). (1984). *Language learning disabilities in school-age children.* Baltimore, MD: Williams and Wilkins.

Wallach, G., and Liebergott, J. (1984). Who shall be called "learning disabled?": Some new directions. In G. Wallach and K. Butler (Eds.), *Language learning disabilities in school-age children* (pp. 1–15). Baltimore, MD: Williams and Wilkins.

Wallach, G., and Miller, L. (1988). *Language intervention and academic success.* Boston, MA: College-Hill Press.

Wang, M., Reynolds, M., and Walberg, H. (1988). Integrating the children of the second system. *Phi Delta Kappan, 69*, 248–251.

Wardhaugh, R. (1985). *How conversations work.* Oxford, England: Blackwell.

Weaver, C. (1991). Whole language and its potential for developing readers. *Topics in Language Disorders, 11*(3), 28–44.

Wechsler, D. (1974a). *Wechsler preschool and primary scale of intelligence (WPPSI).* Cleveland, OH: The Psychological Corporation.

Wechsler, D. (1974b). *Wechsler intelligence scale for children-revised (WISC-R).* Cleveland, OH: The Psychological Corporation.

Wechsler, D. (1981). *Wechsler adult intelligence scale-revised (WAIS-R).* New York: The Psychological Corporation.

Weiss, G., Hechtman, L., Milroy, T., and Perlman, T. (1985). Psychiatric status of hyperactives as adults: A controlled prospective 15-year follow-up of 63 hyperactive children. *Journal of American Academy of Child Psychiatry, 24*, 211–220.

Wellman, B., Case, I., Mengurt, I., and Bradbury, D. (1931). *Speech sounds of young children* (University of Iowa Studies in Child Welfare). Iowa City, IA: University of Iowa Press.

Wells, G. (1981). *Language through interaction.* New York: Cambridge University Press.

Wells, G. (1985). *Language development in the preschool years.* New York: Cambridge University Press.

Werker, J., and Tees, R. (1984). Cross-language speech perception: Evidence for perceptual reorganization during the first year of life. *Infant Behavior and Development, 7*, 49–64.

Westby, C. (1980). Assessment of cognitive and language abilities through play. *Language, Speech, and Hearing Services in Schools, 11*, 154–168.

Westby, C. (1984). Development of narrative language abilities. In G. Wallach and K. Butler (Eds.), *Language learning disabilities in school-age children* (pp. 103–127). Baltimore, MD: Williams and Wilkins.

Westby, C. (1990). The role of the speech-language pathologist in whole language. *Language, Speech, and Hearing Services in Schools, 21*(4), 228–287.

Westby, C. (1991). Learning to talk-talking to learn: Oral literate language differences. In C. Simon (Ed.), *Communication skills and classroom success: Assessment and therapy methodologies for language and learning disabled students* (pp. 334–357). Eau Claire, WI: Thinking Publications.

Westby, C., and Costlow, L. (1991). Implementing a whole language program in a special edcuation class. *Topics in Language Disorders, 11*(3), 69–87.

Wetherby, A. (1986). Ontogeny of communicative functions in autism. *Journal of Autism and Developmental Disorders, 16,* 295–316.

Wetherby, A., Cain, D., Yonclas, D., and Walker, V. (1988). Analysis of intentional communication of normal children from the prelinguistic to the multi-word stage. *Journal of Speech and Hearing Research, 31,* 240–252.

Wetherby, A., and Prizant, B. (1989). The expression of communicative intent: Assessment guidelines. *Seminars in Speech and Language, 10,* 77–90.

White, S., and White, R. (1984). The deaf imperative: Characteristics of maternal input to hearing impaired children. *Topics in Language Disorders, 4,* 38–49.

Wieder, S. (1992). Opening the door: Approaches to engage children with multisystem developmental disorders. *Zero to Three, 13*(2), 10–15.

Wiggers, M., and van Lieshout, C. (1985). Development of recognitions of emotions: Children's reliance on situational and facial expressive cues. *Developmental Psychology, 21,* 338–349.

Wiig, E. (1990). Language disabilities in school-age children and youth. In G. Shames and E. Wiig (Eds.), *Human communication disorders* (3rd ed.) (pp. 193–221). New York: Charles E. Merrill.

Wiig, E. (1991). Language-learning disabilities: Paradigms for the nineties. *Annals of Dyslexia, 41,* 3–22.

Wiig, E., and Semel, E. (1984). *Language assessment and intervention for the learning disabled* (2nd ed.). Columbus, OH: Charles E. Merrill.

Wilcox, J., Kouri, T., and Caswell, S. (1991). Early language intervention: A comparison of classroom and individual treatment. *American Journal of Speech-Language Pathology, 1*(1), 49–62.

Will, M. (1986). Educating students with learning problems: A shared responsibility. *Exceptional Children, 52*(5), 411–415.

Williams, D. (1992). *Nobody, nowhere.* New York: Times Books.

Williams, H. (1983). *Perceptual and motor development.* Englewood Cliffs, NJ: Prentice-Hall.

Williams, J. (1984). Phonemic analysis and how it relates to reading. *Journal of Learning Disabilities, 17,* 240–245.

Willig, A., and Greenberg, H. (1986). *Bilingualism and learning disabilities.* New York: American Library.

Willig, A., and Ortiz, A. (1990). The non-biased individualized educational program: Linking assessment to instruction. In E. Hamayan, and J. Damico (Eds.), *Limiting bias in the assessment of bilingual students* (pp. 241–302). Austin, TX: Pro-Ed.

Wilson, K., Blackmon, R., Hall, R., and Elcholtz, G., (1991). Methods of language assessment: A survey of California public school clinicians. *Language, Speech, and Hearing Services in Schools, 22,* 236–241.

Wolf, M., and Dickinson, D. (1985). From oral to written language: Transitions in the school years. In J. Gleason (Ed.), *The development of language* (pp. 227–276). Columbus, OH: Charles E. Merrill.

Wolff, A., and Harkins, J. (1986). Multihandicapped students. In A. Schildroth and M. Karchmer (Eds.), *Deaf children in America* (pp. 55–81). Boston, MA: College-Hill Press.

Wong, B. (Ed.). (1991). *Learning about learning disabilities.* San Diego, CA: Academic Press.

Wong-Fillmore, L. (1991b). Second language-learning in children: A model of language learning in social context. In E. Bialystok (Ed.), *Language processing in bilingual children* (pp. 49–69). New York: Cambridge University Press.

Wood, D. (1981). Some developmental aspects of prelingual deafness: In B. Woll, J. Kyle, and M. Deuchar (Eds.), *Perspectives on British Sign Language and deafness* (pp. 27–42). London: Croom Helm.

Wood, D. (1986). Aspects of teaching and learning. In M. Richards and P. Light (Eds.), *Children of social worlds*. Oxford, England: Blackwell.

Wood, D., Griffiths, D., Howarth, S., and Howarth, C. (1982). The structure of conversation with 6- to 10-year-old deaf children. *Journal of Child Psychology and Psychiatry and Applied Disciplines, 23*, 295–308.

Wood, D., Wood, H., Griffiths, A., and Howarth, I. (1986). *Teaching and talking with deaf children.* New York: John Wiley and Sons.

Wulz, S., Hall, M., and Klein, M. (1983). A home-centered instructional communication strategy for severely handicapped children. *Journal of Speech and Hearing Disorders, 48*, 2–10.

Zangwill, I. (1910). *The melting pot.* New York: Macmillan.

Zavola, J., and Mims, J. (1983). Identification of bilingual Hispanic students. *Learning Disability Quarterly, 6*, 479–488.

Zeskind, P. (1980). Adult responses to cries of low and high risk infants. *Infant Behavior and Development, 3*, 167–177.

Zeskind, P., and Lester, B. (1981). Analysis of cry features in newborns with differential fetal growth. *Child Development, 52*, 207–212.

Zigler, E., and Balla, D. (Eds.). (1982). *Mental retardation: The developmental-difference controversy.* Hillsdale, NJ: Erlbaum.

Zigler, E., and Hodapp, R. (1986). *Understanding mental retardation.* Cambridge, MA: Harvard University Press.

Zuckerman, B. (1988). Marijuana and cigarette smoking during pregnancy: Neonatal effects. In I. Chasnoff (Ed.), *Drugs, alcohol, pregnancy, and parenting* (pp. 73–89). Hingham, MA: Kluwer Academic.

Zuckerman, B. (1991). Drug-exposed infants: Understanding the medical risk. *The Future of Children, 1*(1), 26–35.

Zuckerman, B., and Bresnahan, K. (1991). Developmental and behavioral consequences of prenatal drug and alcohol exposure. *Pediatric Clinics of North America, 38*(6), 1387–1406.

Zuckerman, B., and Frank, D. (1992). "Crack kids": Not broken. *Pediatrics, 89*(2), 337–339.

Zukow, P. (1984). Criteria for the emergence of symbolic conduct: When words refer and play is symbolic. In L. Feagans, C. Garvey, and R. Golinkoff (Eds.), *The origins and growth of communication* (pp. 162–175). Norwood, NJ: Ablex.

AUTHOR INDEX

SUBJECT INDEX